Health Care Technology
and its Assessment

Health Care Technology and its Assessment

An International Perspective

H. DAVID BANTA

and

BRYAN R. LUCE

Oxford New York Tokyo
OXFORD UNIVERSITY PRESS
1993

Oxford University Press, Walton Street, Oxford OX2 6DP

Oxford New York Toronto
Delhi Bombay Calcutta Madras Karachi
Kuala Lumpur Singapore Hong Kong Tokyo
Nairobi Dar es Salaam Cape Town
Melbourne Auckland Madrid
and associated companies in
Berlin Ibadan

Oxford is a trade mark of Oxford University Press

Published in the United States
by Oxford University Press Inc., New York

A catalogue record for this book is available from the British Library

Library of Congress Cataloging in Publication Data
Banta, H. David (Henry David), 1938–
Health care technology and its assessment: an international
perspective/H. David Banta and Bryan R. Luce.
Includes bibliographical references and index.
1. Medical technology. 2. Technology assessment.
I. Luce, Bryan R. II. Title
[DNLM: 1. Delivery of Health Care—organization & administration.
2. Technology Assessment, Biomedical. W 84.1 B219h 1993]
R855.3.B35 1993 362.1—dc20 93-18467
ISBN 0-19-262297-8

Typeset by
Advance Typesetting Ltd, Long Hanborough, Oxfordshire
Printed in Great Britain on acid-free paper by
St Edmundsbury Press, Bury St Edmunds

Foreword

by Professor Egon Jonsson

The field of health care technology assessment is now almost 20 years old. During this period, we have seen the introduction of many dramatic new technologies, such as the computed tomography (CT) scanner, the magnetic resonance imaging (MRI) scanner, the fibre-optic endoscope, the automated chemistry analyser, and powerful new drugs produced by biotechnology. Thus, I do not question that technology is useful. However, technology is also often (or usually) costly. It has tended to be rushed into use before its benefits, risks, and costs have been understood. This problem, which a number of us began to recognize as early as the late 1960s, became increasingly apparent with time.

I became involved as an economist in the field of health care technology assessment in the early 1970s, as we in Sweden began to be concerned about the value of large investments in health care services. Our first study in technology assessment, done when I was with SPRI, was a cost-effectiveness analysis of the CT scanner, aimed at giving hospitals guidance as to whether or not they would be wise to purchase a scanner. My group then did other studies of health care technologies. While David Banta has sometimes said that I was involved in technology assessment before he was, and in a sense this is true, it is also true that the definitions and conceptualizations developed in the Office of Technology Assessment under David's guidance in the period 1976–1980 gave us important ideas concerning what we were doing and why.

I have been very pleased during these 15 years to have many contacts with David Banta. He first came to Sweden in 1977, seeking to develop a network in health care technology assessment. While we did not meet on that visit because I was away, I invited David to Sweden in 1979 for an International Workshop on Evaluation of Medical Technology. I doubt that either of us could figure out how many times I have invited David to Sweden since then, but it must be 10 or more times for a period of 8 or 9 weeks. David has travelled all over Sweden to lecture, give seminars, or consult. It is no exaggeration to say that he is a familiar figure to health policy-makers and planners in Sweden!

In 1987, David decided to work 50 per cent of his time as a consultant and he asked me if I could use him on an on-going basis. At that time, I chaired the Nordic Evaluation of Medical Technology (NEMT) group, made up of representatives from four Nordic institutions, and we contracted David to write a paper on medical imaging from an international perspective. Subsequently, the Swedish Council on Health Care Technology Assessment (SBU) was formed in 1988, and I asked David if he would be willing to set aside a certain amount of time for SBU's work. During these last years, we have valued David's work and have turned to him several times. He has done reports for us on future health care technology, quality of organ transplants, minimally invasive surgery, and other subjects. He is presently working on international implications of the use of radiotherapy for cancer. He also wrote a report on strategies for health care technology assessment for Sweden. We used the report and summarized it in some of our own documents. When David learned that we did not intend to publish the report in full, he asked if he could seek a private publisher. I was delighted. Thus, SBU is a partial financial sponsor of this book.

I had used the earlier book by David and his collaborators Clyde Behney and Jane Sisk (Willems), *Toward rational technology in medicine*, in courses and seminars in Sweden and found it very useful. However, it became increasingly out of date. I suggested several times to David that he update it. I know others made the same suggestion, since the book was used in courses (that I know of) in New York, Houston, and Rio de Janeiro. David, though, was not content with an updating. He developed, with Bryan Luce, the idea for a quite new and different book, focusing on the international issue of health care technology. It is the first time that I know of, for example, that the problem of less-developed countries has been given reasonable prominence in a book in the field of health care technology assessment. This fact alone makes the book a substantial contribution.

With the development of educational programmes in health care technology assessment, I have no doubt that the book will find a market. It is written in an easy, readable style. It can be read and appreciated by someone with no scientific background. It gives much useful information on what is actually happening in the world. At the same time, someone sophisticated in the field of health care technology assessment will also find much to learn from this book.

I know that David Banta and Bryan Luce are passionately committed to the idea that health care technology assessment should make a difference to the health of ordinary people. Writing this book is a labour of love for both of them. I think that they will achieve their goal of making that difference.

Preface

This book results from more than 15 years work in the field of health care technology assessment. In 1975, when David Banta first joined the US Congressional Office of Technology Assessment (OTA), the term technology assessment had hardly ever been used in the health-related literature. Such terms as 'health care technology' had not been defined.

During those early years, OTA did much to develop the field of health care technology assessment. Many people were involved in this effort, both OTA staff and outside advisors. Two of the first reports from OTA described methods for assessing the social implications of health care technology and for assessing efficacy and safety. In 1978, Banta became head of the OTA Health Program. That year, OTA decided to examine methods of assessing cost-effectiveness analysis. We worked together on that report, with Bryan Luce, who had joined the OTA staff, as senior methodologist on the project.

The diffusion of the computed tomography (CT) scanner probably had more to do with the development of the field of health care technology assessment than any other event. OTA published a draft report on that subject in 1976. The draft was sent out for comments and criticism, and must have been one of the most copied health care reports in history. It came just at the right time. It was the basis for an uncounted number of newspaper and magazine articles. Phone calls came from all over the USA, as well as most European countries, Japan, Australia, and New Zealand. The contacts resulting in this report led to the first development toward a network of those working in the field. In particular, reports by Jonsson in Sweden (1975) and Stocking in the UK (1978) contributed substantially to the new field.

From its modest beginnings in 1975, the field has grown rapidly. There is now an *International Journal for Technology Assessment in Health Care* and an International Society with over 800 members in more than 30 countries. A number of countries, including Sweden, France, and the UK, have national, publicly funded bodies that assess health care technology for the purposes of affecting policy. In 1990, the US Congress established the Agency for Health Policy Research, with a central task of fostering health care technology assessment. That legislation, for example, recognized that the literature in the field of health care technology assessment is burgeoning, but is often not accessible, because it is largely made up of research reports and syntheses published in non-archival literature, often in the form of desktop-published material by the organization that has done the analysis. In 1991, the National Library of Medicine, acting under this same legislative mandate, gave a contract to ECRI, an organization in Pennsylvania, to develop an international clearing house of health care technology assessment information. The database from that effort is now developed and will be continuously updated.

Our own careers reflect the internationalization of the field. In 1985, Banta moved to The Netherlands at the invitation of the Dutch government to study future health care technology. He also became active in consulting on other countries' efforts. During the period following 1985, he was invited to participate in national consultations in a number of countries, including Canada, Venezuela, Brazil, Australia, China, Poland, Romania, and essentially all Western European countries. Bryan Luce joined the international firm Battelle in 1984 and, as director of Battelle's Medical Technology Assessment and Policy (MEDTAP) Research Center, has had substantial international technology-related research experience, especially in evaluating pharmaceutical products and developing methodological guidelines for cost-effectiveness analysis. In 1990, Battelle opened a branch office of MEDTAP in London, which has led to technology assessments and policy studies throughout Europe.

This book is an attempt to describe the field as it exists in the world in 1992. While it draws on many experiences of both of us, a few steps were particularly important. The chapters on methods in the book are derived partly from OTA reports on those subjects, with updating as appropriate—too many individuals contributed to these reports to be acknowledged. The first overall synthesis in this field was done in *Toward rational technology in medicine* by D. Banta, C. Behney, and J. Willems (now Sisk) in 1981. Doubtless, some thoughts of Behney and Willems remain in this book, and we owe them thanks for their enthusiastic permission to use this material as we wish. Reports written by Banta and Annetine Gelijns for the Dutch Steering Committee on Future Health Scenarios in 1986−1987 particularly influenced Banta's thinking on development and timely evaluation of technology. In 1990, the Swedish Council on Technology Assessment in Health Care (SBU) commissioned Banta to develop a health care technology assessment document for Sweden (as described by Egon Jonsson in his Foreword). This led to a report that was, in effect, the first draft of this book. Banta invited Luce to co-author the book and to take primary responsibility for the chapters on health economics, the USA, assessment of prevention, and assessment of pharmaceuticals. Nevertheless, the book in its entirety is a synthesis of the knowledge and experiences of both authors, supplemented by the knowledge of a number of contributors.

The book is organized to give the reader a context for examining issues of health care technology. The first section introduces key concepts and concerns and gives an historical perspective. The second section summarizes influences on technological change in health care. The third section describes the effects of health care technology and methods for evaluating those effects. The fourth section examines several cases from different areas of health care practice to illustrate how technology assessment can be approached. And the final section gives an international perspective and includes chapters on specific countries by special contributors.

All in all, many of our friends and collaborators, and our experiences in different institutions, have made great contributions to the thinking represented in this book. Still, any opinions are our own and do not represent the official policy of any organization with which we are associated.

May 1993   D.B., B.L.

Acknowledgements

The editors gratefully acknowledge permission to reproduce the following figures: **Figure 6** reprinted with permission from *Medical technology and the health care system: a study of the diffusion of equipment-embodied technology*, courtesy of the National Academic Press, Washington, D.C., 1979; **Figures 7 and 16** reprinted in part with permission from Williams and Torrens, *Introduction to health services, third edition*, copyright 1988 by Delmar Publishers, Inc., Albany, New York.

Contents

Contributors

Carlos Cruz National Institute of Public Health, Cuernavaca, Mexico

Gladys Faba National Center for Information and Documentation on Health, Ministry of Health, Mexico City, Mexico

Julio Frenk Director General, National Institute of Public Health, Cuernavaca, Mexico

Chen Jie Deputy Director, Department of Hospital Management, Shanghai Medical University, Shanghai, China

Jaime Martuscelli Center for Technological Innovation, National Autonomous University of Mexico, Mexico City, Mexico

Dennis Revicki Deputy Director, Medical Technology Assessment and Policy Research Center, Battelle, Washington, D.C.

Henk Rigter Professor, Social Aspects of Medical Technology, Institute of Medical Technology Assessment and Department of Public Health and Social Medicine, Erasmus University, Rotterdam, The Netherlands

Jackie Spiby Bromley Health Authority, Hayes, Kent, England

Barbara Stocking Director, King's Fund Centre, London, England

Lars Werkö President, Swedish Council on Health Care Technology Assessment (SBU), Stockholm, Sweden

Tables

Figures

Introduction and summary

If the Lord Almighty had consulted me before embarking upon the Creation, I would have recommended something simpler.

Alfonso X of Castile

The present time is full of challenges and opportunities. Observers often echo the bewilderment of Alfonso X: it is just too complex to deal with. Among the many challenges, that posed by technology and the rapidity of technological change is one of the most pressing.

The field of health care has the same characteristics, including the challenge of rapid technological change. Every country in the world must deal with this challenge.

The philosophy of technology assessment

The field of technology assessment has developed as an aid to policy-making with regard to technology (35,492). Technology is applied knowledge. It is this applied knowledge that allows prevention, diagnosis, and treatment of disease and rehabilitation from its consequences.

The goal of health care is a healthier population. Health care technology assessment is also aimed at this overall goal. Thus, the main purpose of health care technology assessment is to help ensure that medical technologies are safe, efficacious, and appropriately used. Technologies must be as safe as possible to avoid undue harm to health. Technologies must be efficacious, that is, beneficial to health, or they should not be used. And technologies must be appropriately used if health is to be the result.

Still, safety, efficacy, and appropriate use are not the only concerns of technology assessment. Health care costs money. Resources are used in health care that could also be applied, perhaps with greater benefit, in other areas of societal activities. Therefore, it is not enough to know that a health care technology is beneficial in use; one also needs to have an idea that the benefit is worth the cost expended.

Likewise, some technology has social consequences. Technology in the aggregate leads to changes in systems. Systems also lead to technological modifications. At the level of individual technologies, some interventions are associated with significant social and ethical issues. For example, genetic screening and abortion has been controversial in most countries. The provision of intensive care for very small babies and for very old and sick people has been of increasing concern.

Technology assessment exists to provide information. The information provided does not determine the decision made, however. Technology assessment should be seen merely as a tool that may make difficult decisions easier. In most cases, however, important decisions will require judgement, and may depend on power relationships within a society. Therefore, those who hope that technology assessment will make decisions much more rational and much less subjective will be disappointed. Those who fear that technocrats and analysts will become more important than democratically or administratively chosen policy-makers have little to fear.

Historical developments concerning health care and technology

The development of the present relationship between health care and its technology has been a dynamic interaction of funding, institutions, personnel, and the applied knowledge, including machines that embody the knowledge. The development of public health care in the 1800s furnished stable resources for the development of hospitals and the payment of physicians and other providers. The hospital took on its present form following the development of national health insurance and national health services, beginning about 1880. Public funding for biomedical research during this century, but particularly since World War II, stimulated technological development. A technology industry developed in response to the available market and the knowledge that made new drugs and useful machines possible. The hospital had become the major home of health care technology by the early 1900s.

The field of radiology can serve as an example. The discovery of X-rays in 1895 led to the specialty of radiology. By 1900, X-rays were being used to diagnose fractures, gall and kidney stones, foreign objects in the body, and diseases of the lungs. Bismuth was first used in 1896 to make pictures of the gastro-intestinal tract from end to end (555). Departments of radiology were established in the early decades of the century, and they expanded rapidly in the 1920s (653, p. 46). A specialized group of physicians, called radiologists, gradually formed to oversee the process of taking X-ray images and to provide expert interpretation of them. The medical specialty was formally established in the 1930s (652, p. 325).

As pointed out by Russell (586), until fairly recently, governments functioned in health care mainly to promote new technology's development and adoption. By the 1950s, however, the available panoply of technology was broad enough, effective enough, and expensive enough to begin to bring problems to public attention. The result was the development of planning systems to encourage greater efficiency in the use of technology. For example, a number of countries developed standards for volume of use, for the cost of certain volumes of service, and for capacity of certain facilities. Questions of benefits and risks were left to professionals. It was only during the late 1960s that questions began to be raised about those issues.

The need for technology assessment

Technology assessment in health care has developed in response to needs of the system to understand the consequences of technological change in health care. Policy-makers became less content with being asked to have faith in the benefits and costs of health care technology.

Questions were stimulated by a number of highly publicized cases of technology that simply did not work. Perhaps the most classic example was that of gastric freezing (239). In the mid-1950s, a US surgeon developed a device to treat peptic ulcer disease by circulating very cold alcohol through the stomach for the purpose of freezing the stomach to kill acid-producing cells. In 1962, he reported no serious side effects, reduced stomach acid output, and radiographic evidence of ulcer healing. By the end of 1963, 1000 devices had been sold in the USA and 15 000 procedures using the device had been performed. However, reports increasingly indicated patient harm, and even death. The device fell rapidly out of use. Clinical trials published in 1964 showed no benefit. By 1966, the technique was rarely used.

Another much-publicized example is diethylstilbestrol (DES), used for the treatment of pregnancy complications, especially threatened abortion (16). DES was introduced in the late 1930s and was promoted as a treatment for pregnancy complications during the 1940s and 1950s based on a number of badly designed studies. Controlled studies in the 1950s showed no benefit from treatment by DES, but widespread use continued throughout the world. In 1970, a rare type of vaginal cancer was discovered in young women whose mothers had taken DES during pregnancy. Since then, a number of other complications have become evident in both sons and daughters. The drug gradually fell out of use during the 1970s.

Perhaps a more common situation in health care is the effective technology that is overused. The computed tomography (CT) scanner may serve as an example. After its introduction in 1972, the CT scanner diffused into use extraordinarily rapidly. Radiologists and other physicians were beguiled by images unlike any they had ever seen. Surely, such images would improve treatment and health status. However, such assumptions were not necessarily borne out. CT scanners, while indisputably beneficial for some problems, were used very frequently in situations where little benefit could be expected, such as chronic headache (502,503). While the present situation with CT scanners is not known, mainly because they are now considered a fundamental and essential tool for medical diagnosis, the likelihood is that they are used in even more situations where benefit is doubtful or very unlikely.

Such cases showed policy-makers that depending merely on health care professionals to assure benefits from health care technology was insufficient as a strategy. Simultaneously, the costs of health care began to increase rapidly in response to a number of factors, including technological developments.

Technology assessment developed (and continues to develop) incrementally, in response to the needs of the hour or the year. Thus, the 1970s was the time of concern about efficacy and safety. The early 1980s saw increasing concern about costs and cost-effectiveness. At present, more and more interest is expressed in social and ethical considerations. Programmes have begun to proliferate. More and more assessments are carried out. The result is a confusing plethora of studies and an incomplete coverage of new and existing technology. No country has yet succeeded in developing a coherent system for assessing health care technology. No country has succeeded in developing a strategic approach to health care technology assessment.

Present and future needs for a strategy

The central point is that, today, technological change in health care is extremely rapid and will likely continue to accelerate. To the extent that these technologies are well assessed and prove to be highly effective as well as cost-effective in combating disease, reducing disability and extending life, this trend is desirable indeed. The problem is that the capacities to innovate and develop technology have far outstripped society's ability to assess them in order for rational decisions to be made about its appropriate use. In the absence of adequate assessments, suboptimal decisions are made, leading to gross inefficiencies, or at least to marginal ineffectiveness and sometimes even harm. If present circumstances continue, many technologies will never be adequately assessed before they are replaced by new technologies (42).

Decision-makers who are in the firing line within the health care system find themselves in a very difficult position regarding technology purchase, adoption, insurance coverage, and use. Patients pressure physicians and physicians pressure administrators to purchase or to pay for the latest innovations. Yet, hospitals, insurers, sick funds, and all levels of government in each country are under increasingly tight budget constraints. Thus, decisions concerning technology must be made almost under duress, especially since the information base is so inadequate. These observations pertain not only to dramatic new and often very costly innovations; it is a particular problem for incremental advances of existing technologies (90).

In the absence of impartial assessments, how will the decisions about replacement be made? In response to the capacity of industry to innovate? In response to the claims of certain medical specialists? In response to concerns about increasing budgets? Or is it possible that replacement can be at least partially decided on the basis of well-validated information on benefits in relation to costs?

One of the great challenges societies face is that a complete system for assessment would require monitoring of the entire universe of health care technology, future, new, and existing; evaluating each technology at various parts of its life-cycle, and doing multiple evaluations to assure correct results and coverage of all potentially important effects; summarizing the information so that it would be usable to policy-makers, health care providers, and the public; and furnishing the information from the evaluations to all those who would need it at that point in time (39).

Such a system is not possible or necessary. Neither the money nor the trained people are available for such an effort, nor will they be in the foreseeable future. And if they were, would it be wise to indiscriminately carry out such a complex of activities? Resources are limited for health care. Resources are even more limited for technology assessment. This means that choices must be made.

Thus, the reason to develop a strategy is based in part on the need for setting priorities. Assessment resources must be used in the best possible way to meet society's needs. Systems for setting priorities range from informal consensus methods to highly technical data-driven methods.

Another reason for a strategy is to ensure that information is available when it is needed for policy-making.

Elements of a strategy for health care technology assessment

The tool of a strategy for health care technology is a systematic process of information development, dissemination, and use. The goal is to produce information needed to assist the most important health care decisions. A strategy or system for health care technology assessment includes attention to four discrete, also mutually reinforcing tasks:

(1) identification of technologies needing assessment;

(2) collecting data on the selected technology;

(3) synthesizing the data collected;

(4) disseminating the information resulting from the synthesis.

The system must also take into account the society and the values of the society and the individuals who live in it, including possible different values between different groups, such as providers and consumers or different ethnic groups. The goals of health care technology and health care technology assessment need to be made more specific within such a context. In addition, a strategy needs to consider the demands of important groups for information, as well as resistances to the implications of such information. Perhaps above all, a strategy needs to consider the existing and future health care policy contexts and work to develop information helpful within those contexts.

Section I BACKGROUND ON HEALTH CARE TECHNOLOGY

A society's technology is a critical part of that society. Technology affects all aspects of human life. One could almost say that technology is what defines humanity. The development of technology and its application is surely one of the critical factors that separates man from other animals.

Health care technology is one of the most important forms of technology in society. Everyone has some experience with health care technology, through birth, ageing, illness, and death, both personal experiences and experiences of family members. Health care technology touches every individual directly.

Society's investment in health care technology is one measure of how that society values its members. One can also examine relative investments to understand the priorities of a society. One country will invest more heavily in children; another in elderly people. One country will emphasize primary care and prevention; another will invest heavily in specialty care.

This Section presents some background material on this critical area, beginning with key definitions and concepts. The second chapter of the Section presents an historical perspective on health care technology and health care technology assessment.

1. Important concepts in health care technology assessment

The ability to face unprecedented situations by using the accumulated intellectual power of the race is mankind's most precious possession.

Arthur E. Bestor

Technology is a central force in modern society. It affects diet, work, and use of leisure time. And it certainly has had an enormous effect on health care.

Technology has become controversial, in part because of its very power, in part because of undesirable side effects, and in part because of its high costs (29,221). Overall, though, technology is controversial because it is pervasive. It is impossible to escape technology. In fact, modern life seems inconceivable without technology (519,539).

Is technology good? Or is it evil? Is there a technological imperative? Is technology an autonomous force? In the terms of this book, technology is merely a tool. Technology can be developed or not. It can be used or rejected. Thus, the spirit of this chapter is to define technology as an important force in human life, one that should be examined critically so that informed choices can be made concerning its role and use.

1.1 Definition of technology

Technology can be simply defined: '. . . the systematic application of scientific or other organized knowledge to practical tasks' (275). Jacques Ellul refers to the 'ensemble of practices by which one uses available resources in order to achieve certain valued ends' (215). This definition, in its breadth, emphasizes the pervasiveness of technology.

The term 'technology' is sometimes taken to be synonymous with physical objects such as machines. Mesthene (462) states:

The meaning of technology includes more than machines. As most serious investigators have found, understanding is not advanced by concentrating single-mindedly on such narrowly drawn yet imprecise questions as 'What are the social implications of computers, or lasers, or space technology?'. Society and the influences of technology upon it are much too complex for such artificially limited approaches to be meaningful. . . . We have found it more useful to define technology as tools in a general sense, including machines, but also including linguistic and intellectual tools and contemporary analytic and mathematical techniques. That is, we define technology as the organization of knowledge for practical purposes. . . . Its pervasive influence on our very culture would be unintelligible if technology were understood as no more than hardware.

The relationship between science and technology is complex. Technology is not merely applied science. New scientific knowledge often results in new technology, but new technology also contributes to scientific knowledge. 'The vikings who built ocean-going ships knew absolutely nothing about physics, and modern aeroplanes have to be tested in wind tunnels and in many other ways, as it is quite impossible to deduce their performance from the laws of physics' (762, p. 40). For that reason, 'applied knowledge' seems a more accurate term than 'applied science'. Technology can develop from empirical observations and even from trial and error, when the underlying scientific principles are poorly understood.

1.2 Health care technology

Given a broad concept of technology, health care technology may be defined as 'the drugs, devices, and medical and surgical procedures used in health care, and the organizational and supportive systems within which such care is provided' (487). Thus, a cardiac monitor is a technology. At the same time, the intensive care unit, one of whose component parts is a monitor, is itself a technology.

The medical biologist, like any scientist, seeks 'true knowledge', and is often little concerned about application. The clinical researcher seeks technological knowledge that is, application. The clinician practises. Research on the scientific level and research on the technological level have a fairly close relationship. Still, it is not possible to deduce the success of a new technology by knowing the scientific facts of the field. Therefore, it is important to test practice empirically. 'Clinical practice must not be regarded as applied biological medicine, and it is necessary to adopt the empiricist approach for the solution of clinical problems' (762, p. 43).

Technology needs to be classified to allow generalizations about its different types. Clearly, preventive technology is different from therapeutic technology, for example. A useful system for classifying health care technology distinguishes it on two dimensions: medical purpose and physical nature.

Medical purpose

1. A diagnostic technology helps in determining what disease processes occur in a patient.

2. A preventive technology protects an individual from disease or prevents its extension.

3. A therapeutic technology provides treatment for a disease that is sometimes curative, but more often gives symptomatic or functional relief but does not address the underlying problem.

4. A rehabilitative technology is for the purpose of compensating for a functional problem or assisting a person with a disability to rise to a higher level of functioning.

5. An organizational or administrative technology is used in management and administration to ensure that health care is delivered as effectively as possible.

6. A supportive technology is used to provide patients, especially those in hospital, with needed services, such as hospital beds and food.

Physical nature

1. A drug is any chemical or biological substance that may be applied to, ingested by, or injected into humans in order to prevent, treat, or diagnose disease or other health conditions.

2. A device is any physical item, excluding drugs, used in health care, and may range from a machine requiring a large capital investment to a small simple instrument or implement.

3. A procedure is a combination, often quite complex, of provider skills or abilities (technique) with drugs, devices, or both.

Drugs and devices are products; without the involvement of humans, that is, both users and providers, they are of little benefit. The key issue, then, concerns the skill and knowledge of the users. A surgical procedure, for example, involves the use of scalpels, clamps, and drugs against infection; the key to the procedure, however, is the surgeon's actions. A drug involves a diagnosis, even if made by a lay person, and is an attempt to apply diagnostic technology and treatment technology to approach a health care problem. The context of health care, including the skills and knowledge of the users, is a critical part of technology often overlooked (230).

1.3 Empirically developed technology

The subject of this book is scientific medicine and technology that has resulted from science, engineering, and technological development activities in research institutes, medical schools, and industry. There is still, however, a body of empirically developed technology whose history and place have not been well-described. Historically, empirically developed technology has been important. For example, midwives used ergot to contract the uterus as early as the 16th century, but it was not accepted by physicians until 1808 (183, p. 15). Lessons from lay midwifery could still contribute much to medical practice, and probably the same is true for much of medicine.

This area of practice has come to be called 'traditional medicine' in less developed countries and 'alternative therapy' in industrialized countries. Technologies offered in alternative therapy include acupuncture, homeopathy, magnetic and electrical diagnosis and therapy, manual therapy, and special diets (42). In addition, use of psychological techniques, such as imagery, in diagnosis and therapy is spreading. In some cases, these alternatives are sought because of lack of access to services. In some cases, they are sought because they may be more personal or human than medical services. In some cases, they are sought because they have a powerful placebo effect. But empirical technologies can also turn out to be effective. Until (and if) biomedical science is perfected, the test for application must be: does it work? Methods of determining workability (or effectiveness) will be discussed later in this book.

1.4 Concerns about health care technology

Present-day concerns have been eloquently summed up by Wulff *et al.* (762, p. 11):

People have lost their naïve belief in technological progress which—with intermissions—has characterized our culture since the industrial revolution, and instead they want to control the development. In other words, it is realized that new scientific results and new technologies are not an end in themselves, but only a means to improve life, and that realization must of necessity lead to a debate about moral values and, among doctors, to an interest in medical ethics.

This age is characterized by the most rapid technological change in history. The rapidity of change makes it difficult to understand, even for experts. No-one can understand the implications of change in all areas of society.

Anticipating the rapidly growing armoury of future health care technology, many important issues can be recognized. Who is to assure safety? Who is to examine efficacy (or effectiveness)? Will the costs of the technology be bearable by society? Will technology be used, not only effectively and efficiently, but also humanely? How will the caring function fit into the health care system of the future? Which tasks will be performed by machines, and which tasks will be kept within the domain of people?

The value of 'life at any cost' is already being seriously questioned. Grave ethical questions surround many technologies, especially those applied at the beginning and the end of life.

Elderly people are kept alive on machines when they might prefer to die. Smaller and smaller babies, often with potential for severe mental and physical handicaps, are kept alive. Infertile couples undergo a great amount of intervention, and the women take powerful drugs whose long-term effects are not known, in attempts to have children. Technology gives an increasing number of powerful tools, but society may not be wise enough to know how to use and control them.

With moves to limit resources for health care, other serious problems are becoming apparent. The population of the developed world is ageing, and rates of chronic diseases are increasing. Technology has much to offer to many of these people. But available resources mean that all cannot benefit maximally from the new tools. Many problems of equality and equity in access to health care are apparent. Conflicts will continue to grow between individual rights and demands and collective decisions.

These concerns indicate an inevitable expansion in evaluation, planning, and control of health care. The alternative is to turn health care over to the market, to 'privatize' it. That is surely an avoidance of responsibility. The technological challenges of today and the future force continued changes in the legal and policy structure of any country.

1.5 Some preliminary conclusions

In this chapter, a few of the concerns that will be the theme of this book have been introduced. In summary, one might say that medicine has a 'paradigm' crisis (397). The idea of the Cartesian paradigm will be introduced in the next chapter. A paradigm is, simply stated, a collective term for all that the practitioners of a particular scientific discipline take for granted (762, p. 2). Medicine has functioned historically, and very much in this century, according to a paradigm based on the body as a machine and the generalizability of solutions based on empirical knowledge. This paradigm is increasingly unsatisfactory.

This book will not propose a new paradigm. The only contribution to a new paradigm here is to emphasize that evaluation and assessment in a scientific and statistical sense have not been sufficiently integrated into the medical paradigm. That situation is changing, though, and will probably change more rapidly in the future. This book will consider methods to accelerate such a change.

2. Historical perspective on technology in health care

. . . he is acknowledged as a good doctor because he meets the deep but unformulated expectation of the sick for a sense of fraternity.

John Berger

It has been said that though God cannot alter the past, historians can; it is perhaps because they can be useful to him in this respect that He tolerates their existence.

Samuel Butler

Historically speaking, the health care system has had little effective technology. The health care system was not designed to provide effective technology to sick people. The system instead provided care to people with problems. Gradually, effective technology did begin to enter practice, but even today many possibly ineffective practices remain common.

This chapter will consider some of the historical forces that led to the present situation. Although the history of evaluation and assessment is relatively short, it too will be presented.

2.1 History of technology in medicine

The history of medical science and health care technology may be divided into three periods:

(1) an early period of slow accumulation of medical knowledge through description and empirical observation, which began even before the ancient Greeks and ended with the beginning of modern scientific thought as described by Descartes in 1637;

(2) a period of relatively rapid development of knowledge, primarily during the 1800s and early 1900s;

(3) the modern era of the biological revolution, the development of machine-based technology, and the appearance of extended longevity and corresponding rapidly increasing rates of chronic disease.

Before the ancient Greeks, diseases tended to be attributed to supernatural causes. Hippocrates, the father of modern medicine, recognized disease as part of nature. Still, developments were impeded by dogma until Vesalius began his careful observations of human anatomy in the 19th century (555, pp. 13−16). As anatomy developed as a discipline, physiology—the study of normal function—became possible. In 1628, for example, William Harvey published his observations on the circulation of the blood that laid the basis for modern physiology and its relation to anatomy (625, pp. 25–31).

The classification of disease was a major contribution of the early stages of scientific medicine. In the 17th century, Thomas Sydenham put forward the view that diseases should be classified into a finite number of conditions. By the 18th century, this idea was accepted, and Morgagni was able to describe relationships between clinical illness, findings at autopsy, and pathological changes (625, pp. 121–126). The invention of the microscope made it possible to examine pathological changes in cells (625, pp. 13–14). Virchow developed a dynamic view of disease based on findings made possible by such tools as the microscope (555, pp. 78–80). However, it was not until the early 19th century that physicians in France began to examine patients physically and then after death correlate findings at autopsy with the physical signs.

Therapy was limited during the early history of medicine. Treatment with drugs is one of the oldest therapies, but less than two dozen effective drugs were known before the year 1700. Surgery was also common, and spread further with developments in anatomy (625, pp. 261–266).

The principles of modern science were laid down in 1627 by René Descartes. Descartes' principles included separating mind from body and studying the biological organism as a mechanism or machine (762). Because of the power of this Cartesian paradigm, the 17th century saw 'the emergence of a new faith in the potentialities of human initiative' (681, p. 661).

The Cartesian paradigm made it possible to intervene in human disasters, including disease. Under the influence of this paradigm, medical science developed rapidly during the 1700s and 1800s. The modern technology of diagnosis might be said to have begun with Auenbrugger, who developed percussion, the striking of the body with the fingers to produce sounds that give information about organs within the body (625, p. 226; 555, pp. 20–22). In 1816 Laennec extended the physical examination further, with his invention of the stethoscope to listen to sounds within the body (555, pp. 23–44). Reiser (555) has described the subsequent development of many of the diagnostic tools of medicine, including the ophthalmoscope (1850), the thermometer (early 1700s), the blood pressure cuff (1876), the electrocardiograph (1901), and the laryngoscope (1857). The development of chemistry as a tool for diagnosis began with analyses of the urine for sugar in the late 1700s (555, p. 133). The microscope had a profound effect on diagnosis, beginning with studies of the normal human body, and later leading to the field of bacteriology and its advances in the control of infectious diseases in the late 1800s (555, pp. 82–90). The discovery of X-rays in 1895 and its rapid spread into practice made 'looking into' the living human body possible for the first time, and inaugurated the field now known more and more as medical imaging.

The sanitary revolution of the 19th century, a systematic intervention in the physical environment to make it safer, was built on ecological approaches to disease prevention begun by the Greeks (625, pp. 289–293). The knowledge of the cause of infectious disease gained by Pasteur, Koch, and others, made hygiene even more effective.

The development of vaccines to prevent disease was a great advance. Jenner is usually given credit for the first medical use of cowpox to prevent smallpox in 1796 (625, pp. 285–288). In the late 1800s, Pasteur weakened organisms to produce vaccines, including the well-known vaccine for rabies. The isolation of viruses in 1935 and their subsequent growth in cell culture made possible the development of vaccines for poliomyelitis, measles, rubella, and influenza.

Developments in surgery were facilitated by bacteriology. Lister demonstrated that he could prevent infection by applying disinfectants to the surgical wound and its dressing. With the discovery by Davy that nitrous oxide was an effective narcotic, and the demonstration by Wells in 1844 that the gas made extraction of a tooth painless, the development of modern surgery had begun (625, pp. 266–268).

Developments in chemistry stimulated the beginnings of modern pharmacology. The development of pharmaceutical technology was slow in ancient times, but accelerated in the 19th century (395). Organic chemical substances such as morphine were isolated from plants. Dosages, side effects, and effects on disease were studied. In 1860, salicylic acid was synthesized from coal tar (625, p. 248). In 1911 Ehrlich demonstrated that Salvarsan, the 'magic bullet', was an effective treatment for syphilis (625, pp. 248–249). Discovery that the red dye, prontosil rubrum, protected animals from streptococcal disease led to the introduction of sulfa drugs in 1936 (419). Penicillin was introduced in 1943, followed by streptomycin. With the development of modern drugs, the revolution in health care was truly established.

Drug delivery systems also developed slowly over the centuries. Intravenous injections were first performed in the 17th century. The first pill machine was developed in the 18th century and pill coating began in the 19th century. Rectal suppositories were first manufactured in 1762. In 1852, the first syringe was constructed, and intramuscular and subcutaneous injection began. Sterile fluids in glass ampoules for subcutaneous injection were first made in 1886. Multiple dose injection vials were not made until 1922, when insulin became available. Surprisingly, the first aerosol product was not introduced to the market until 1950. Sustained dosage drugs were introduced in 1952. Methods of mass production of pills also changed rapidly in the period following World War II. Finally, in 1975 the results of transdermal therapy were presented for the first time (395).

Despite this long history, effective therapies were rare until recently. In 1980, Beeson (56) compared treatments recommended in a 1927 textbook of medicine to those recommended in 1975. Beeson rates the value of 60 per cent of the remedies in 1927 as harmful, dubious, or merely symptomatic; only 3 per cent provided fully effective treatment or prevention. In the interval, effective regimens increased seven-fold and dubious ones decreased by two-thirds.

The period since World War II has seen the most rapid development of health care technology in history. Since 1950 there has been an explosion of medical knowledge. The discovery of the structure of DNA set off a true biological reaction. Available laboratory tests have expanded dramatically. New imaging devices such as computed tomography (CT) scanning, introduced in 1972, and more recently, magnetic resonance imaging (MRI) and positron-emission tomography (PET) have radically changed the process of diagnosis. New operative technology has made such procedures as open-heart surgery relatively safe, and surgery combined with other disciplines such as immunology has led to an era of organ transplants. Overall, the period is most characterized by an extremely dramatic development of machines, as human actions such as monitoring vital functions, mixing substances together to observe reactions, and measuring myopia (short-sightedness) have been embodied in electronic and mechanical devices. At the same time, advances in such fields in electronics and biomaterials have made such technologies as cardiac pacemakers possible.

Despite this rapidity of change, the next 40 years will probably see even more rapid change (42). While advances may be seen in many areas, two are dramatic enough to highlight. One is computers, which now are found in almost all complex devices and are used widely in both administrative and clinical functions. The other is the new biotechnology, the result of the discovery of the structure of DNA, which is now beginning to result in a panoply of approaches to prevention, diagnosis, and treatment that were not possible previously.

2.2 Historical roots of technology-dependent health care

This section will touch lightly on the historical roots of some of the major forces seen in today's health care systems.

Cartesian thought. Cartesian thought certainly set off the development of modern technological medicine, which has had many benefits. But Cartesian thought has had significant, and increasingly negative, consequences. The mechanistic Cartesian view has led to much wasted effort and money and has fostered the hospital-based, specialized system of today. Cartesian thought tends to focus on what is tangible and understandable and to ignore the more complex variables that cannot be quantified, such as social and behavioural factors. It fosters an approach that leads to coronary care units and coronary bypass surgery rather than programmes to prevent heart disease.

The profession of medicine. In early years, physicians had few effective tools, they often had poor pay and prestige, and they often worked part-time. As technology has developed, and medicine has become more effective, they have seen their sense of profession rise, along with their income and prestige.

Today's medicine is highly specialized and subspecialized. The development of medical specialties has historically been very much related to the development of medical knowledge and health care technology, especially since the 19th century (555). The development of the ophthalmoscope in 1851 was a stimulus to physicians to specialize in the eye; in 1881, the Ophthalmological Society of the United Kingdom was founded (653). In 1855 the laryngoscope began to interest certain physicians in diseases of the upper respiratory tract, and the British Laryngological and Rhinological Association was founded in 1888 (653). Abdominal and gynaecological surgery developed rapidly in the 1880s, due to the development of operative techniques, antisepsis and anaesthesia (652). The specialty of radiology developed in the early 1900s, following the discovery of X-rays in 1895 (652,653). Clinical laboratories became important in the late 1800s, following the expanding use of the microscope in diagnosis and pathology beginning in about 1870, and leading to the establishment of the specialty of pathology in the early 1900s (386).

While specialization is obviously important and necessary, one result has been that physicians tend to concentrate on the technical aspects of care and to ignore 'the patient's inner world' (442). The traditional method of medical diagnosis is intended to be strictly objective. In general, health care today does not aim to help the patient understand the meaning of illness or to deal with anxiety or moral and spiritual problems (762).

Medical education. In ancient Greece, physicians learned their profession by apprenticeship. Although that tradition continues today, the emphasis on apprenticeship began to diminish somewhat as the universities began to develop in the Middle Ages and medical instruction became more formal (625, pp. 300−304). In the decades after the Flexner Report in 1910 in the USA, medical education gradually changed to its present form: hospital-based, with a heavy emphasis on biomedical science and technology presented by a full-time faculty who are themselves biomedical researchers and medical specialists. However, medical students generally are not taught the scientific method (362). Rather than being taught to doubt and to question, the student is taught belief.

Organization and financing of health care. In the Middle Ages, physicians usually practised alone and rarely had a connection with a hospital. The knowledge of the cause of infectious diseases and a lessening of the fear of infection in hospitals combined to encourage their use. The development of social insurance and public support for health care facilitated transition to a health system covering the entire population on a compulsory basis, beginning in Europe in the late 1800s. For the first time, in some societies a minimal standard of health care was available to all.

These developments provided a ready home for the newly developing technology. To an extent, centralization of technology was necessary, and an institutional base for the large capital investments was often essential. Subsequently, technology had a great effect on the organization of institutions. Hospitals now generally have radiology departments, laboratories, and blood banking. Intensive care units and dialysis centres are related to specific technologies. Today, less invasive technology is encouraging care to move from the hospital to the outpatient setting.

The emergence of the drug and device industry. The development of pharmacology in the 1800s and the increasing possibilities of synthesizing drugs led to a drug industry. The Civil War in the USA provided an impetus because of the associated sharp growth in the need for drugs. E.R. Squibb & Sons, Sharp and Dohme, Parke, Davis & Company, and Eli Lilly were all founded about that time. During the late 1800s, a variety of machines were made to fabricate tablets, giving a technological base to the growing industry (395). Insulin and the development of vitamins gave the industry new products in the 1900s (444, p. 10). World War II stimulated further changes, as the industry made a transition from supplying bulk drugs to supplying pills and capsules. The development of penicillin, and its introduction to the market in 1948 (395), and the subsequent development of broad-spectrum antibiotics encouraged a number of new companies to enter the market. Between 1951 and 1960, more than 3800 new products and dosage forms were introduced into the US market (444).

The development of the industry has had profound effects on health care practice. The great benefit has been equipment and drugs that generally meet acceptable standards of safety, as compared with the ad-hoc situation of the past when each practitioner might make his or her own drugs. At the same time, the industry has become a powerful force in the health care system.

With recent economic problems and the need for economic development (employment, exports), criticism of the industry has tended to be muted, enhancing the influence of the industry in policy and practice decisions.

Government support for biomedical research. Prior to World War II, biomedical research was largely a private endeavour or was funded by such sources as private foundations. World War II led to the co-ordination of research efforts in the USA, and the National Institutes of Health (NIH) were formed in the 1940s. The NIH grew phenomenally during the 1950s, and has continued to grow despite budget deficits in the USA.

By 1980, expenditure on biomedical research in the USA was about US$6.5 billion, or US$3584 per million dollars of gross domestic product (see Table 1). At the same time, expenditure in Europe also grew rapidly, so that more than 35 per cent of world expenditure on biomedical research in 1980 was from European countries. Sweden alone invested US$288.1 million, or 4500 per million dollars of gross domestic product, one of the highest rates in the world. By 1990, US investment had risen to $22.6 billion (479).

One result of this government support was an increase in medical school faculty members. Medical schools concentrated more on research and less on teaching, and teachers became more involved in research. The results included a fantastic growth in knowledge, a corresponding growth in technology, and an educational system already described.

Table 1. Domestic funding for biomedical research and development (BMRD), OECD Countries, 1980.

Country	Domestic BMRD (million US$)	GDP (million US$)	BMRD per million $ of GDP	BMRD as % of all R&D	BMRD % of total
USA	6 504.9	2 598 960	3.584	10.4	45.2
Japan	2 447.6	1 004 009	3.495	12.1	17.0
Germany	1 578.9	583 099	3.883	12.1	11.0
France	885.1	490 864	2.577	9.9	6.1
UK	778.5	432 067	2.578	8.2	5.4
Italy	549.0	416 202	1.890	16.4	3.8
Netherlands	322.5	123 930	3.721	14.0	2.2
Switzerland	297.5	70 676	6.034	18.0	2.1
Sweden	288.1	91 763	4.500	17.0	2.0
Canada	282.8	244 351	1.656	12.6	2.0
Belgium	143.3	88 857	2.306	12.1	1.0
Australia	94.1	145 070	922	7.1	0.7
Spain	91.6	220 428	594	—	0.6
Denmark	82.7	46 897	2.537	18.0	0.5
Norway	72.1	44 299	2.326	12.5	0.5
Finland	46.3	43 964	1.506	10.3	0.3
Portugal	16.3	37 638	619	15.0	0.1
New Zealand	16.1	20 275	1.153	—	0.1
Ireland	8.3	17 650	676	6.5	0.1
Total	14 405.7				100.0

Source: modified from ref. 621, Table 1, p. 18.

2.3 Historical view of assessment in health care

Throughout recorded history, physician assessment has had an important role in the selection of therapy. Most studies, however, utilized personal and anecdotal information (70). The single most important problem with this early research was lack of a control or comparison group to ensure that the observed effect was, in fact, due to the intervention.

Credit for carrying out the first controlled clinical trial goes to John Lind, who tested a number of cures for scurvy in 1747. Lind's trial gave powerful evidence for the efficacy of lemon and orange juice in the prevention and treatment of scurvy. In perhaps the first example of officials ignoring expert advice well-founded on evidence, the British Navy did not supply its ships with lemon juice until 1795 (399, pp. 139–140).

Statistics and probability techniques were used in the 18th century in support of medicine and public health. For example, Cotton Mather reported in 1721 that in the Boston smallpox epidemic of that year more than 1 in 16 persons who were not inoculated against the disease died, but that only about 1 in 60 who were inoculated did so (624).

Quantitative evaluations in the late 1800s demonstrated that many interventions were not effective. This led to a decline in the confidence of the public in medicine. However, the research of Pasteur brought a whole panoply of new methods in health care practice, and evaluation played its part in their acceptance, especially for public health interventions. For example, before 1900, clinical trials of diphtheria antitoxin demonstrated its effectiveness in preventing diphtheria (70). In 1914, Goldberger and his colleagues tested the effects of dietary changes on persons with pellagra in two institutions. In one of these institutions, wards were divided into those whose residents were given the experimental diet and those whose residents were given the regular diet. The trial gave dramatic evidence of the effectiveness of the dietary treatment (70).

These early assessments were not well-designed, however. It was not until Bradford Hill formulated the principles of the randomized controlled clinical trial in the mid-1930s that scientific assessment began to be accepted. The first randomized, controlled, double blind study was directed by Hill and tested a vaccine for pertussis (whooping cough). Hill also collaborated with Daniels in developing a randomized clinical trial of streptomycin in tuberculosis, published in 1948 (70). In recent years, a great literature on the subject of the design and implementation of clinical trials has developed (496) and a journal, *Controlled Clinical Trials*, is entirely devoted to the subject.

The development of drug and biological products has been a great stimulus for assessment. In 1938, the US Federal Food, Drug, and Cosmetic Act was passed, requiring that the safety of new drugs (and vaccines) be demonstrated before they could be marketed. The 1962 amendments to the Act added the requirement that efficacy be demonstrated by well-controlled trials. All Western countries now require evidence of efficacy and safety before drugs can be marketed. Some European countries, including Sweden, the UK, and The Netherlands, have standards essentially as high as those of the US Food and Drug Administration (FDA).

After World War II, the concept of establishing the efficacy and safety of all technologies grew, and was given a tremendous impetus by the publication of Cochrane's *Effectiveness and efficiency* in 1972. Funding for clinical trials grew in the USA, especially through the National Institutes of Health. By 1975, the NIH funded 95 clinical trials of preventive interventions at a cost of $21 million (487, p. 73). This may be contrasted with the investment of $62 million in 575 trials of therapies.

In recent years, there has been an increased interest in outcomes research, especially in the USA. Outcomes research is essentially the application of technology assessment within regular clinical practice. It is an effort to discover what medical practices work for whom under what conditions.

Financial costs have also long been a consideration in assessment. In 1667 Sir William Petty suggested transporting people out of London for the summer months, at government expense, in order to increase the probability of their survival. He calculated that every pound spent would return 84 pounds to society (70). Almost 2 centuries later, Lemuel Shattuck used the same return-on-investment argument in Massachusetts, to promote public health measures.

Cost-benefit and cost-effectiveness analyses (CEAs) are developments of the 20th century (see Chapter 9). In 1920 Dublin and Whitney examined the cost of years of life lost due to tuberculosis and concluded that the loss of a year of life for all people who died of tuberculosis represented a national loss of US$26.5 billion (70). CEA began to be prominent in Western society as expenditure on health care has grown and as the role of government in health care expanded during the 1960s and 1970s. The growth in the number of CEAs in health care began in the mid-1960s (214). Still, CEA has had relatively little effect on either policy or practice (497,718).

Notwithstanding the increased emphasis over the years on assessment of medical practice and its technologies, there is a great deal that is never assessed adequately. Drugs are subjected to the most comprehensive assessment, but even they are generally assessed early in their life cycle and on limited populations for highly specific conditions under strict protocols. Actual medical practice seldom conforms to the conditions of the study. Devices and diagnostics tend to be tested more for safety than for efficacy and to diffuse widely before adequate assessment is done. Medical and surgical procedures generally creep into practice without any formal testing or oversight.

Why has evaluation not been sufficiently integral in medical technology development and use? Lambert (399) suggests three main reasons historically: (1) reverence for authority and tradition; (2) lack of effective remedies; and (3) the relationship of doctor and patient, and the need for both to believe that planned interventions will be successful. This indicates that clinical experience must be considered limited in its utility and that controlled trials and statistical techniques are essential to assure validity of statements concerning benefits of health care technology.

2.4 Conclusions

Today's health care provider has a great arsenal of tools to choose from in preventing, diagnosing, and treating disease. The support for evaluation has not grown rapidly enough to assure sound evaluation of all of these tools. In addition, physicians have been slow to accept the results of scientific evaluations as a guide to practice, as will be demonstrated in Section II.

Ordinary patients obviously have a great stake in their health care. With increased questioning of the value of medicine, and increased concern about health, people are becoming more involved in determining the shape and nature of their care. Assessment results can be of substantial help in such determinations. Not only can assessments be helpful to individuals, but they can also be used by organized groups. One important future development in health care seems certain to be increased involvement of the lay public in health care decisions.

Section II THE DEVELOPMENT AND DIFFUSION OF HEALTH CARE TECHNOLOGY

Observers of developments in health care often comment on health care technology as if it suddenly appears, confounding decision-making and planning (657). Seen in this way, health care technology is always unexpected. Or at least, it develops so rapidly that it is impossible to anticipate.

In fact, technological development is made up of a prolonged sequence of activities. The knowledge that makes technology possible accumulates over decades and even centuries. (It is often forgotten that diagnostic technologies such as the CT scanner would be of little use without the knowledge of anatomy and pathology that was developed from the time of the ancient Greeks.) First, theoretical research and the sum of previous experience form a background or conceptual base. Then basic empirical research provides a framework of knowledge about the mechanisms involved in natural processes, discovers points in those processes that are susceptible to technological intervention, and suggests strategies for technological development. Applied or mission-oriented research is then directed to applying this basic knowledge to a practical purpose and to demonstrating the feasibility of the proposed technology.

This process may be illustrated by the development of the CT scanner (see Fig. 1). The CT scanner was a revolutionary diagnostic device, combining X-ray equipment with a computer and a cathode ray tube (or other imaging device such as a video screen), to produce images of cross sections of the human body. Modern advances in the fields of X-ray instrumentation, computers, and mathematics were all necessary to produce it (53,54). The earliest X-ray films depended on the exposure of film to X-rays to measure the amount of radiation that passes through different parts of the body. Tomographic techniques, beginning with mechanical methods, overcame to some extent the two-dimensional nature of the X-ray and showed objects in a particular plane. William Oldendorf, a Los Angeles neurologist, first used a nuclear detector as part of a tomographic device. Simultaneously, instrumentation developed that made measurement of radiation easier. Mathematics made it possible to reconstruct images from large sets of data. In 1917, Radon showed that a two- or three-dimensional object can be uniquely reconstructed from the infinite set of all of its projections. However, producing mathematical models capable of doing such reconstruction depended on the development of modern computers.

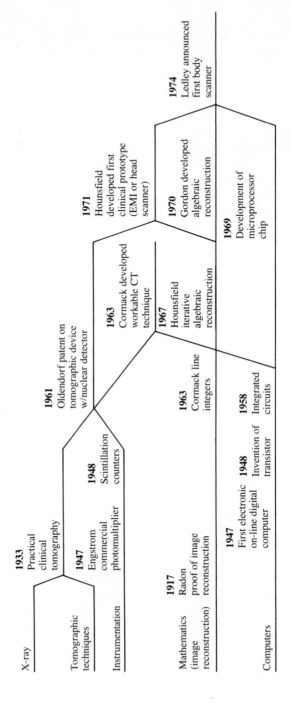

Figure 1. Development of the computed tomography (CT) scanner (source: 53).

Cormack, a physicist, built the first workable CT instrument and patented it in 1961. However, his work received little or no attention from the medical community. Hounsfield, working in the Central Research Laboratory of EMI in London, developed a scanner that produced its first crude pictures in 1967. A prototype instrument was installed in Atkinson Morley Hospital in London in 1971. Results of initial evaluations were reported in 1972 (8), and the first commercial models were installed in 1973, with the first in the USA at the Mayo Clinic (25). Figure 2 shows the diffusion of the CT scanner in several countries. The first scanner made images only of the head, but a body scanner was marketed by Pfizer in about 1974. A number of companies scrambled to develop scanners. The CT scanner became a national policy issue in the USA and Sweden in 1976–1977, and subsequently has been an issue for policy making in every country. Ultimately, the large companies such as General Electric, Philips, and Siemens, as well as several Japanese companies, have come to dominate the world market for CT scanning (23,24,200,502,503).

The development of a particular drug also encompasses many years, often decades, of research (279). One major line of research involves the physiology of the human body and the biochemistry of the living cell. A second line of research involves the disease process itself and the micro-organisms that cause

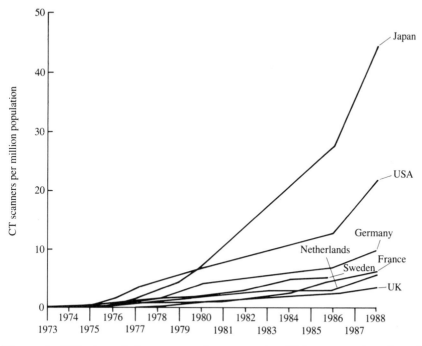

Figure 2. Diffusion of the computed tomography (CT) scanner in selected countries.

disease. A third involves research into the chemistry of the compounds. Once these three streams of research are matched, a clinical research programme can be contemplated.

The case of a pure medical or surgical procedure is considerably different, although no less important (279). Although these innovations may also have a long and rich history of early discovery, they tend to appear on the medical scene more quickly via independent research physicians, either medical or surgical specialists. A case study may appear in a leading medical journal and the physician may be asked to give talks and to conduct grand rounds. Useful or at least interesting innovations diffuse informally from these pioneers and from opinion leaders. These innovative technologies are somewhat more difficult to detect in an early stage in the life cycle in order to consider an assessment. However, many medical and surgical procedures include drugs, diagnostics, and devices.

The specific case of the CT scanner and the general case of a new drug illustrate the complexity of the process of development of a health care technology. Yet in the case of the scanner, there was ample time to anticipate the implications of the scanner, even if evaluations had only begun in 1973. In the case of the drug, there is at least several years during large-scale human trials when broader assessments could be contemplated, planned, and conducted. A lead time of 5 years is ordinarily ample for evaluation and policy-making. However, a procedure may be identified only one year or less before it begins to diffuse.

In this section, the processes of research and development and of adoption and use of health care technology will be described. The purpose of this section is to develop a framework for policy-making and for evaluation of health care technology.

3. The development of health care technology

... many shall run to and fro, and knowledge shall be increased.

Book of Daniel, Chapter 12, Verse 4

Science simply operates on the faith that knowledge is good and ignorance is something to overcome. You can't really vindicate this faith empirically. It is a faith.

Isadore Rabi

A new technology results from a long and complicated set of activities. In summary, this can be referred to as the process of technological change. This process covers the wide range of interacting events by which technology evolves over time, and includes not only scientific activities, but empirical observations, and is based not only on rational experimentation but on serendipity.

3.1 Basic and applied research

New or improved technology is generally described as developing through a process that includes basic research, applied research, and targeted development (492). Basic research is thought of as being aimed at understanding nature, or developing knowledge. It is a phenomenon-oriented activity. Applied research is thought of as leading to manipulation or control of problems. It is a goal-oriented activity. As Lewis Thomas said, '. . . surprise is what makes the difference' between the two (682, p. 118). The targeted development of a new technology begins when knowledge derived from basic and applied research is sufficient to support the effort.

In reality the process is far less systematic and more complex and dynamic than the model above implies (281). The developments in the various stages often occur simultaneously and not sequentially. Various feedback loops also exist between these stages. For instance, recent technological developments such as positron-emission tomography (PET) scanning may lead to new insights into the functioning of healthy and diseased organs. In addition, the boundaries between these stages are fluid. There is a large area of research that can be very difficult to classify as basic or applied.

Theories of innovation emphasize different aspects of the process. Some studies stress the importance of the right conditions, others emphasize the characteristics of the innovator (individual or organization), and others refer to the influence of serendipity. Trial and error is an important part of the process, and blind alleys and mistakes are common. Generally, it is important to recognize that uncertainty and variability are important characteristics of the process of technological change.

3.2 Development of specific types of technology

Certain developments in health care technology depend on biomedical research, whereas knowledge is imported from other fields for other health care technologies (e.g. physics, engineering, chemistry, or mathematical modelling). The traditional boundaries between various fields of science and between science and technology are not as fixed as they once were. Examples can be found in the emergence of a biotechnology industry, the coupling of robotics and psychobiology in the analysis of vision, and the merging of optics, solid state physics and cellular biology in the creation of flow cytometry.

The innovation process is substantially different for drugs, devices, and procedures (279,492). Drugs and devices are developed largely within industry, undergo technical testing for safety, and must meet regulatory standards, for example.

3.2.1 *Development of pharmaceuticals*

The link between basic biomedical research and drug development is often clear. Drugs develop from a basic knowledge of organic chemistry, pharmacology, and human pathophysiology.

The drug discovery process in modern times has usually been carried out by multidisciplinary teams and is often a long trial-and-error search. Serendipity has played a large role in this area, as indicated by the experience of Fleming's discovery of penicillin. The discovery of tranquilizers was the result of the observation that certain antihistamines depress the central nervous system. The medical literature is still full of clinical experiences of the use of drugs for innovative purposes.

Random screening has been another technique of drug discovery in this century (295). For example, Lederle Laboratories tested 103,000 available chemical compounds in search of a drug against tuberculosis, finally discovering one useful drug. Such trial-and-error processes may play a smaller role in the future of pharmaceutical developments due to deeper insights into molecular biology, development of computer-assisted design of drugs, and the use of receptor screens (65,279). For example, basic research in biochemistry and bacteriology has permitted the prediction of successful strategies for synthesizing some antibiotics. The drug Tagamet was developed by SmithKline scientists' attempts to design a molecule to lock onto a receptor site at the cellular level to block the action of histamine (295).

To the present, the private pharmaceutical industry has been the primary source of discovery of new drugs (295). Still, new drug discoveries are dependent on the stock of biomedical knowledge. As drug design becomes more planned, this dependency will increase, emphasizing the importance of publicly-funded basic research.

The drug industry is truly international, and while development is dominated by large multinational firms, there are also thousands of small companies.

Perhaps the most dramatic discovery of the latter half of the 20th century in terms of drugs has been the use of the new biotechnology, especially recombinant DNA techniques, both for research and for the synthesis of new compounds (488). The biological revolution is now beginning, and great numbers of new drugs can be expected to appear on the market (42). Improved understanding of the nervous system, the endocrine system, the immune system, and of cancer is the result of decades of research. The study of receptors, substances on the surface of cells that control interactions between a cell and its environment, has led to an improved understanding of how natural body chemicals interact with their receptors. The new drugs will result from this developing knowledge, as well as from the ability to synthesize substances that could not be made synthetically before. Drugs will be more specific and will more often be natural products such as peptides and proteins.

The drug industry is also beginning to use computer-aided design to develop new drugs. The structural design assistance currently provided by computers in synthesizing molecules will be expanded in the future. As computers and graphics improve, these techniques will also improve. The ability to model a molecule's effect on cells of the body will be of great importance in the future.

In addition, active research on delivery systems is presently seeking new ways to deliver drugs. Delivery systems such as pumps and reservoirs are already in use. In the future, polymer injections, delivery by aerosol, microencapsulization, and use of liposomes are examples of likely delivery methods. In addition, controlled release drugs are capable of improving the efficacy/safety ratio for many chemicals.

A critical consideration in drug development is regulation (599). Almost all countries regulate drugs for efficacy and safety. In general, after a chemical entity is developed, the company must apply to the government for permission to test it in humans. After safety studies and clinical trials are carried out, the industry must present the data to the government. If the evidence is convincing, the drug is approved for marketing. This approach has been important in protecting the public from unsafe and ineffective drugs, but it is also expensive and time-consuming. The process in the USA takes from 7 to 10 years for successful drugs (295). Given that many possible drugs are not approved for marketing (only about 10 per cent are approved), the cost of developing a marketable drug was estimated as US$231 million in the USA in 1987 (173).

None the less, the market for drugs is very attractive, with high profits to the industry, and is likely to remain so because of the value that consumers and physicians put on drugs.

In 1974, Silverman and Lee (628) summed up the changes brought by the modern era of drugs. These observations are still relevant today:

1. In place of relatively few drugs, there are thousands of products.
2. The locale of drug discovery has changed remarkably. Since 1938, most new drugs have been discovered by teams of scientists working in drug industry laboratories.
3. The new drugs are usually both very powerful and far more toxic than the products of the past.
4. The impact of new drugs on the public health has been extraordinary.

3.2.2 *Development of medical devices and equipment*

Research in biomedical sciences such as physiology and anatomy also provides knowledge that permits development of devices for diagnostic, preventive, and therapeutic purposes. Basic bioengineering research contributes to the knowledge base underlying medical device development (279). However, the situation is quite complex for devices. For one thing, much of the research that leads to the development of devices is performed outside the biomedical research sector in such fields as physics, chemistry, and electronics. For example, computers are used in co-ordinative and administrative activities and chemical testing devices are used in ancillary activities such as those of the clinical laboratory. In addition, device development often is not as dependent on new knowledge, as is true with drugs, but on the application of already-existing knowledge.

In addition, innovation in medical devices is commonly based on engineering problem-solving by individuals and small firms (568,683). One frequent model is the clinician who defines a need and develops the initial innovation, either from his or her own knowledge or in collaboration with an engineer (568). Later, a manufacturer acquires the invention and engages in commercial development. Between 80 and 100 per cent of the ideas for scientific device innovations have been found to come from users, often physicians (702). A recent study in the UK found that in half of British medical innovations, a prototype was developed and produced by a user. In only four of 34 cases was the innovation developed by a manufacturer who performed market research to determine the nature and magnitude of the potential need and then developed a product to satisfy the need (617). The pattern, then, is that a user usually develops a prototype device and then transfers it to a small firm. If the device is successful, it often is transferred to a larger company, either by purchase of the patent or takeover of the small company (702).

The US Office of Technology Assessment has developed a series of inventors' vignettes that give interesting insights into this innovation process. A number of them have been included in a book published by the National Academy of Sciences (213).

The successful development of devices requires a combination of expertise in both the biological and the physical sciences (139). Biomedical engineers have achieved some spectacular successes in recent years, but numerous difficulties beset their work. One is that most physicians are not trained to collaborate effectively with engineers to solve problems, or even to recognize the possibility of a technological solution. Few individuals have sufficient training in both biology (or medicine) and engineering to work alone. Also, in a marketplace oriented to profits, medical device manufacturers may develop and overproduce equipment of questionable utility or fail to support the development of types of equipment that are needed. Finally, engineers and physicists are trained to think in terms of physical performance characteristics and technical precision, but often do not think about the effect of new equipment on the health of populations or individuals.

Medical devices are generally not as highly regulated as are drugs, and in some countries are not regulated at all. The USA has a programme that regulates all devices for efficacy and safety, and other countries such as Canada and Japan scrutinize devices. In Europe, little regulation of devices is carried out except for devices using radiation, implants, and those concerned with sterility. Nevertheless, test institutes such as TNO in The Netherlands often examine devices, and national programmes and hospitals may delay purchase until the results of such an evaluation are known.

The period since World War II has been a period of rapid change in medical devices. Many new devices have been introduced—available devices number in the thousands. Many of these devices automated existing functions; that is, they embodied human knowledge and skills in equipment, such as monitoring devices. Much of this equipment has been on a large scale, required sophisticated users, and needed a considerable capital investment. New generations of devices that are appearing are on much smaller scale and, through the incorporation of computers, are much easier to use.

While device development does not seem likely to continue at the same high rate, such areas as neural prostheses, biomechanics and biomaterials, biosensors, and artificial organs will continue to grow (42,683). With the ageing of the population, these applications will become more important.

The medical devices industry is also a high profit enterprise (495). Growth prospects look good, and new firms continue to enter the marketplace. This helps to assure continued rapid innovation.

3.2.3 Development of procedures

Procedures are combinations of medical and surgical techniques with drugs or devices or both. This means that their development is particularly complex and may depend on research and development in several different fields. For example, it was more than 50 years before animal experimentation on kidney transplantion led to a clinical procedure in people (254). Techniques develop largely from knowledge gained from empirical, clinical experience. Thus, advances in techniques depend on skilful and creative physicians and encompass thousands of small incremental changes in medical practice, which diffuse in unstudied ways. During the initial stages of development, the procedure itself and the practitioner's skills and expertise evolve, so that risks and benefits may change considerably (279).

Barnes (50) reviewed developments in surgery during the period 1880 to 1942, and illustrated the empirical development of procedures. In a time of limited biological knowledge, a number of procedures to treat such conditions as constipation and problems of the peripheral nervous system were developed and widely used, but ultimately proved to be worthless. Clinical studies presenting optimistic results were especially lacking in control groups. Barnes feels that advances in biomedical knowledge and collaboration between such specialists as internists and anaesthetists with surgeons has reduced the 'individualistic and singlehanded characteristics of surgical performances in earlier times'. Still, he concludes, 'We must at least consider the possibility that our knowledge, compared with that which our surgical heirs will have, is as incomplete and as short of the ultimate truth as the knowledge of earlier surgeons in relation to our present understanding'.

One could argue that the rapid changes in medical devices have perhaps made the situation worse. While the technology is unquestionably better, it often depends on a skilful user (230). Since physician performance is generally unregulated, much uncontrolled experimentation goes on in the guise of standard care. The rapid developments in hip-joint replacement can be cited as one example of a great many possibilities.

3.3 Societal support for technology development

The relationships between science and society are obviously complex, and include such factors as the image of science, the inquisitiveness of a particular society, the perceived needs for scientific discoveries in certain areas, available resources, both financial and intellectual, and the already existing system for scientific discovery in each country. One critical area to consider is how science is supported.

In all countries, basic research is primarily supported by public funds; that is, by government. It is carried out largely in universities and research institutes.

The private sector, on the other hand, concentrates on applied research and technology development, and industry accounts for most of the support in this area. In the health area, industry concentrates on the development of drugs and medical devices.

Medical and surgical procedures are developed primarily in large academic medical centres, and little is known about these processes (279). Such development is often funded by patient care funds, by government, or by a mixture of the two.

The commercial private sector responds primarily to profit (446, p. 20). When there is profit to be found or anticipated, as in the development of many diagnostic devices or therapeutic drugs, the private system works fairly well.

Technological research and development and health insurance have a mutually reinforcing relationship (722).

When insurance coverage is widespread and offers rewards for a certain diagnostic or treatment area, financial signals are sent to investors to develop technologies. To the extent that these technologies are cost- and quality-increasing, demand for insurance grows, which in turns sends positive signals to R&D markets. Cost-based insurance payment systems send signals to develop virtually any technology regardless of cost as long as a quality increase is expected. Prospective payment systems and fixed budgets change these incentives dramatically and encourage cost-decreasing technologies. They also send signals to decrease R&D for technologies that may not be associated with profits. One example is the cochlear implant for hearing-impaired persons. The 3M Company discontinued research on the multichannel cochlear implant model because of hospital disincentives under the DRG law that went into effect in the USA in 1983 (373). In Europe, budgetary systems have slowed the diffusion of minimally invasive therapies, undoubtedly slowing R&D investments in this area in Europe (24,28).

In effect, the two systems that produce scientific knowledge and health care technology seem to function somewhat autonomously and the relations between these systems are not clear-cut. The development of health care technology often seems to have little relation to important health care needs, except where those needs translate into reimburseable demands. So, for instance, pressing needs such as home care and rehabilitation technologies, prevention, treatments that might be effective for a small number of people, and technologies that might be particularly useful in developing countries receive little investment (34,42,133). An important question, then, is why only some technologies of those that are scientifically feasible are developed. The answer is certainly a combination of 'science-push' and 'market-pull' factors. The market for technology reflects human needs in some way, of course. At the same time, certain technologies are favoured without a clear connection to immediate and important human needs. University hospitals, with user populations of specialized clinicians and researchers, for example, make a ready-made market for new sophisticated devices, and this market is often targeted by industry (72). And pressing health needs do not necessarily lead to investments in technological development, especially when the market is uncertain, as in the case of drugs for tropical diseases.

There are several public policy options available when needed products would not otherwise be developed by industry due to a potentially low return on investment (279). A long-standing policy concerns patent law, which in effect conveys on the inventor a monopoly to market the product for a given period of time, for example, seven years. Patent terms have been widely debated in many countries, and have been extended in some such as the USA, to compensate somewhat for the long development time due to safety and efficacy testing required by national registration authorities. A second policy concerns what has been termed 'orphan drugs', potentially important drugs that may not be developed due to the small size of the market. In this instance, for example in the USA, companies are allowed a longer patent life when a drug is classified as having orphan status.

In comparison with the development of scientific knowledge, technological development is more directly affected by society. Biological knowledge can lead to many types of technology, but selection occurs. To some extent, technology is similar everywhere because of rapid communication between countries, but cultural differences persist. These cultural differences are expressed in subtle ways, but the most direct is probably through the marketplace, since the development of drugs and devices is largely a private activity in Western countries.

3.4 Conclusions

Overall, societal support for technology development seems wise. Technology offers much hope for the future. If society loses faith in research as a tool for progress, much will be lost and may be impossible to replace. Societies have supported research because of this faith in research and knowledge development. The failures of medical science and technology should not be allowed to obscure the fact that past, present, and future progress depends largely on support for technological change.

4. The adoption of health care technology

To write prescriptions is easy but to come to an understanding with people is hard.

Franz Kafka

Figure 3 illustrates the processes of development and diffusion by the well-known sigmoid curve. This curve relates the percentage of potential to actual adopters. This curve does not convey the dynamism of the diffusion process, and thus may not give sufficient insights into diffusion itself. It is particularly useful, however, in visualizing the policy framework affecting technology. Policies have been developed that deal with several stages in the life cycle of any health care technology.

Simply stated, diffusion begins when the technology is used on people. The first use is when the technology is tested on human subjects. This area encompasses a range of activities from first human use to large-scale controlled clinical trials. Usually, first human use reveals problems that require modification of the

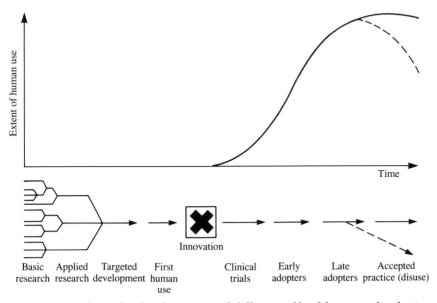

Figure 3. A scheme for development and diffusion of health care technologies (source: 492).

technology or further research. First human use is fairly easy to identify. However, it is not so easy to see when a technology ceases to be experimental and is established as worthy of widespread use.

Once the testing/experimental phase is completed, diffusion has two phases: the initial period when an individual or institution decides to adopt an innovation, and the subsequent period, encompassing the many decisions about how (and how frequently) to use it. Historically, adoption has been studied much more than use. Formal government policies have also dealt much more with adoption than with use. This is unfortunate in some ways, because the goal of public policy is to optimize use of technology. At the same time, it is much easier to control adoption than to influence use. The general pattern is adoption, followed by increasing use over time. A machine which has been purchased may still be underused. Overuse, too, is part of diffusion.

This chapter will deal with the stage of adoption. In some ways, separating adoption and use is an artificial separation, especially when dealing with procedures where adoption and use mingle. Nevertheless, adoption and use are different, especially when dealing with drugs and devices. Thus, this chapter tends to focus on the decisions concerning purchasing or providing a specific technology, particularly a product, while Chapter 5 tends to deal with physician procedures, whether they include drugs and devices or not.

4.1 Diffusion of some specific technologies

The diffusion of the CT scanner was described in the Introduction. Figure 4 shows another classic diffusion curve, that for the cardiac pacemaker in the USA. This again follows the sigmoid diffusion curve. As shown in these curves, initial diffusion is generally relatively slow. This is interpreted as indicating caution (573, p. 188). Then, as experience accumulates, more providers adopt an innovation, until it is in widespread use and the diffusion curve has flattened. Slow diffusion can also indicate government intervention.

Diffusion of health care technologies does not always follow the sigmoid curve. One major departure from this model occurs when diffusion reaches a high rate almost immediately after the technology becomes available, as in the case of chemotherapy for leukaemia in the USA, shown in Fig. 5. This pattern has been called the 'desperation-reaction model' (715,717). A first phase of rapid diffusion seems to occur because of the provider's sense of responsibility to help the patient and their mutual desperation. Later, evidence of efficacy and safety may influence diffusion, and the technology may diffuse further or fall from use. This case illustrates how the aggregate behaviour of many desperate patients and physicians may result in the extensive and premature diffusion of technologies that are incompletely developed, not effective, or possibly even dangerous. Another example is that of gastric freezing, which was widely used in the 1960s to treat peptic ulcers, until it was found to be ineffective and dangerous (see Fig. 6) (239). The different ineffective surgical procedures that

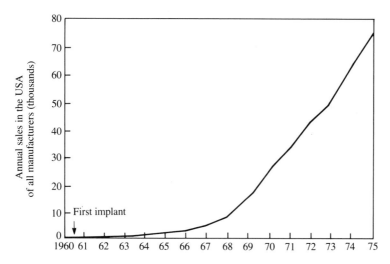

Figure 4. Diffusion of the cardiac pacemaker in the USA (source: 492).

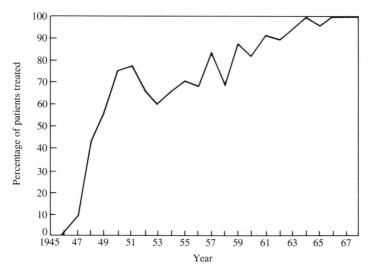

Figure 5. Diffusion of chemotherapy for leukaemia in the USA (source: 492).

were performed as a treatment for coronary artery disease before by-pass graft surgery was begun can also be cited (542). Finally, transplants, particularly the early heart transplants, fit this desperation-reaction idea (254).

Technology tends to have a life cycle. Over time it becomes obsolete and falls out of use or is replaced by a newer technology. For example, the technology

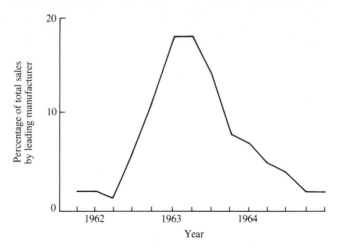

Figure 6. Diffusion of gastric freezing machines in the USA (source: 239).

of respirators and rehabilitation centres for polio victims disappeared rather quickly when polio vaccine came into use (682). When technologies are found to be of limited value, they are abandoned. Many surgical procedures have been developed and then abandoned as ineffective or relatively ineffective. A more recent example is extracranial—intracranial by-pass surgery for strokes, widely done since the late 1960s, which has been found to be ineffective (199).

It is difficult to describe diffusion in a way that conveys the dynamism of the process (37,299,716). Diffusion is made up of hundreds, perhaps thousands, of individual decisions. Research that attempts to discover the reasons for diffusion must summarize these many decisions in a way that makes the process look simpler than it in fact is. Few technologies have been studied, and many of these have differing patterns of diffusion and different factors that seem to be of importance in influencing the diffusion. Most studies have dealt with drugs or medical devices, and little is known about the diffusion of medical and surgical procedures.

Perhaps the most important point about diffusion, then, is that there is no theory or model that can be applied confidently to all technology. At the same time, a number of factors have been identified that influence diffusion.

A common situation is that a prestigious clinical researcher makes a discovery that seems to merit rapid diffusion. The typical behaviour is not to demand a careful evaluation. Rather, a common response is to state that the innovation should be available to anyone. It is common for such researchers to approach the media, and then patient demands make it increasingly difficult for policy makers to say 'no'. Practitioners do not generally have time to carefully review the literature, so prominent statements by well-known specialists, combined with patient demands or requests, may influence them greatly. When industry is involved in promoting the technology, the forces for its rapid diffusion are even greater. This complex situation is becoming even more complex with the growing commercial involvement of medical institutions.

4.2 Problems of adoption of new technology

Many observers have noted that health care practitioners often do not incorporate new medical knowledge into practice or that they misuse it (241,300). Technologies believed or proven to be efficacious are often slow to gain acceptance (182,293). Technologies that are questionable, and sometimes those that have been shown to useless, continue to be used (47,50,239). Some dangerous technologies that have turned out to be useless, such as the use of diethylstilbetrol (DES), have been widely adopted in some countries (16).

The variations in practice from one area to another, or from one country to another, are surprisingly large (526,727). Useless technology may be abandoned in one community, but continue to be used in another.

These observations point out that while biomedical science is truly international, technology is less so. Technology is subject to local standards and regulations, local reimbursement/pricing policies, local consensus, and local norms. In part, this is because physicians and other practitioners are trained to rely on their own judgement and experience. In part, however, this is because culture is inextricably interwoven with health care practice (303).

A major problem for a practitioner is uncertainty. He or she must deal with variations in disease and symptoms, variations in the performance of technology, a rapidly changing health care environment, especially medical knowledge and technology, as well as dealing with an unpredictable human being who has complaints and seeks rapid relief (303). Practitioners use various means to deal with these uncertainties (380). One is 'coherence', insisting that an observation makes sense within the practitioner's own framework of understanding; this holding onto pre-existing beliefs in the face of evidence is one of the reasons that practitioners sometimes reject efficacious therapies (293). Another means is staying within the local consensus or following the lead of a respected professor or senior colleague (278,303,429). Specialization helps a practitioner reduce uncertainty since it narrows the range of problems to be dealt with while also allowing one to limit one's perspectives. Finally, technology itself contributes to the easing of uncertainty, especially if it is a modern device that seems to give certainty in diagnosis. Eddy (209) has referred to the physician's tendency to act: 'when in doubt, do'.

4.3 Communicating information about new technologies

Before adoption can occur, knowledge about a technology must be communicated to a potential adopter. Little research has been done on the transferring of information from those who develop information to those who may use it.

Much of the information on communication that exists deals with drugs. Studies have indicated that physicians generally learn about a new technology from direct mail advertising and personal visits from industry representatives. However, the decision to buy or prescribe the technology seems to depend on more professional sources, such as colleagues or medical journals (6,370). Research on drugs led to the description of a two-step model, in which information flows initially to physicians who are opinion leaders. Through informal channels, the opinion leaders then transfer information to their followers (673).

Academicians often express dismay that practitioners do not use the scientific literature more effectively in their clinical decisions. Greer (303) has found that clinical physicians have limited trust in the scientific literature. They consider that it is biased because of the commitment of academicians to new technology and pressures on them to publish results. Practitioners continue to be conservative and wait for more convincing evidence of efficacy. Indeed, analyses of the biomedical literature have shown that early reports are often more optimistic than is justified in the light of later experience and research (239,286,763). One problem with the published literature is the long time delay before a study is published. In addition, the scientific literature is not addressed to practice needs (404). It does not report effectively on indications for use of a technology, limitations, safety problems, and factors in the testing situation that may explain success. Fletcher *et al.* (246) note a decline over time in articles dealing with clinical observations that would be helpful to practitioners. Young (764) found that researchers involved in clinical trials felt no responsibility for translating their findings into terms appropriate for clinical practice.

It is likely, therefore, that national and international conferences play a significant part in decisions of practitioners (25). At a clinical meeting, practitioners, especially specialists, can actually meet the innovators and assess for themselves their credibility (303). In addition, they can ask about specific factors not appearing in published work that may be key for success. However, this is only information, and may or may not lead to a decision to try out a new procedure. The actual decision to adopt depends on more than information transferred from the specialized medical centres.

Information is generally transferred by opinion-leaders (660). As Lohr *et al.* (429) say: 'In general, professional colleagues are considered more potent legitimizing agents than any other single influence, and the most effective force for physicians' adoption of medical innovations is professional, face-to-face contact with recognized peers.'

This formulation goes a long way towards explaining the adoption of new practice behaviours (159,211,605).

4.4 Factors influencing adoption

4.4.1 Characteristics of the technology

Recent literature on technology tends to stress the importance of knowing that it is efficacious and safe (487,350). Earlier literature, on the other hand, tended to assume that new technology was good and focused on characteristics of the technology that hastened its adoption: relative advantage over previous methods, compatibility with the adopter's values, complexity of understanding and using the innovation, ability to be tested on a limited basis, and observability or visibility of the results to others (673). Technologies that are thought to increase effectiveness in patient care tend to be adopted rapidly. On the other hand, if the technology is very complex or is not compatible with existing patterns of care, its diffusion is likely to be slower. Such a technology may require new skills or may involve a large number of people of diverse backgrounds, which makes it more difficult to adopt.

The CT scanner, described in the introduction to this Section, exemplifies a technology with many of the characteristics expected to speed adoption (23,25). The scanner was compatible with existing radiological practice, producing easily readable pictures of areas of the body previously not very accessible. Compared to other procedures, the CT scanner was associated with less discomfort and risk for the patient. In addition, it was a very profitable procedure, at least in the USA (502,503).

4.4.2 Characteristics of the adopter

The adopter of a large technology is usually an organization, especially a hospital. The literature, however, has mostly centred on individuals, either practitioners or those acting within institutions.

Research on individuals has tended to focus on drugs. Physicians with a higher level of training and a higher level of participation in the medical community more readily adopt a new drug (673). The nature of physicians that accept or reject new technology is very important, because physicians continue to have a large degree of autonomy as valued professionals (302). At the same time, many other clinicians are now involved in health care. Clinicians accepting an innovation tend to be more specialized. Well-established specialties tend to be more conservative; newer specialties with less tradition are more innovative (660).

Within organizations, adoption has generally been associated with members and administrators who have a higher level of training and a more cosmopolitan outlook (299,369,370). Decision-making within organizations is spread among subgroups who have different interests. All researchers agree that physicians are key decision-makers. Some researchers portray physicians as medically conservative, resistant to change, and sceptical of innovation (136,665). Others have stressed physician dominance in the formulation of hospital policies as explaining their decision-making processes and have emphasized that physicians often hold a consensus that overall capacity of the institution should be increased (316). A number of analyses have tended to confirm that hospitals must cater to physicians' desire for new technology (299,350,370,586,657).

Greer's studies in the USA and the UK have clarified this issue. She found that physicians are not homogenous, but can be classified into different categories tending to have a common view on technology. In the USA the categories were:

(1) community physicians, concerned primarily with patients seen in offices;

(2) community specialists, who are largely office based, but who emphasize a specialty oriented to hospital services and technologies;

(3) referral physicians, who restrict their practice to specialized procedures and are very dependent on the hospital;

(4) hospital-based physicians, who are entirely dependent on the hospital and typically have no private patients.

Hospital-based physicians are dependent on technology, readily accept new technology, and, because of their proximity and their commitment to a particular hospital, greatly influence decision-making in hospitals. Radiologists are members of the last group, which helps to explain the great growth in imaging capabilities in hospitals during the last decades (298,300,301).

The role of the administrator in these decisions has grown as hospitals have become larger and more complex (531,613). Administrators, like physicians, are a diverse group. Some are eager to acquire new technology, whereas others are more conservative. Clearly, the ability of administrators to influence hospital decisions increases as these institutions become more complex.

Large institutions buy new machines before smaller institutions, and university hospitals with concentrations of specialists especially accept new technology early. The decision to adopt can be greatly influenced by a few individuals, sometimes called opinion leaders or product champions (303,660). Product champions can be either individuals or one specialty group, pressing for the adoption of a particular technology. Generally speaking, radiologists functioned as product champions for medical imaging technologies.

Few studies have dealt with technology, especially equipment technology, in the out-of-hospital setting. This is unfortunate, for such technology is beginning to move rapidly into clinics and practices. Knowing more about this process is a challenge for future research.

By the 1990s, decisions to purchase or reimburse certain classes of new technology were increasingly being made by specialized committees, at least in the USA (90). Hospitals have two main types of committees. Technology assessment committees review decisions to purchase capital-intensive equipment and other technology-oriented expenditures, for example, cardiac catherization laboratories. These committees tend to be more concerned with prudent purchasing issues: is the expenditure a wise business investment for the hospital, rather than whether the investment is safe, efficacious, and cost-effective for society. Thus, these committees tend to be dominated by proprietary concerns related to hospital financial issues and the medical technologies themselves are treated similarly to non-medical technologies, such as computerized billing systems. Hospitals in health maintenance organizations (HMOs) in the US and European hospitals have similar committees with similar procedures for capital-intensive technologies. On the other hand, hospital drug formulary committees are concerned strictly with decisions regarding which drugs are purchased and made available to the medical staff. These committees are much more sophisticated in terms of assessing the relative safety, efficacy, and cost-effectiveness of a new drug compared with alternative drugs (90).

In the USA, HMOs and insurers also have technology assessment committees for insurance coverage decisions (90). These committees limit their concerns to major expensive new technologies, including medical and surgical procedures. Although they report that cost and cost-effectiveness are not criteria for acceptance, it is clear that only expensive technologies are assessed for their relative clinical advantages.

In Europe, institutions and insurers still tend to make decisions in an *ad hoc* manner (78,79,387,657). However, there is a trend toward making such decisions explicit, as will be described in Section V.

4.4.3 *Characteristics of the environment*

External factors affecting technology adoption are certainly important (25,39). Many of the factors mentioned so far are difficult or impossible to affect. Environmental factors such as financing, planning, and so forth are often easier to manipulate. National policy, therefore, tends to focus at this level.

Ideally, evaluation for efficacy and safety would be a central part of the process of adoption of technologies. However, formal evaluations in themselves have generally been found to have little impact (238,496). Why? The answer is complex, but one reason seems to be that evaluations are seldom done early enough in the development of a technology in order to have results available in time to influence adoption. Overall, relatively little information is available on efficacy and safety, and even less on cost and cost-effectiveness. Few outside the medical profession understand the extent to which practice is based on custom rather than science.

Diffusion has been found to be associated with a variety of factors aside from those mentioned. One important question is the relationship between technology and human health needs. Is technology autonomous, in search of a problem, or is it diffused to meet clear needs? The answer to this question is complex and has not been well-examined. It seems almost beyond question that technology is directed to the solution of human problems. In a sense, the relation between health care technology and human health problems is obvious. Technologies are addressed to the prevention, diagnosis, or treatment of disease. Perhaps the question would be clearer if it were stated as follows: Do important health needs determine the diffusion of technology, or does technology diffuse because of other factors? What is surprising in this context is that so much use of technology appears to be discretionary. Rates of use of technology vary remarkably from country to country and in small areas within countries, even after the rates of use are adjusted for age differences (604). Differences as large as twenty-fold have been found for such conditions as hysterectomy, urinary tract stones, medical back problems, and cataract excision (441).

What is the relation of societal values and patient preference to patterns of diffusion? This is another question difficult to answer. Clearly, society values technological progress. In fact, both physicians and patients often seem overly optimistic about the benefits of technology. But scepticism seems to be growing, and the public shows signs of wanting to have more systematic input to decisions about health care technology. In some cases where ethical concerns are important, as in prenatal screening and *in vitro* fertilization, consumers have been actively involved in discussions concerning diffusion (517,554).

It is obviously important for policy-makers to understand such factors so that policies can deal with the situation as it is in the 'real world'. However, directly manipulating these system factors is difficult. Factors in the environment that could be manipulated are of more interest, but the research on them is limited.

Society is obviously involved in controlling and channelling technological development. The public investment in research not only indicates the broad interest in knowledge development, but supports the public's right to know and influence. The major tool, of course, is government policy, and the major approach used so far to control technology is patent policy, tax policy for R&D investment, and regulation. Drugs and devices are regulated for efficacy and safety. Planning laws in some countries and some US states require approval before certain large technologies can be purchased, and cost-effectiveness is now being considered in several countries (164,320,327,511,512). The Canadian Province of Ontario and the Australian national government have both proposed regulations to require pharmaceutical firms to submit cost-effectiveness data developed from a prescribed methodological design as part of the drug approval applications. Quality is regulated by some government programmes. Obviously, programmes that prevent adoption of drugs and medical devices until they have been shown to be efficacious and safe influence their adoption. However, available research does not show much effect on diffusion from other regulatory programmes.

Probably the greatest force affecting diffusion of technology in an open system, such as those of The Netherlands and the USA, is payment (39,586). Payment for health care services through insurance mechanisms shows the society's general faith in the value of health care technology. However, the public and policy-makers increasingly question the value and cost-effectiveness of health care services. This scepticism is promoting change, including changes in the methods of payment. A much-publicized experiment in the US State of

Oregon has proposed that priorities are established for coverage in Medicaid, the state-funded medical poverty programme, based on a combination of cost-effectiveness data and value preferences stated in town meetings (205). Norway has also developed a priority list of services and The Netherlands is discussing priorities, an implicit recognition of limited resources.

Adoption of technology is fostered by third-party payment for health care services and is hindered by self-payment (233,586). Cost reimbursement to hospitals and fee-for-service payments to physicians have been associated with acceptance of new technology (586). Large profits are often built into re-imbursement for new high-technology services (24,25,487). Russell (586) found that the adoption of cobalt therapy and electroencephalography occurred more quickly in hospitals where the level of insurance coverage was higher and proceeded more rapidly as the level grew. On the other hand, global budgets or prospective budgets slow adoption (657).

The nature of the market for hospital services may also influence adoption of technology. Russell (586) found that hospitals in more concentrated markets were less likely to adopt open heart surgery, for example. Thus, competition among hospitals can also be an important force in the adoption of technology (25).

While health planning programmes in the USA have been found to have limited effect on technology adoption (25,596), regulation of rates of payment has been found to slow technology adoption (67,461). Joskow (367) examined the effects of different factors on the diffusion of CT scanning and found that only rate regulation had a clear constraining effect. In addition, different financial incentives within payment systems affect technology adoption. For example, Weisbrod (722) noted a retardation in the diffusion process following implementation of the US Medicare DRG prospective payment system in 1982. The new system pays hospitals a flat rate per admission rather than reimbursing costs, as it had been doing.

4.5 Conclusions

Overall, little is known about the influences on adoption of health care technology. Still, enough is known to point to the importance of public policy mechanisms in attempts to rationalize technological change. However, whatever public policy mechanism is used, whether it be regulation of market approval, reimbursement, or planning, better information from technology assessment is required for rational and efficient choices to be made.

Most countries have realized the importance of financial incentives and are grappling with policy changes to neutralize these important forces. European countries have moved toward fixed budgets for health care or global budgeting for hospitals (28,657). The important question now is how to improve processes of choosing which technologies to adopt.

5. Use of health care technology

I simply do not believe that when technology is injected into the medical system, it necessarily does what it is supposed to do, relieve human suffering. One of the reasons it does not achieve this is that medical personnel very often do not know how to be human.

Alan Sheldon

Be not swept off your feet by the vividness of the impression, but say, 'Impression, wait for me a little. Let me see what you are and what you represent. Let me try you'.

Epictetus

You can't always get what you want, but if you try, sometimes you get what you need.

The Rolling Stones

In the past, use of technology has received relatively little attention either from policy-makers or researchers. Regulatory programmes and explicit decisions within health care systems have tended to focus on the adoption stage. However, the recent focus on outcomes research in the USA is beginning to change this situation.

Adoption and use of technology have been separated into two chapters for several reasons. One is that no general relationship between adoption and use has been observed. Obviously, technology must be acquired to be used. However, adopted technologies are used at very different rates. Availability of a technology has been observed to increase use in the case of laboratory services and surgery (25). On the other hand, many pieces of equipment tend to be used under capacity.

Whereas the adoption decision can involve many different types of health care workers, the use decision is usually made by the physician. In the case of drugs or medical equipment, a prescription or order by a physician is usually required. In the case of a medical procedure, the physician's skill is a critical part of the technology. Thus, this chapter focuses more on the role of the physician than do other chapters.

5.1 Problems in the use of health care technology

The use of health care technology is obviously addressed to patient needs. Patients consult physicians. Sick patients are admitted by physicians to hospitals. Home-bound, chronically sick patients and those in nursing homes receive care under doctors' orders. During these encounters, technology is used as an integral part of the attempt to diagnose or treat disease or to ameliorate its consequences.

Within the complex health care system of clinicians, institutions, technology, and government interventions, it is crucial to remember the purpose of the enterprise: to promote or restore health to individuals. Ideally, then, patient choice should be respected, although there are often difficulties in practice. Few health care decisions are absolutely clear-cut. In prescribing a treatment for cancer, for example, a surgical treatment might give a slightly better chance of survival but more mutilation, while radiotherapy might give a lower chance of survival but might leave the patient with a better quality of life (439). Surely, the physician has no right in such cases to impose his or her own value systems on the patient. But information that is available indicates that patient choice is quite often not respected or even elicited. For example, a survey of European countries showed that few institutions give women a choice in birth position or whether or not certain procedures are carried out around the time of childbirth, even when these procedures have not been shown to be of value (753).

Ideally, technological decisions would involve clinical services given in a context of patient choice. However, the broader environment obviously limits and channels those choices. If a certain machine is not available in the country, or is too limited in numbers, a choice of another service must be made. This is particularly pertinent today, when governments and other policy-makers are attempting to rationalize the diffusion of technology. Such methods as technology assessment are attempts to make choices more rational in the aggregate. An important challenge is how to promote patient choice while at the same time making technological diffusion more rational.

Given that the purpose of technology appears to be relatively clear, it is surprising that use varies so dramatically—that use of technology appears to be so often discretionary. Wennberg and Gittelsohn (729) observed that the rates of common surgical procedures such as tonsillectomy, hysterectomy, and appendectomy in similar areas in New England varied by as much as 300 to 400 per cent. Subsequently, beginning with publications in 1982, such variations in use were documented internationally. Surgical rates were found to be higher in the USA than in the UK or Norway, but the degree of variability in the rates was approximately the same in all three countries, even after age- and sex-standardization (441). The greatest differences between countries was with tonsillectomy, which had a rate of 289 per 100 000 in the USA, 172 in the UK, and 64 in Norway. McPherson *et al.* stress the role of professional uncertainty in these variations. They felt that the procedures with little variation in use, such as herniorrhaphy and appendectomy, are those for which there is a consensus among physicians concerning their appropriate application.

Research on variations in use has now expanded rapidly in a number of countries, and a wide range of technologies have been studied, including admission rates to hospitals, lengths of stay for different diagnoses, cervical smear examinations, psychiatric services, certain drugs, and certain X-ray examinations. In 1984 the Copenhagen Collaborating Centre (CCC) was established to support and facilitate research concerning regional variations in health care. The CCC has published two extensive bibliographies of research in this area (143,144).

The problem revealed by variations in use is that practitioners are not aware of optimal use of technology, either because the evidence does not exist or because it is not utilized. At the same time, the intensity of use of technology has increased greatly. In the USA, laboratory and radiological services alone were found to account for up to 25 per cent of total bills in some hospitals (474). The average number of some diagnostic and therapeutic services provided per patient grew by over 500 per cent between 1951 and 1971, while length of stay dropped by as much as 40 per cent (609). These trends have continued into the 1990s. Patients and physicians alike tend to equate more intensive medical and health care with better care. In the absence of evidence, and without active policy interventions, care will merely become more and more intensive as new technology is developed.

Much use of technology seems to be discretionary and unnecessary. For example, previously recommended long hospital stays have been found to be unnecessary for uncomplicated myocardial infarction and post-delivery patients (343). Hospitalized patients in Rochester, New York, who were subjected to greatly increased use of laboratory test procedures or intensive care, showed no greater improvement than a control group not receiving these services (304). Additional care may actually be harmful to patients. Needless surgery, excessive drugs, or invasive procedures can cause iatrogenic disease (390,606). Unnecessary tests can also cause harm, especially through false-positive results, since such results can cause undue anxiety as well as lead to more invasive studies. Furthermore, test results are often ignored by physicians, implying that tests were not needed in the first place (474). A major problem is that appropriateness of use is often not known because of lack of information on efficacy and effectiveness (see Section III).

Variations in use indicate that much use of technology is socio-economic and cultural. Different groups in the population are treated in different ways. For example, Greenberg *et al.* (296) found that treatment of patients with lung cancer varied according to their marital status, medical insurance coverage, and proximity to a cancer-treatment centre. Patients with the same stage of cancer who were married were more likely to be treated with surgery, for example. Private insurance coverage was associated with higher rates of treatment: surgery, radiation, and chemotherapy.

5.2 The physician and technology

5.2.1 *Professionalism and technology*

As prestigious professionals, physicians have a high degree of autonomy. Society has granted physicians and other professionals such autonomy in part as a way of ensuring quality of services. At the same time, professionals fight to gain and keep autonomy over their work. In fact, autonomy is one of the basic factors in what makes up a profession. 'Control by an occupational group over its technology is what basically distinguishes a profession from other groups' (633, p. 161). Such control and autonomy is confirmed by government decisions, such as physician licensing and requirements for prescriptions for drugs. Studies of use of medical technology in Europe have shown continued dominance by physicians (657).

One of the implications of such control over technology is that the cost of health care, as well as the benefits, is largely under the control of physicians. It is a physician who decides who should be admitted to hospital, how long the person will stay, what tests will be performed, and what drugs will be prescribed. Physicians' decisions result in expenditures far beyond their own incomes, therefore. Data from the USA indicates that the average total expenditure obligated per physician exceeded US$400 000 in 1980 (181), and a simple extrapolation suggests that that figure rose to $992 000 in 1992.

Other groups of health workers are now seeking to emulate physicians in gaining immunity in order to control the conditions of their work. With the development of multiple groups of specialized workers in health care, outside control is increasingly difficult.

Part of the 'social contract' that gives the physician autonomy as a professional is that he or she is expected to act as the agent of the patient against any competing interest. In a situation of full financial coverage of health care, the physician has every reason to use a potentially beneficial technology, especially if the risk is small, despite costs or other societal implications. Clinical diagnosis and treatment are complex, and involve considerable uncertainty. Physicians in training are particularly prone to handle uncertainty by ordering excessive tests and procedures (474). In general, however, physicians believe that patient care will be improved by the use of technology. All these factors tend to lead to increased costs, which in turn lead to public policies that threaten physician autonomy.

Nevertheless, physicians continue to have high prestige in all countries, accompanying their status as important professionals, which means that they tend to be deferred to. They act politically to gain and maintain prerogatives. In health care systems, physicians tend to be administrators and other important decision-makers.

5.2.2 *Specialization and technology*

The growth in medical specialties is one of the most important phenomena of modern health care and one that has great consequences for the use of technology. In reality, the relationship is a very dynamic one. The development of new technologies has been one of the main forces leading to the establishment of medical specialties, as described in Chapter 2. Technology promotes the development of specialties; specialties in turn promote and use their technology.

Still, the growth of specialties has been moulded historically more by professional and economic interests than as a response to real needs (652). Mechanic estimated that a relatively small proportion of physicians—perhaps 15 or 20 per cent—could meet the need for consulting specialties in the USA (453, p. 48).

Of course, much specialization is not only natural in a technological world, it is necessary and desirable when it helps to improve quality of care (230). Misgivings have arisen, however, about the orientation of medical education and the numbers of specialists trained, especially in the USA. Medical education depends on hospital-based clinical training dominated by a full-time faculty of specialists. Medical education involves the socialization of those entering the medical profession to accept and emulate that model. Students are trained to rely on and to use specialized technologies housed in large hospitals and to pursue specialty practice, with its higher prestige and income (362). Physicians associated with teaching hospitals use more resources for the same type of patient— more consultations, laboratory tests, X-rays, and other diagnostic procedures (474).

In summary, specialization is generally associated with increased use of technology. A specialty is generally involved with a specific technology that it believes in and wants to apply. The payment system generally rewards specialists and the public seeks specialty-oriented health care. These forces have both positive and negative consequences in addition to limiting the ability of policy-makers to influence the use of technology.

5.3 Organization of health care

The growth of medical technology has stimulated the development of large and complex institutions. In part, these institutions merely house the technology, often making it available on a regional basis. In part, the large capital investments that have been required for technological development could only be made by large and complex institutions.

5.3.1 Technology and organizations

The hospital is the most important social institution involved with health care technology. It is the centre for the expanding technology of health care and it serves the sickest people. Medical and surgical specialists tend to orient their practice towards hospital services and procedures. Indeed, modern medical practice is unthinkable without specialized hospital services.

Literature on the adoption of medical technology by hospitals was reviewed in the previous chapter. Although little work has been done on the implications of hospital structure or size on technology use compared with adoption, the hospital must have such influences. In a time of increasing concern about excessive services, the administration of hospitals often takes action to lower costs per case. This is especially true for hospitals operating under constrained budgets, either from global budgets or from set fees per case, such as DRGs.

The literature does not show clearly what the effect of the organization of non-hospital services is on the use of technology (37, pp. 84–85). However, in the USA, health maintenance organizations have been shown to have lower hospitalization rates and lower rates of certain types of surgery than free-standing hospitals (434). This tends to confirm that organization itself may have effects on the use of technology, but it is difficult to separate such effects from those of payment mechanisms, discussed below.

5.3.2 Bureaucratization and technology

As medical practice has become increasingly institutionalized and specialized, it has also become increasingly bureaucratized (452). The administrator makes more of the important decisions, and politicians and lay boards, as well as various committees, have more influence.

Scientific management and bureaucratic functioning are in considerable conflict with professional norms as applied by physicians (369). The bureaucratic model sees health care as an economic good that should be provided in an economically efficient manner, instead of as a service that should be provided by a professional group committed to high quality and ethical practice. The bureaucratic organization calls for a hierarchy of authority, while the professional prefers a high degree of discretion and informality. Thus, clashes of culture can and do occur.

One important aspect of the institutionalization of practice is that it dilutes the physician's commitment to the interests of the patient (257,258). Physicians practising in institutions tend to be more oriented to their peers, while physicians practising alone are more patient-oriented (258). On the whole, economic efficiency is not in the individual patient's best interest, although it may be in the best interest of the collective of patients. The physician in the organization comes under pressure to satisfy organizational needs. One of these needs, for example, may be to avoid 'unnecessary services'. On the other hand, since technology is usually associated with increased prestige, growth of an institution, and often increased income, the physician may also come under pressure to use certain services (474). In addition, patients themselves assert pressure on physicians to use the latest technologies available.

The institutionalization of medicine is also related to a loss of the caring function in medicine, and must then be related to public dissatisfaction with present-day medicine. The organization relieves the physician of continuing responsibility for the patient. Failures of the organization are harder to attribute. Accountability may be lessened or lost. The pressures for efficiency tend to lead to a system that rewards good management or the ability to cope with a large work load rather than humane and interested health care practice.

The bureaucratic organization has great theoretical advantages in an era of limited resources, but the physician's commitment to the patient may conflict with the rationing and control of the technology of medicine. Thus, the promotion of solutions to the problem of overuse of technology through organization may lead to increasing dehumanization of health care, as well as dissatisfaction within the medical profession. In addition, it is not fully clear the degree to which managers are ready to take on a role of limiting health care technology. This argues for caution in implementing organization strategies, even though they are one of the most powerful tools available to policy makers.

5.4 Liability for malpractice

Malpractice is often cited as a reason for using technology, particularly diagnostic tests such as clinical laboratory tests and X-rays (69,348), which presumably make the diagnostic process more reliable (so-called 'defensive' medicine). A specialty that has been a target for malpractice suits in the USA is obstetrics (581). The desire for a 'perfect baby' has led to lawsuits when babies are born with injuries, and the resulting fear of liability has led obstetricians to use electronic fetal monitoring (678) and contributed to a higher rate of Caesarean section (593). Although the problem of malpractice is most visible in the USA, its occurrence is increasing in Europe as well. In the USA, the original malpractice system was established to protect patients from and indemnify them for acts of medical negligence. However, with time, awards have been made to provide compensation to victims of medical accidents, even if there was no negligence (198). This philosophy has led to a proliferation of malpractice suits in the USA. In the UK, partly for this reason, it was decided to keep malpractice closely based on the negligence concept (421). None the less, there is a worldwide trend towards compensating the victims of medical and technological injury (190, p. 362). For example, in the UK, malpractice has been increasing at the rate of 75 per cent per year (69).

Starr (647, p. 445) points to the growth of bureaucratic practice and the resulting weakening of the doctor–patient relationship as a key cause for malpractice. Since medicine has been more highly organized in Europe and other areas of the world, this explanation will not necessarily hold everywhere.

5.5 Payment for health care services

Probably the greatest force affecting the use of technology is the system of payment, with its built-in incentives. Payment for health care services through insurance mechanisms and health care budgets shows society's general faith in the value of health care technology. Payment can be used not only to discourage use, but to lead to more rapid or widespread use. For example, if the level of payment is set well above the cost of providing the service, the provider has a strong incentive to provide the service. If the payment is lower than the cost, the provider will be cautious in using that technology.

Rises in health care costs and a degree of scepticism about the benefits of health care technology is promoting change, including changes in the methods of payment. The adoption and use of technology is greatest in countries with liberal payment policies. It is no accident that costs in the USA are the highest in the world. In many ways, medical technology has fuelled these costs due to the historically low restraint within the payment system. The US experience can be contrasted with that of the UK, which has been one of extreme budget constraint, low cost, and relatively slow technology adoption and use. Most other countries fall between these extremes.

In the USA, payment to hospitals has historically been cost-reimbursement, and physicians are generally paid fee-for-service. Both of these methods encourage the use of technology. The US Congress realized this fact and has changed the basis of hospital payment in the US Medicare Program to a prospective system based on diagnosis-related groups (DRGs), which has most likely slowed the diffusion of technology to some extent. The DRG payment system is now being considered for adoption in several European countries, such as France and The Netherlands, because of its impact on use.

Payments also give incentives to use certain technologies. At the moment, high-technology diagnostic and curative services are generally reimbursed at well above cost levels, while prevention and rehabilitation are reimbursed at lower levels, if at all (474). Insurance funds and governments are beginning to realize such facts, and the situation may change (7,37,67,499,586,706). In the USA, prospective budgeting is spreading through such mechanisms as preferred provider organizations (PPOs), managed care, and selective contracting with physicians and hospitals.

Weisbrod (722) argues that prospective payment schemes encourage, at the margin, health care institutions to reduce cost rather than improve quality. He notes that the cost/quality tradeoff is particularly problematic when it is costly (or difficult) to observe changes in quality. He cites examples of increased use of 'disposables' in hospitals (516,575) and decreased lengths of stay as a direct result of the DRG system. In both instances, there is little evidence of quality decrease, but neither has been studied well. On the other hand, prospective pricing mechanisms can foster easily observable quality increasing activities such as improved amenities in hospitals. US hospitals compete actively by providing gourmet meals and much nicer accommodation for patients and guests.

Relman (556) has pointed to commercial interests of physicians in certain services as promoting conflicts of interest. For example, if a physician owns a laboratory or X-ray equipment, he or she may over-use it if there is profit in such use. Such commercial involvements have been growing, at least in the USA.

5.6 Industry promotion of its products

Industries spend a great deal of money and effort promoting their products. This is particularly true of the drug industry. In 1970, the Commissioner of the Food and Drug Administration estimated that the drug industry spent around US$4000 per US physician a year promoting their products (628). Promotion is generally 11–25 per cent of sales (122). In The Netherlands, it was estimated in 1991 that the advertising budget for drugs was 20–24 per cent of company budgets (195).

Most of the promotional money spent by the drug industry is used to support 'detail' men and women who visit physicians, pharmacists, and hospital purchasing agents. In the USA in 1978, industry supported an estimated 25 000 such individuals (628). In 1983, 55 per cent of company promotional budgets in the UK paid for sales representatives, enough to ensure one representative for every 8 general practitioners (59). Since physicians do not have the time to keep up with the professional literature, and lack the training to critically examine it, these detailers can have a large influence on prescribing habits (628, p. 50). When physicians were asked to list the most important sources for information on new drugs, 68 per cent specified detail men and women (183, p. 274). Drug promotional activities include free samples, gifts, financial support for medical conventions, exhibits at medical conventions, and advertisements in medical journals. Repeated examinations of drug industry advertising have shown that it is not reliable (628,705). In particular, drug advertising gives only positive information about the drug (122). In addition, prominent experts are retained as consultants by drug companies, and sometimes promote drugs without identifying a financial interest. The industry defends its promotional practices as bringing useful drugs to the attention of physicians, making possible mass production, and lowering production costs (628, pp. 50–51).

The issue of financial relationships between the pharmaceutical industry has been extensively analysed (84,124,227,635). Gifts to physicians raise ethical problems. They may threaten the physican's role as patient trustee, shifting the balance between self-interest and altruism (124). In the USA, professional associations have become increasingly involved in this issue. For example, the American Surgical Association has deemed it unethical for a surgeon to accept a material reward for participating in product promotional activities not related to a professional service (84).

Promotion of pharmaceuticals is even more important in less developed countries (319). Many developing countries have one sales representative to every three physicians (630). Silverman has carried out studies in Latin America, Africa, and Asia during the 1970s, comparing information in the US Physician's Desk Reference to claims made for the same products in the developing countries. Silverman found glaring differences between the promotion of selected prescription drugs in the US and other countries, with claims of efficacy broader in the developing countries, while the information on side effects and contra-indications often did not appear. Sometimes exaggerated claims were made for potentially dangerous drugs, such as chloramphenicol (an antibiotic) and 'tissue building' anabolic hormones (627,630). Silverman found the situation improved in 1984, but the problem still persisted (629). By the late 1980s, the multinational companies were more willing to restrict claims of efficacy and to disclose major hazards, but domestic firms had not changed their practices (409). In 1992, the US Office of Technology Assessment found that the problem of labelling was still quite serious (57). Promotion in developing countries is more serious than in industrialized countries because sources of information are much more limited.

At the same time, it should be noted that the drug industry is the largest single supporter of controlled clinical trials. In the USA, it was estimated that US$750 million of the total US$1.1 billion invested in clinical trials in 1984 was spent by the drug industry (350). The industry reports that it has been increasing its investment in developing new drugs, from 11.7 per cent of sales in 1980 to 15.9 per cent of sales in 1990 (535).

In addition, the industry supports educational seminars and other educational activities, such as scientific meetings. These are both valuable and biased, sometimes subtly, sometimes blatantly. Such industry sponsorship is more intense in European countries such as Sweden than in the USA (731).

The equivalent system for medical devices has not been thoroughly described. None the less, it certainly exists and from personal observations has many of the characteristics of the drug promotional system. Because of the capital expense of many devices, however, the promotional activity is focused more toward institutions than to individual physicians. Advertisements in recent medical journals include offers to have a sales representative visit an institution to demonstrate and explain certain pieces of medical equipment.

The health care industries have well-organized trade associations that lobby nationally and internationally on their behalf. One has the impression that the industry is more powerful now than in past years, as economies weaken and governments seem often more responsive to arguments concerning jobs, profits, and exports than to arguments concerning health and quality of care.

Industry promotion is effective. In the opinion of a medical journalist, 'drug industry marketing strategy is often much more effective than scientific information' (3). In a survey of UK general practitioners, 58 per cent mentioned a sales representative as the source of information for new products that they prescribed (15).

5.7 The general public and use of technology

The public also demands use of technological services. Patients often associate advanced technological procedures, diagnostic tests, and drug prescription with good health care (474). For example, Marton *et al.* (450) found that nearly two-thirds of patients felt that a better doctor would order more tests when evaluating a patient's problem. Patients thus often equate technological sophistication with high-quality care.

Every physician is familiar with the patient who demands a certain diagnostic procedure or a special treatment. This tendency is stimulated by the growing media coverage of new technology. The 'miracles' of modern technology are now often described in newspapers and lay periodicals, leading to immediate demands for new procedures. The case of laparoscopic cholecystectomy, described in Chapter 14, is an example of a technology that has diffused extremely rapidly into practice around the world despite surgeon resistance because of media reports and resulting patient demands for a less-invasive alternative (24,28).

This phenomenon also applies to medical periodicals. The lay press scrutinizes each issue of prestigious publications for newsworthy material. The *New England Journal of Medicine* has a policy to embargo press coverage of stories under the release date, to give physicians a chance to evaluate an article for themselves before stories in the press cause patients to embarrass them with demands for unfamiliar treatments (557). This is a serious problem, because journalists seldom do even the simplest form of assessment of the validity of statements by medical and scientific experts (3). An example was a study published in the *New England Journal* in 1988 of the benefits of taking small amounts of aspirin in the prevention of myocardial infarction. The article, and the accompanying press coverage, apparently stimulated many questions to physicians and pharmacists in the USA, and probably many people began taking aspirin who should not do so (558).

Increasingly, health care technology is promoted directly to the public, and not through physicians and other providers. In the USA, an anti-allergy drug was advertised in the *New York Times* and *Chicago Tribune*, and other newspapers in 1987 (134). There are a number of problems with such advertisements, including their truthfulness. In particular, studies have shown that even if advertisements of drugs are honest, those reading them tend to remember potential benefits much more than risks. The drug industry would like to promote public demand for more drugs. However, societies until now have decided that physicians have the responsibility for diagnosing disease and prescribing a treatment. This direct promotion is probably not in the public interest (134).

The business and investment communities also follow closely and act upon reports of new studies, in the press and elsewhere. In June 1986, for example, the *New England Journal of Medicine* published results of a clinical study indicating a superior quality of life with a new antihypertensive medication (147). The price of the manufacturers' stock (a major pharmaceutical firm) was reported to have increased by 10 per cent due to the report. In January 1991, an article in the *Journal of the American Medical Association* (210) reported that same drug to be highly cost-ineffective relative to competitors. The *Wall Street Journal* carried a major story covering this study. Also, virtually any hearing of the Food and Drug Administration on a major new technology, particularly a biotechnology, has reporters and investment counsellors crowding the hearing room.

Another example is a recent series of Battelle studies in the USA and France estimating the future potential health and economic benefits of medical technological innovations and improvements in lifestyles (12,91,92). The findings, widely reported in the press, were that the most promising areas were pharmaceutical products and public health efforts to change unhealthy lifestyles.

In the USA and throughout the industrialized world, there seems to be almost as much public interest in the cost of new technologies as in their medical promise. Due to the high budget impact of health care on governments, hospitals, insurers, and even general industry, the prices and costs of new technologies are coming under increased scrutiny. Policies are being developed in all societies to constrain the prices and the adoption and use of new technologies.

Thus, society at all levels—the medical profession and health care community, insurers, the consumer, the business and investment sector, the press, and governments—are intensely interested in medical technologies. They love them on a personal level, and are worried about them on an institutional or societal level. Much of this concern could be alleviated with appropriate policies for assessment.

5.8 Technology assessment and use of technology

The other force that is of great interest to policy-makers is the assessment or evaluation of technology. However, as noted, aside from mandated premarket studies, most assessments are done when the technology is already in widespread use, so they have had limited effect on diffusion. Patterns of use are often established before evaluations are completed. It is therefore important to evaluate early.

Does technology assessment affect physician behaviour? The evidence is imperfect and difficult to interpret (496). It will be reviewed in Section III of this book.

5.9 Conclusions

The tendency in public policy has been to focus on technology adoption and to use regulation as the main tool in attempting to channel technological change. This approach has demonstrably failed. Increasingly, financial incentives are being developed and used for optimizing technology adoption and use. A combination of assessment and education for professionals, along with a financial system that rewards cost-effective practice, seems to be the model for the immediate future. This new approach seems to have considerable potential, but in itself it requires further research and evaluation.

However, the public is largely forgotten. Given the difficulties of changing the health care system, with its many vested interests, perhaps a direct approach to the public would be of benefit. None the less, ultimately there is no easy solution to problems of rapidly diffusing health care technology in a climate of increasingly strained resources.

Section III ASSESSING HEALTH CARE TECHNOLOGY

The adoption and use of health care technology should be based on well-validated information on its benefits and risks first and foremost. In many cases, information on financial implications is also necessary. In some cases, analysis of the social and ethical dimensions of a particular technological area may be helpful to decision-makers.

Such information can be produced by a process that has come to be known as technology assessment, developed because of general societal concerns about technology and its effects. The field began formally in about 1965 in the Committee on Science and Astronautics of the House of Representatives of the US Congress. Through hearings and studies, the Committee described the need for new approaches to anticipating and controlling the consequences of technological change (130,157). One important result of the Committee's work was the development and passage of the Technology Assessment Act of 1972 (Public Law 92-484), establishing the Office of Technology Assessment (OTA) as an agency to serve the Congress. OTA's work has gone far to develop the field and to demonstrate its importance and its relevance to responsible policy decision-making.

Technology assessment is seen as a comprehensive form of policy research that examines short- and long-term social consequences (for example, societal, economic, ethical, legal) of the application of technology (19,130,492). Thus, technology assessment is an analysis of primarily social rather than technical issues, and it is particularly concerned with unintended, indirect, or delayed social impacts. The goal of technology assessment is to provide policy-makers with information on policy alternatives, such as allocation of research and development funds, formulation of regulations, or development of legislation.

Technology assessments have been completed in virtually every area of technological change, from examining global warming to the placement of nuclear missiles. As health care technology became an important policy issue, primarily because of the rising costs of health care, it was natural to attempt to apply these developing ideas to it. The US National Academy of Sciences published a report in 1973 that examined the implications of four technologies: *in vitro* fertilization, choosing the sex of children, retardation of ageing, and modifying human behaviour (138). The National Institutes of Health carried out an assessment of the totally implantable artificial heart in 1973 (478). In 1975, the US Congress developed a health programme in the Office of Technology Assessment. That may be said to be the birth of the formal field of health care technology assessment, although studies had begun simultaneously in Stockholm (366).

To assure that assessment information is available to the appropriate decision-makers at the time it is needed, many believe that a policy concerning technology assessment is needed at the national level. The first chapter of this section (Chapter 6) describes the structure of such a system in more detail. Chapter 7 discusses efficacy and safety and its measurement and estimation. Chapter 8 discusses the evaluation of costs, including cost-effectiveness, cost-benefit and cost-utility analysis. Chapter 9 presents the techniques, methods, and state of the art of measuring the effects of health care technologies on the quality of life. Chapter 10 introduces social consequences of health care technology and their evaluation. And the final chapter of this section, Chapter 11, discusses some concepts of quality of care assurance.

6. A system for health care technology assessment

It is disgraceful in every art, and more especially in medicine, after much trouble, much display, and much talk, to do no good after all.

Hippocrates

Knowledge is of two kinds. We know a subject ourselves, or we know where we can find information upon it.

Samuel Johnson

Effective planning requires information on which technologies are beneficial and how beneficial each is. It requires that technologies be applied to important health care needs. It requires an idea of how much each technology will cost. It requires some idea of the social context of the technology: will it be acceptable to patients, does it challenge ethical systems, will physicians and other providers use it? The consequences of technological change must be well understood. The goal is to identify important developments and to assess their implications. Ultimately, such information could be used in making policy decisions.

Decisions about today's technologies should be made today. Decisions about tomorrow's technologies should be made as early in their respective life cycles as is reasonably possible. Both existing and future technology can be dealt with in a system of health care technology assessment.

6.1 What is technology assessment?

Technology assessment arose because of general social concerns about technology. As already described, one result of reports and discussions in the US Congress was the formation of the US Office of Technology Assessment (OTA) in the Congress in 1972.

Technology assessment is a form of policy research that examines short- and long-term social consequences (for example, societal, economic, ethical, legal) of the application of technology (19,130,131). The goal of technology assessment is to provide policy-makers with information on policy alternatives.

In 1975, OTA established a health programme, formally beginning the field of health care technology assessment. Within the broader context of technology assessment, differences with health technology were recognized. The first was the goal of health care: to improve health. In addition, health care technologies are often small and discrete, as compared to huge investments in industry, defence, or energy. The impact of health care technology depends on its pervasiveness: it touches virtually everyone's life. Therefore, as it has developed, health benefits of technology have been the main focus of health care technology assessment, with increasing attention to financial costs over time. The main application of health care technology assessment has been to make specific decisions within specific policy areas, to be discussed in Section 6.2.

It is important to realize, however, that the field of technology assessment encompasses much broader studies. The diffusion of technology needs more research. The role of technology in society and the health care system should be better understood. The public role, and the public's understanding of technological issues, need to be taken into account. Technology assessment should develop in such a way as to shed light on these broader questions.

6.2 Using technology assessment in public policy mechanisms

As described in earlier chapters, there are a variety of public policy mechanisms dealing with health care technology (35). Governments fund health-related research and development. Drugs are regulated for efficacy and safety. Medical devices are similarly regulated in some societies. Physicians are licensed to practise medicine and in the USA they may become board-certified in medical specialties; hospitals and other facilities are licensed and accredited; health planning bodies sometimes regulate technology. And payment policy may be the most important determinant of technology use. Payment for health care services by sickness funds and insurance companies means that patients and physicians use technologies either free or at a small cost to themselves. Hospital, regional, provincial, and even national budgeting systems severely constrain technology acquisition.

Using technology assessment as an aid to decision-making in these programmes is a relatively new idea. Only in the area of drug regulation is evidence concerning the technology systematically collected and used as an important determinant in decision-making. And in this case, it is mainly used for the initial market introduction and labelling, but not the ultimate use of the drug.

Each policy mechanism, each regulation, each decision concerning payment and payment levels, could be improved by using the best available information on a technology or a group of technologies. The actual information needed varies from programme to programme. In the area of drug regulation, scientific evidence on safety and efficacy is the main need; economic and social implications play relatively little part in the decisions. In regulation of facilities, efficacy and safety are important, but costs and efficiency are also key variables; cost-effectiveness analysis can be very helpful at this stage. A number of countries engage in price regulation of new technologies. In other countries, prices are determined by the manufacturer or the market. In a truly competitive market, prices will ultimately approximate to the costs of production, but the medical market is far from a truly competitive market. For manufactured technologies, patents are awarded to encourage investment in R&D, which may permit monopolistic pricing except where pricing is regulated. Nevertheless, in all cases, prices should be reasonable and commensurate with the benefits provided.

Today, a serious problem in using technology assessment as an aid to decision-making is that information from assessments is often not available when it is needed. Assessments are generally not done with strategic purposes in mind. Ideally, assessments should be done in phase with the life cycle of a particular technology. Thinking of the life cycle of a technology in five stages may help clarify this point:

(1) future technology—technology not yet developed;

(2) emerging technology—technology prior to adoption;

(3) new technology—technology in the phase of adoption;

(4) accepted technology—technology in general use;

(5) obsolete technology—technology that should be taken out of use.

This scheme can make some of the decision points obvious. If a future technology is a drug or device, industry must decide whether or not to commit resources to develop it; must then decide if it wants to market and promote it; and must ultimately decide whether to maintain, alter, or discard it. If a new drug is to be marketed, the drug regulatory system must decide if it is to be allowed on the market. If the new technology is to be used in practice, someone must decide whether to provide it, purchase it, or pay for it. Decisions must also be made to stop providing obsolete technology. Hospitals must decide whether to purchase, and practitioners and their patients must decide whether to use, the technology. Finally, accepted or existing technology needs to be reviewed for new uses and modifications or the possibility of obsolescence.

If the technology is a medical or surgical procedure, there are fewer decision points (although complex procedures often involve drugs and devices). Procedures are not regulated and industry is not directly involved. The main decisions, then, are institutional and practitioner decisions to provide the technology and payment decisions. The policy mechanism that can affect procedures is then the payment or budget mechanism.

To affect the diffusion of technology in a constructive way requires attention to the needs for information. Information needs differ for different technologies, but they also differ according to such factors as the stage in the life cycle and the importance of the technology for society. One important stage in the life cycle of a technology is before it has actually been developed or evaluated: when it is an issue for the future. There has, none the less, been relatively little research concerning future health care technology.

One scheme to integrate technology assessment into planning processes is shown in Fig. 7 (231). The planning process starts with the burden of illness, considering how much is modifiable by technology. The technology is assessed in controlled circumstances, those in need are identified, and community effectiveness is estimated. The cost of a programme is put in relation to its benefits. All information is then combined synthetically to arrive at recommendations on facilities planning and diffusion of technology.

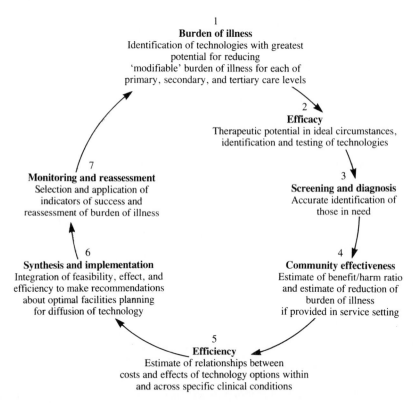

Figure 7. The technology assessment iterative loop (source: 231).

6.3 A system for assessing health care technology

A complete system for technology assessment of all new health care technology would monitor technological change at all different stages of technological development and diffusion. The following assessments would be part of its activities.

1. *Prospective assessments*. Certain technologies expected to be important—in terms of costs, impact on health, or impact on the health system—could be assessed before they are developed. This is a speculative type of assessment that is concerned primarily with social effects of the technology. The attempt is to identify technology that is likely to develop. A project in The Netherlands examined five technological areas prospectively: neurosciences, lasers, vaccines, genetic screening, and home care technology. One conclusion was that expanding opportunities in human genetics raises social issues such as discrimating against people with certain genetic susceptibilities for jobs or insurance (41). The suggestion was to make the use of genetic tests for this purpose unlawful. Another conclusion was that technology can help make home care more possible and more cost-effective (34). Strategic investments in this area of R&D could give great returns to society.

2. *Assessments for efficacy and safety*. Traditionally, these assessments are early in the life cycle. At present, only drugs and biologics are systematically examined for efficacy and safety. Many technologies come into widespread use without such assessments. Policies could be used to slow technological diffusion until such evidence was available. In addition, the system for identifying future technology would alert policy-makers when it was nearing readiness for diffusion, and assessments could be required or funded at that point. It is also necessary to assess efficacy and safety as the technology diffuses. The technology continues to improve, and it is used for ever-broadened indications. Therefore, an iterative process of assessment is necessary (48).

3. *Assessments for cost-effectiveness*. When data are available on efficacy, cost-effectiveness calculations can be made. In many cases, cost data can be collected during early clinical trials. Cost-effectiveness studies can be done at any stage in the life cycle, but are probably most useful before widespread diffusion (154,188).

4. *Assessments after diffusion*. When a technology has diffused widely, generally little attention is paid to it. However, there are a number of reasons for examining a technology at this stage after it has been widely accepted. The costs of the technology tend to come down over time. Medical devices may become easier to handle because of the manufacturer's modifications. The usefulness of the technology may be quite different in the community compared with its usefulness in the university hospital. A different group of people may receive the technology. Indications may be broader: the technology may be used

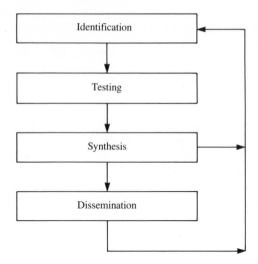

Figure 8. A process for developing and disseminating health care technology assessments (source: 489).

with less severe cases of the disease or with older or younger people. The providers may be less (or more) skilful. Patients may be less prone to follow the advice of physicians.

In some cases, important technologies would be examined prospectively and then examined iteratively (48). In other cases, only a few studies to demonstrate efficacy and safety might be necessary. The number and type of studies would be determined by the importance of the technological decisions to be made and by the resources available for assessment. Such assessments should be done without preconceptions. The technology might be encouraged; the assessment might show that it is valuable enough to be diffused very rapidly. The technology might be discouraged, or it might be left alone to diffuse without active policy intervention.

Such a complicated set of activities requires a systematic approach. A system or process of technology assessment may be viewed as an interdependent and non-discrete flow of four types of actions (see Fig. 8).

1. Identification: monitoring technologies, selecting those in need of study and deciding which to study.
2. Testing: conducting the appropriate data collection and analysis.
3. Synthesis: collecting and interpreting existing information and the results of the testing step, and, usually, making recommendations or judgements about appropriate use.

4. Dissemination: providing the synthesized information, or any other relevant information, to the appropriate persons who use or make decisions concerning the use of health care technologies.

A system for assessing health care technology should include all of these actions. This is not to say that one institution must carry out all of these actions. The system could be made up of a number of subparts. However, the system should be coordinated and integrated.

6.3.1 *Identification*

A decision to conduct technology assessments must be preceded by the identification of technologies that are candidates for assessment and the setting of priorities among candidate technologies. Some identification of technologies is already carried out routinely. For example, the process of regulating drugs requires that all drugs be registered before they can be marketed. Thus, a complete list of present drugs is available, and some information on future drugs is available through this mechanism. A similar process exists for the introduction of major devices and diagnostic technologies in the USA, especially for invasive devices.

A technology that is a discrete medical procedure is unregulated. Examples include renal dialysis, gastrointestinal endoscopy, and heart transplantation. Some information is available through health planning mechanisms and special studies. However, this information covers only a small part of the universe of new and existing health care technology. In addition, new or expanded uses of existing drugs, devices, and diagnostic technologies are often not identified.

Without a rather complete list of technologies, priority setting is severely hampered, since priorities can only be set among technologies that are already known. Thus, although priorities may be set for carrying out health care technology assessments, these are necessarily imperfect. Priorities for assessment might include beneficial technologies that are neglected or technologies that are suspected to be useless or dangerous. Technologies that are, or are expected to be, either expensive or widely used could also be given priority. For new technologies, potentially important advances should be given priority so that they could be assessed rapidly. For old technologies, syntheses of available knowledge can indicate if the technology has been well-tested or that it might be obsolete.

Priority setting has received increasing attention (180,208). Eddy (208) summarizes criteria used by several different organizations in setting priorities. Eddy also developed the Technology Assessment Priority-Setting System (TAPSS) for the Methods Panel of the Council on Health Care Technology of the Institute of Medicine (IOM). TAPSS is a quantitative model that combines data on the population affected, the economic importance of the technology, and the impact of an assessment on the health and economic outcomes for a population. Eddy recognized that his model does not provide precise answers, but states that it is 'more accurate and accountable than attempting to perform the entire exercise implicitly and subjectively'. Phelps and Parente (537) have developed an alternative approach to quantifying priorities in this field.

The development of the 'effectiveness initiative' in the USA has stimulated a great deal of work on setting priorities, especially that funded by the new Agency for Health Care Policy and Research (see Chapter 20). The US Institute of Medicine (IOM) has done much of this work (427). In 1990, Lara and Goodman (401), working in the IOM, invited a large set of interested groups to nominate candidate technologies and conditions for assessment. As part of the effort, the report described an ongoing process for ranking specific candidates for health care technology assessment. The process was applied to the candidate technologies and 20 high-priority candidates were selected. Subsequently, priorities in such areas as breast cancer (424), myocardial infarction (451), and hip fracture (426) were defined.

The most extensive attempt to develop an analytic model was done by a committee of the Institute of Medicine (180). The model incorporates seven criteria with which to judge a topic's importance. It combines scores and weights for each criterion to produce a priority ranking for each candidate topic. Using the model also requires judgements by a panel, data gathering by programme staff, and review by a national advisory council. The model was tested during 1991.

The development of quantitative models seems a helpful step in the field of health care technology assessment. However, all priority-setting programmes also include human judgement. This is important both because of the inherent limitations of the models and because health care technology assessment is itself part of human and political processes (38).

6.3.2 *Testing (data collection)*

This step includes stimulating, requiring, funding, or conducting studies and collecting data. Testing can and often should be done at various stages in the life cycle of the technology.

The assessment of future technology is limited (39). The technology does not yet exist, so its effects cannot be directly evaluated; nor are its costs known. Thus, only limited data collection can be done. One example would be to collect data on existing health care practice that the technology is destined to change and then model the difference that a particular technology might make. Or perhaps the most important data collection done at this stage would deal with social effects. If a technology were identified as being potentially very important for the societal or the health care delivery system, it might be desirable to monitor its progress systematically or periodically. The first stage might be a thorough analysis of what could be projected concerning its potential costs, legal, economic, and other relevant implications, and so forth.

Under an ideal model, all technologies would be tested for safety and efficacy before they come into widespread use. In practice, that goal is only achieved in the area of drug regulation. Otherwise, the testing of technologies for benefits by well-designed studies is done less often than desirable (487) (see Chapter 7).

It would be desirable to collect information on technology costs and economic consequences of the use of specific technologies. As already noted, benefit is only one part of what the policy-maker needs to know. Benefit at what cost is the most important question. Once the technology exists, cost data can be collected. For example, early clinical trials can include collection of cost data; such a step has been proposed by Culyer (153) and Drummond and Stoddard (188) (see Chapter 8).

Social evaluations can also be done early in the diffusion of a technology. As the technology begins to be used, the early results can be very important. Ethical implications that could only be speculated upon may become clear. The technology may challenge certain important societal beliefs. It might be that early in the diffusion of a technology is the most important time to collect data on its social effects. For example, in organ transplantations, there may be an unanticipated socio-economic imbalance whereby upper-class patients tend to be the donor recipients while lower socio-economic class individuals or minorities may tend to be the donors. However, there is no clear-cut and accepted method to evaluate social effects, so several studies by different investigators would often be necessary (see Chapter 10).

Once the technology is in the clinical inventory, studies are less frequently done. One critical question concerns how the technology is actually used in practice. Efficacy information has usually been collected in well-controlled studies in academic situations—what might be called 'ideal' circumstances, with good facilities, well-trained health care providers, and highly motivated staff. The results in this kind of study may have little relation to the benefit at the community level. More studies of the real-life situation with technology are needed. This has been called the 'effectiveness' of technology (487), and is a key target of the new thrust for medical outcomes research in the US.

Overall, insufficient data collection on health care technology is done for many technologies. Clinical trials of technology are funded by different sources as part of applied research; however, the amounts of money are small relative to the economic and health consequences of their use. Few cost-effectiveness analyses or other economic studies are funded, although their numbers are increasing (214).

6.3.3 Synthesis

Synthesis is a critical part of technology assessment (447,758), involving a critical analysis of the results of testing (available data from preclinical to clinical experience, epidemiological studies, and experiments) and all other available and relevant information. It often takes the form of judgements or recommendations (743). Synthesis of the information generated during the testing phase of the assessment process is necessary to provide a responsible basis for decisions made on the technology. Since policy-makers and others are not trained in the study of design and interpretation, presenting the raw data may be of little use. Nevertheless, the data needs to be used to develop informed decisions. The main purpose of synthesis, then, is to make knowledge relevant to policy. Synthesis reports can be used in such decisions as whether or not to pay for a given technology, and can be used to examine quality of care (121).

The advantage of synthesis is that it provides focused, user-oriented information at a relatively low cost (447). If done carefully, with attention to limitations of knowledge, synthesis can both guide technological decision-making and research to answer important questions (743).

A cost-effectiveness analysis that does not involve the prospective collection of data is essentially a form of synthesis. So is a consensus meeting that draws on available studies as the basis for conclusions.

For policy-makers such as health planners, insurers, and health care providers, synthesis is almost synonymous with assessment, and this is generally appropriate. To them, assessing a technology does mean examining available information, summarizing and analysing it, and arriving at a judgement. Without this step, there is no assessment. Synthesis might be considered as the most important step in the assessment process for their purposes.

Synthesis varies quite a lot from one part of the life cycle of a technology to another. For future technology, the only information readily available may be that generated by scientific studies. Early in the diffusion of a technology, only limited information on benefits and costs is available. Later in the life cycle, much more information is available. This is one reason, perhaps, that most assessments that have been done have dealt with older technology. It is surely true that information collected later in the life cycle of a technology will be more accurate (763). This is not an argument for waiting, however. Decisions must be made during the critical stages of the diffusion of technology, and they should be based on the best information that can be developed. If mistakes are made in early assessments, they can be corrected if assessment is developed as an iterative process.

The most widespread method of synthesis continues to be the literature review (508,756). However, a literature review inevitably expresses the preconceptions and biases of the people who carry it out (471). Methodological problems in individual studies are often ignored or distorted. A report from the UK states, 'Basic scientific principles are frequently disregarded, and, as a result, reviewers and their readers may be misled by biases or random errors that are similar in size to the likely effects of the technologies being reviewed' (4). Increasingly, good assessments make use of meta-analysis techniques, a quantitative process that combines results of scientific studies, weighting studies by design characteristics (290,508,594). Thus, double-blind studies with large samples are given more weight than unblinded smaller studies.

One specific problem is gaining access to existing information. Reliance on easily searched bibliographies such as MEDLINE of the US National Library of Medicine can result in reviewers missing 50 per cent or more of the relevant articles (118). In 1992, neither 'technology assessment' nor 'health care technology assessment' were subject headings in the MEDLINE system (291). Reviews that rely only on published information may be misleading since the results of published studies may not be representative of the totality of relevant studies (172). It is also a specific problem that negative results tend not to be published, while positive results are (116).

Cost-effectiveness analysis can also be very useful in synthesizing data (497). The number of such studies has been increasing steadily in the clinical literature since the 1960s (214,718). They attempt to compare the net health and economic consequences of technological innovations. However, they suffer from a lack of clear methodological standards, which can lead to potential bias in findings (189,190,214).

Group decision-making methods are very popular synthesis techniques. They seek to evoke expert opinion to aid decision-making. The National Institutes of Health Consensus Development Program, described later in this Chapter, is an example (351).

Decision-analysis is a method of analysing medical decisions (720). The method begins from a set of symptoms or a definite health problem and develops a decision tree to show alternatives. Each decision is then assigned a probability, based on such data as expected outcomes following treatment. The entire process of diagnosis and therapy, or part of it, can then be evaluated mathematically.

The problem is that policy decisions often have to be made within a limited time. It is often not possible to go through an elaborate and time-consuming data-collection process. The policy-maker needs to have access to what is known. Any synthetic document should present this information, but should also indicate the limits of knowledge.

One possibility that seems promising is a method of non-quantitative synthesis involving a literature review, expert reviews of draft material, revision(s) of the draft, and development of policy options or recommendations. This method is used by the US Office of Technology Assessment and by such organizations as the Dutch Health Council. A synthesis of effectiveness of interventions in pregnancy and childbirth, based on identification of RCTs, is also exemplary (117), as is a synthesis of research on common diagnostic methods (641). This method can also be combined with meta-analysis, if time and data are available. Another method that can be used is formal decision analysis. The NIH Consensus Development Program has explored the use of decision analysis models to assist panelists in consensus groups (350,525). Decision analysis has also been used in a synthesis of information on appropriate use of diagnostic imaging (440). As the number of studies in any discipline increases, quantitative methods of synthesis will become more important (403).

Another type of synthesis leading to standards for appropriate use has been developed by the RAND Corporation in California (87,121,242,328). A detailed literature review is carried out and presented to a panel of experts. After examining the literature, the experts rate different indications for a given procedure. A procedure is deemed appropriate for a given condition when the benefits of performing the procedure outweigh the risks by a sufficient margin such that it is worth doing and preferable to alternatives.

A type of synthesis that is gaining great visibility, especially in the USA, is developing practice guidelines, also sometimes referred to as practice policies or practice parameters (236). Guidelines are being actively developed by physician organizations, insurance companies, government agencies, and others. Eddy (206) defined practice guidelines as 'recommendations issued for the purpose of influencing decisions about health interventions'. Guidelines can be voluntary or mandatory, they can be flexible or rigid, and they can be coupled with rewards and penalties, such as financial penalties. Eddy (204) is sceptical about the value of guidelines as a control procedure because of the need for information on outcomes and on patient preferences, both of which are lacking. Practice guidelines might improve quality of care and avoid malpractice, but evidence that they do in fact lead to such improvements is lacking (277,333).

The general lack of data means that conclusions will often only be supported by uncontrolled clinical data (22). Such tentative conclusions, reached with the help of experts, should be better than policy decisions reached after advice from one or two specialists. It is important to emphasize that technology assessment is an iterative process, often giving tentative conclusions that may need alteration later (48). In the long run, the most important issue in synthesis is the validity of the results (350). Does any synthesis method reach the right answer? More research is needed on methods to ensure that the results of a synthesis are unbiased and based on the best available data.

6.3.4 *Consensus conferences*

Consensus conferences are part synthesis, part group decision-making. Since this model is now being used by a number of countries, it will be discussed separately.

The National Institutes of Health (NIH) inaugurated its consensus development programme in 1977, and by the end of 1991 had conducted more than 80 conferences. The goal is to bring together various concerned parties—physicians, consumers, ethicists, etc.—to seek consensus on the safety, efficacy, and appropriate conditions for use of various health care technologies (357). Judgements are intended to be based on the available scientific evidence. The consensus development process is designed to produce a written document, called a 'consensus statement', that can be accepted by clinicians, researchers, and the public. The statement is supposed to identify what is both known and not known about the technology.

A panel of experts is selected by the NIH to hear presentations by the leading medical researchers addressing a specified set of questions. After a two-day meeting, the panel spends the evening of the second day drafting a statement intended to address the questions. The next morning, the consensus statement is read to the audience, which is invited to comment. The conference concludes with a press conference. A few final changes may be made in the statement, and then it is released to thousands of organizations and individuals and is published in leading medical journals.

The NIH consensus conference model has inspired a number of European countries to hold their own conferences. The Netherlands, Sweden, the UK, Denmark, and France have held conferences, and all intend to continue to do so. Each country, however, has developed a model specific to its own needs. This section will describe some of those differences.

In the NIH model, the focus is efficacy and safety of the technology. The audience is primarily composed of physicians, although implicitly it is specialized physicians and researchers. The NIH does not want to become involved in policy issues such as regulation, planning, economics, or reimbursement (350, p. 132). In other countries, this focus is considered too narrow. In Denmark, for example, a health care technology is only socially acceptable when it is available to all persons who need the procedure (96). Therefore, access to the technology is as important as its theoretical benefits. Inevitably, then, financial costs and other considerations are a central issue.

Consensus conferences have been held in Sweden since 1982, beginning with a conference on the artificial hip. The Swedish method follows closely the one developed by the NIH (106). However, in Sweden the panels are broader than in the USA, resulting in a focus that is not so narrow. Conferences examine broader impacts, including societal, organizational, ethical, and economic issues. The target group for the statements include physicians, politicians, administrators, and the public. Statements are published in professional journals and are extensively covered by the lay press, radio, and television.

In The Netherlands, consensus conferences are organized by the medical profession itself. The meetings are used for the development of criteria and standards for good medical practice (110). Subsequently, these standards can be used as the basis for audit procedures in hospitals.

In the UK, conferences also follow the US model closely, but panels are not experts. They represent a range of interests, including consumers. The hope is to foster a societal discussion. The questions put include cost and other aspects, but the panels do not receive sufficient information to consider 'competing demands for services' (658).

Although the NIH reports are publicly available, the focus is on the role of physicians. In other countries, the public has played a larger part (699). In Denmark, for example, experts are purposely excluded from the panel, although a panel will include distinguished physicians, as well as administrators, economists, and public representatives (96). The report is disseminated widely, especially to the policy-makers, including Parliament. Consensus conferences in Denmark, then, are seen as part of a democratic process of dealing with technology.

Some evaluative studies of consensus development are reviewed later in this chapter. The US Institute of Medicine (292,351) has made suggestions for improving the NIH programme, and has also developed standards for any programme of consensus development. The standards include one important in the context of this book: 'Prior to a consensus development conference, programs should provide an ordered and categorized compilation or synthesis of research reports and related evidence . . .' (292, p. 150).

There are other consensus-type activities to assist in technology decision-making. For example, the State of Oregon in the USA has employed population-based consensus meetings to set priorities for decision-making on public preferences for priority setting (205,494,723). In addition, physician organizations in the USA poll their members to reach expert consensus on the appropriate use of technologies.

The former director of the Office of Medical Applications of Research (OMAR) has also developed an alternative to consensus conferences, called a 'forum', which addresses some of the criticisms given below (533). Two key points in the forum are that a thorough synthesis of existing literature is always required in advance and that the forum method does not attempt to force consensus from the participants.

6.3.5 *Dissemination*

Dissemination of health care technology assessment information is generally done in a rather passive way. The main vehicles are the medical scientific literature and meetings (4). This presents a number of problems:

(1) the scientific literature is oriented to research studies, not to synthesis;

(2) there are large time lags in publication of studies;

(3) physicians and others do not necessarily carefully keep up on the literature;

(4) the medical literature often presents studies that purport to give data on efficacy and safety but which are not based on rigorously controlled studies;

(5) the journals have little interest in cost or other social effects.

A number of studies have examined the quality of the biomedical literature (9,232,246,285,294,541,591,603,733). Kohn (391) has reviewed the subject of fraud and error in science and medicine and concluded that it is more widespread than it should be. These studies, in sum, have shown that reports on research in the literature, even in the best journals, are not totally reliable and often do not conform to generally accepted statistical methods. This problem could be made worse by increasing industry support for studies, if care is not taken. Nevertheless, as a technique of scientific communication, the biomedical literature has proved its utility many times over. The issue here, however, is the dissemination of information to policy-makers and practising physicians, who are not able, for reasons of time and training, to analyse the results of studies.

This problem is compounded by the explosion in the number of articles and journals. The 'publish or perish' syndrome is still spreading throughout the world, resulting in a continual expansion in numbers of articles printed, with no apparent improvement in the quality of information available. The large number of journals has made the development of computerized indexing systems such as the US National Library of Medicine's MEDLINE system necessary (118,508). These systems, however, give limited information on the usefulness of particular articles for defined purposes. One major problem is that journals require such brevity that one cannot assess the methods and weaknesses of studies to critically analyse them.

Little attention has been paid to effective distribution of information. This would require making contact with the intended audience and convincing the audience of the importance and validity of the information. Dissemination as part of a technology assessment process should be designed to influence behaviour. An important aspect of dissemination is convincing physicians to modify their behaviour. Professional organizations and continuing education courses can play an important role.

In the USA, effective dissemination strategies have been mandated for all major outcomes research studies funded by the Agency for Health Care Policy and Research (AHCPR).

Better methods are needed to communicate information about health care technologies to physicians, researchers, and policy-makers (508). There has been little research on methods for engaging in effective dissemination or for evaluating the success of dissemination (680). What is clear is that available good information is not well-used, for example, in determining good medical practice.

6.4 Impact of technology assessment results

The questions often asked, quite reasonably, are 'What is the effect of carrying out health care technology assessments? Do patterns of care change? Are new policies developed?'.

The prior condition for technology assessment having an impact on either health policy or health care practice is, obviously, that its results must be used by decision-makers. What is not so simple is identifying and measuring such use. Furthermore, many assessment programmes are not able to insist on change; they may only reach conclusions or give recommendations, which tends to weaken their impact.

Possible positive results of technology assessment would be to allocate health resources more efficiently; to affect the adoption and use of medical innovations; to hasten abandonment of ineffective therapies; and to resolve controversies about competing treatments. Technology assessment may be most useful when either the relative benefit of a new treatment is uncertain or the relative benefits of existing therapies are disputed.

There are two basic types of uses of technology assessment: (1) direct, programme-oriented uses, such as in the use of RCT results by the Food and Drug Administration (FDA) in its regulation of drug approvals; and (2) indirect, non-mandated ones that arise from technology assessment as part of an information strategy. In the latter case, the information generated affects the behaviour of decision-makers independent of any mandated use or sanctions for not using it.

There is little debate about the effects of direct uses of technology assessment information. In the FDA programme, for example, the approval of a new drug depends on the availability of assessment information. The FDA approves a research plan; the industry conducts clinical trials and submits the results to FDA; FDA carries out an assessment of the results of the trials; and FDA approves and disapproves the new drug. There is little doubt that the process of assessment has a great impact.

Another example from the USA concerns the Diagnostic Related Group (DRG) system for hospital reimbursement under Medicare, established in 1983. This system moves toward a fixed budget, which gives technology assessment a greater possibility of assisting in policy decisions about which technology to provide and with what intensity (500). The DRG legislation set up a Prospective Payment Assessment Commission to advise on overall rates of payment under the DRG programme and on rates and content of specific DRGs. The Commission was also given a wide-ranging mandate to assess and make recommendations concerning health care technology. This is a direct tie between technology assessment and input to decision-making in a health care service programme. The DRG programme has clearly affected change in the patterns of technology adoption and use in the USA (722) and technology assessment certainly has had an important role in this change.

Increasingly, technology assessment is used as part of decision-making in insurance programmes. In The Netherlands, as already mentioned, cost-effectiveness analyses of heart and liver transplants and *in vitro* fertilization were performed with support from the Dutch Sick Funds Council to determine whether coverage should be granted (77). The resulting analyses affected the policy debate, although they could not be said to have determined the outcome (578,579).

Other examples of cost-effectiveness studies directly affecting policy are relatively scarce, although they may be increasing, especially in Europe. Another Dutch study examined cost-effectiveness of simvistatin for treatment of hypercholesterolaemia (449). The results of this study were presented to the Dutch drug-pricing authorities and reportedly affected the pricing decision (448).

A specific example of technology assessment and its impacts concerns preventive services, particularly vaccines, in the US Medicare programme. Since its inception, the Medicare programme has not included coverage for prevention. The Congressional framers were mainly concerned about providing coverage for hospital care and were apparently worried that preventive activities such as health education could not be limited. They were perhaps also sceptical about the benefits of prevention. In 1978 the Office of Technology Assessment analysed the cost-effectiveness of the (then new) vaccine against pneumococcal pneumonia (506). One result found a cost-effectiveness ratio in those 65 years of age and older of $1000 per healthy life year gained, generally considered to be a good return in health care CEAs. Congress responded and amended the Medicare law to cover pneumococcal vaccine in 1981. In 1984, OTA updated its original analysis (509). It estimated that 20–25 per cent of all people over age 65, or 6.6 million people, had received the vaccine. The result was an estimated monetary saving for Medicare (if subsequent non-pneumococcal medical costs were excluded). The OTA also studied the influenza vaccine in 1981 and found it to be a net medical benefit and money-saving when used in the population over the age of 65 (489). In 1987 the Congress amended the Medicare law to cover the influenza vaccine as well. Congressional decision-makers found the results of these analyses useful, and both House and Senate committees requested the OTA to examine other preventive measures applicable to Medicare (504). In October 1988, the first of these reports, on screening for glaucoma in the elderly, was published, indicating that costs for such a service would be high and benefits uncertain. The analysis showed that the cost of identifying and confirming a case of glaucoma would be between US$2000 and US$16 000 (507). Subsequent reports dealt with cholesterol screening (409) and screening for colorectal cancer (491).

The Swedish Council on Health Care Technology Assessment (SBU) is committed to evaluating its results carefully. After a report on pre-operative routine testing was published in 1989, a questionnaire was used to evaluate the situation before the report was completed and was repeated in the same hospitals both in 1990 and 1991 in order to evaluate the impact of the report and the activities that have followed. The evaluation in 1990 showed a significant decrease in routine pre-operative testing which continued in the 1991 measurement. The savings in economic terms, besides the increase in quality of care, was 50 million crowns per year, or 5 times the yearly budget of SBU.

The Quebec Conseil d'evaluation des technologies de la sante (CETS) commissioned an evaluation of its reports in 1991. Ten reports were selected, and a wide range of policy-makers, clinicians, and administrators were asked about the impact of the reports in semistructured interviews. Eight of the 10 reports had a noticeable impact on policy, six on the organization of care and two on clinical practice. The financial impact of these reports was found to be considerable. The evaluation found that the political choice of the agenda was important, in part because available resources allowed assessment of only 5–10 per cent of technologies needing assessment.

Another example of technology assessment studies having an impact on policy was the Blue Cross Blue Shield-sponsored study by Eddy on cancer screening (207). Eddy modelled the cost-effectiveness of multiple cancer screening policies. His results were adopted by the plan.

Expenditures for unproven or unnecessary health care technology can be prevented by the use of technology assessment results. The US National Center for Health Care Technology, which had a budget of US$4 million in 1980, commissioned studies that showed that its advice saved the Medicare programme hundreds of millions of dollars annually. A Harvard School of Public Health analysis (83) estimated 10-year savings from non-reimbursement of four medical procedures. The procedures and estimated savings were as follows: endothelial cell photography, US$130 million; dialysis for schizophrenia, US$146 million; hyperthermia, for cancer, US$272 million; and radial keratotomy for myopia, US$477 million. The UCLA School of Public Health (696) estimated savings from non-reimbursement of three items: home use of oxygen, US$6–20 million; telephonic monitoring of cardiac pacemakers, US$87–97 million; and plasmapheresis for rheumatoid arthritis, US$10 000–15 000 million.

Naturally, there is always a problem of implementation of technology assessment results. A National Institutes of Health study of coronary bypass graft surgery led to the suggestion that 25 000 grafts done in the USA in a given year were unnecessary; if these could have been avoided, the monetary saving would have been more than US$400 million in 1981 alone (350, pp. 64–66).

The more difficult area of assessment to evaluate concerns its impact on health care practice decisions (496,350). There is little literature on technology assessment itself. However, the impact of randomized clinical trials (RCTs) on practice have been studied. The literature is of two general types: one begins with the results of specific RCTs or the results of RCTs in a specific area, such as hypertension, and examines whether physicians are aware of the results or what their treatment practice is; and the other starts with medical practice, either through literature reviews or by questionnaires, and determines how well practice agrees with the results of appropriate RCTs. Most authors conclude that the impact of RCTs on health care practice has been less than optimal and that their impact is exceedingly slow to develop.

In one of the earliest articles on this subject, Chalmers concluded that physicians' practice in the 1950s and 1960s was often at odds with data from trials (119). McGrady came to the same conclusion in a 1982 survey of family practitioners (438). Christensen *et al.* reviewed 65 RCTs on treatment of duodenal ulcers and compared the results to recommendations in medical textbooks; they found that RCTs had little influence on the recommendations (125). Tygstrup *et al.* (692) concluded that the results of RCTs have little effect on gastroenterological therapy.

On the other hand, Moskowitz *et al.* (468) reviewed RCTs of alcohol-withdrawal treatment. They concluded that such treatment using drugs had been established as superior to that using only a placebo. In this case, practising physicians were using the treatment that the RCTs had shown to be effective.

Stross and Harlan (665) found that only 28 per cent of family physicians and 46 per cent of internists were aware of the results of a major multicentre study using photocoagulation to treat diabetic retinopathy a year after the study had been published. Their study shows that even the results of well-conducted large-scale studies must be brought explicitly to the attention of physicians or the results will not affect practice.

Cancer treatment raises other problems. Thousands of cancer-therapy RCTs have been generated by combining chemotherapeutics along with radiotherapy and surgery. Given that the probability of success is low in cancer research and that most trials use few patients, a large proportion of the results obtained are probably false-positive results (496). The consequence is that many ineffective treatments may be applied because clinicians do not have adequate information.

Treatments for breast cancer are the commonest subject of RCTs in cancer, and the impact of those trials has been felt. Rockette *et al.* (570) conclude that RCTs have contributed substantially to treating primary breast cancer in its early stages, and that clinical management of breast cancer has changed in other ways as a result of the trials.

In the area of heart disease, a number of interventions have been well-studied in North America, Europe, and Australia. From the beginning, studies on hypertension have had a major effect on health care practice. The results of a major clinical trial were known by 40 per cent of family practitioners within 2 months of publication (496). Coronary artery bypass graft (CABG) is another technology that has been much studied; the trials have generally had a significant impact on clinical practice, although certainly less than desirable (243). In recent years, the sponsoring agency for studies has tried to develop a strategy to bring the information to the attention of physicians. For example, the Coronary Drug Project trial of cholesterol-lowering drugs led to a marked reduction in pre-scribing of Clofibrate in the USA, enough to pay for the trial itself (415). How-ever, little research has been done on methods of information dissemination, so little is known about the best methods.

There have been a number of efforts to educate physicians to modify their patterns of use of health care technology (735). Several programmes have shown initial reductions in ordering retests, for example, but long-term effects have not been evaluated (474). An extensive education effort in Rochester, New York, appeared to curtail the ordering of diagnostic tests (305). A number of studies have assessed effects on ordering treatments. An educational pro-gramme concerning appropriate therapy for urinary tract infections resulted in improved prescribing behaviour and significant cost savings (389). Educating physicians on the cost of services was found to reduce the ordering of laboratory tests, X-rays, electrocardiograms, electroencephalograms, and hospital charges per patient (256). Wennberg *et al.* (730) demonstrated a reduction in rates of surgical procedures in high-use areas when physicians were informed of the facts.

One area of apparent success is that of skull X-rays, where active attempts to reduce use have been carried out, since Bell and Loop's classic paper suggesting great overuse and lack of benefit (58). Strategies have been developed to identify high-benefit and low-benefit patients. One such rule was developed in the USA by a special radiological commission, which recommended that any patient with serious neurological signs after a head injury should have a CT scan and that skull X-rays should not be done (684). Use of such decision rules have been associated with a 50 per cent decrease in the ordering of skull films (684). A more comprehensive effort to change ordering of diagnostic imaging was developed at the Harvard Medical School. The intervention was a daily meeting between radiologists and ward physicians to discuss the appropriateness of ordered imaging procedures. One intervention ward was compared to three control wards, and decreases in ordering were observed in most imaging procedures, ranging from 19 per cent decreases of chest films to a 70 per cent decrease in upper gastro-intestinal series. Because this system was very labour-intensive, the investigators developed a computer-based decision system to provide feedback to the physician concerning planned imaging procedures. The system is being evaluated (450).

The consensus conference model has been extensively evaluated, especially in the USA. Wortman examined the process of consensus development as carried out by the NIH, raising a number of criticisms, including the use of evidence in the consensus process (756). Wortman and Yeaton (758) have suggested that all consensus conferences could be based on a formal synthesis document, for example. The NIH does not consistently include experts on methodology in its panels, and it generally does not do a complete literature review (756,757). Apparently, none of the consensus programmes that have recently been initiated in Europe carry out an independent literature review (96,110,699). In some cases, recommendations of NIH consensus panels have not been based on the best experimental evidence (350, p. 133). The RAND Corporation carried out an evaluation of the effects of consensus conferences, but also analysed the content of consensus statements, pointing out, for example, that they tended to have an academic and scholarly tone that might not be ideal to appeal to practising physicians (368).

In its evaluation of the effects of the NIH Consensus Program, RAND studied physician behaviour in areas related to 12 recommendations put forth by four consensus panels concerning surgical management of primary breast cancer, the use of steroid receptors in breast cancer, Caesarean childbirth, and coronary artery bypass surgery (376,393). Care was studied during 24 months before and 13–24 months after each consensus conference in 2770 patients in ten hospitals in the state of Washington. Results showed little effect on physician practice, despite modest success in reaching the target audience. For six of the 11 recommendations analysed for level of physician compliance, the level remained at less than 50 per cent, even after the conference. For other recommendations, practice already conformed rather closely to the recommendation. Recent studies do show increases in prescribing patterns of drugs recommended in NIH consensus statements (375).

In Sweden, the effects of the first five consensus conferences on health policy and administration were evaluated by a questionnaire and interviews with leading politicians and administrators. More than half of the respondents indicated that they had found the statements from one or more conferences to be of practical value. In some cases, statements had a direct effect on political decisions (106). The effects of the first four conferences on physicians were also evaluated. The main target group was defined as hospital-based physicians in supervisory positions within relevant clinics. A mail survey was sent to 1668 physicians, and 86 per cent responded. Awareness of a particular consensus conference was high. According to 7–10 per cent of the respondents, a consensus statement had changed clinical practice. However, most physicians said that there had been no change, because the consensus statement reflected clinical practice prior to the conference (361).

In The Netherlands, too, the effects of consensus conferences have been evaluated (224). Conferences on blood transfusion policy in hospitals, melanoma of the skin, prevention of bed sores, and diagnosis of deep vein thrombosis were assessed by documents, interviews, and questionnaires. The evaluation showed that most physicians were aware of the findings of the conferences and applied them in practice. For example, in the case of bed sores, the consensus document advised against many traditional forms of treatment, including ice, warm air, bandaging, local ointments, and soaps. Two years later, a survey showed that the majority of the centres had adapted and modified their practices.

In the outcomes research initiative by the US government, the last (but not the least) of several major objectives required of the large, often clinically-research-based study teams is to develop innovative and effective dissemination strategies. The goals are to learn what works in real clinical practice and cause change to improve that clinical practice. However, an overall statement by Thier (680) is pertinent: 'The state of the art of information transfer in this field must be considered primitive'.

The central point seems to be that information itself is not enough (375). Any programme based on this strategy must also pay attention to such factors as the context for the use of the technology, as discussed in this chapter. In the opinion of a medical journalist, education and financial penalties together are perhaps the best way to change physician behaviour (436).

In summary, based on limited literature, one can conclude that technology assessment has had a limited, but apparently increasing impact on clinical practice. Consensus conferences seem to have had substantial impact in some areas. The most recent developments are the new mandates for cost-effectiveness information for pricing, coverage, and reimbursement decision-making. These will surely affect policy and practice. Finally, technology assessment bodies have begun to evaluate their impacts, so undoubtedly more information will be available in the future.

6.5 Conclusions

Technology assessment of health care practice seems a necessary policy tool in this modern age. Still, existing programmes are relatively few in number and their resources small. This indicates the necessity that they plan their own activities carefully. A systematic approach to such activities is thus necessary.

The advantages of a system for identifying and assessing health care technology seem obvious. Policy decisions would be improved with better information. Society's resources would be better used. Are there dangers in such a process? The main danger is that innovation could be slowed. If mistakes were made, this slowing could be inappropriate. This is one advantage of the iterative approach proposed here: mistakes could be corrected. In any case, a cautious approach is called for. None the less, it seems clear that developing a system such as that sketched in this chapter offers important advantages.

7. Evaluation of efficacy and safety

All who drink of this remedy recover in a short time, except those whom it does not help, who all die. Therefore, it is obvious that it fails only in incurable cases.

Galen

[The shift to statistical methodology] replaces the concept of inevitable effect by that of probable trend.

Jacob Bronowski

Efficacy (benefits) and safety are the basic starting points for evaluating the overall utility of a health care technology. If a technology is not efficacious, it should not be used, and if its efficacy is unknown, statements about its overall value cannot be made. In addition, efficacy and safety data are needed to evaluate the cost-effectiveness of a technology (see Chapter 8). Neither the need for a technology nor its appropriate use can be established without good information on efficacy and safety.

Health care systems and the policy-makers are, or should be, concerned about efficacy and safety because of their role as protectors of the public health. In addition, the policy-makers have specific roles in the development and use of health care technology. Because public funds pay for health care, policy-makers have a responsibility to make good decisions in health care.

Efficacy and safety have been keystones of medical practice since its beginning, as indicated by the quote from Galen above. However, the standard has been an intuitive one, or based on logical deduction from scientific knowledge of that particular time (762). The scientific evaluation of safety and efficacy is a relatively recent development, as discussed in Chapter 2. This area of research has been given a great impetus by the prominence of effectiveness or outcomes research since the late 1980s (728).

7.1 Problems with efficacy and safety

Many technologies are not adequately assessed before they come into widespread use. It was estimated in 1978 that only 10–20 per cent of all procedures used in medical practice had been shown to be of benefit by controlled clinical trials (487). With the accelerating rate of technological change in health care, the present situation may be worse.

A number of technologies have come into widespread use and then been shown to be without benefit. Gastric freezing for peptic ulcers (239) and diethylstilbestrol (DES) for pregnancy complications (16) are two examples. A number of operations as a treatment for coronary artery disease had been in fairly widespread use without evidence of benefit before coronary artery by-pass grafting was shown to be efficacious (542).

A commonly used technology without evidence of benefit is electronic fetal monitoring (EFM). EFM enables evaluation of the fetal heart rate during labour in relation to uterine contractions and facilitates detection of certain types of abnormal patterns (47). EFM was first marketed in about 1968 and quickly spread into use in delivery rooms around the world. It is presently beginning to diffuse into less developed countries such as China. In 1976, the first controlled clinical trials of EFM were published, showing no benefit to either mother or baby. These trials have largely been ignored by the obstetrical community. By 1988, nine trials had been completed, including two very large ones, one in Dublin and one in Texas, still without clear evidence of benefit (677). In 1988, the US Preventive Services Task Force made the following recommendation: 'Fetal heart rate should be measured by auscultation . . . in . . . labor. Electronic fetal monitoring should not be performed routinely on all women in labor. It should be reserved for pregnancies at increased risk for fetal distress' (697). Nevertheless, EFM seems to continue to be standard practice.

This case illustrates a common problem, probably more common than lack of benefits. A technology is developed and has certain benefits, especially for those with a severe form of a particular disease. When the benefits seem relatively clear, the technology diffuses into use, but is used with more and more indications and also with different conditions, without further evidence of benefits. The result is a widespread use of technology in situations where it is probably not efficacious, or where it has a very low level of benefit. The computed tomography (CT) scanner is a good example. It is commonly used on people with headache and no other problems, although it is known that it is very rare to find abnormalities in such a case (487). Some common technologies that are often overused in a similar way include laboratory tests; many X-rays; gastro-endoscopy; many surgical procedures, including tonsillectomy, hysterectomy, and appendectomy; intensive care units; many drugs (antibiotics are a dramatic example); and many procedures in obstetrics, such as Caesarean section. It is particularly difficult to assure when newer diagnostic methods replace the old ones (212). Obviously, overuse of diagnostic and therapeutic procedures can have profound implications for effectiveness, safety, and financial costs.

Balancing efficacy and safety can be a difficult problem. The example of retrolental fibroplasia (RLF), a cause of blindness in babies, is interesting (631). RLF was first recognized in Boston in 1941. By the late 1940s, an epidemic of RLF was recognized in the USA, and to a lesser extent in other countries. The disease was seen in premature infants who had been placed in intensive care after birth. Gradually, evidence accumulated that oxygen supplements were responsible for the problem and attempts were made to limit oxygen. The rates of onset of RLF fell. With the growth of neonatal intensive care in the 1970s, which included oxygen supplementation, the survival rate of very small premature infants increased, but the rate of RLF also increased dramatically. However, in the 1980s, the oxygen hypothesis appeared to be too simple, and further research was needed to determine the role of oxygen in the genesis of RLF and in the levels of oxygen necessary to sustain life in premature newborns. This question is still not settled (631, pp. 178–179).

Safety problems seem much more common than is recognized in the clinical situation. More than 3 million infections are acquired each year in US hospitals, afflicting 1 in 18 people admitted to an acute care institution (315). In one study of 815 consecutive patients on a general medical service in a teaching hospital, 36 per cent experienced an iatrogenic illness, most arising from drugs or invasive procedures (650).

7.2 The concepts of efficacy and safety

Efficacy and safety have been defined many times (487). In these definitions, four factors can be identified: benefit to be achieved, medical problem giving rise to the use of the technology, population affected, and conditions of use under which the technology is applied. Efficacy may be defined as the probability of benefit to individuals in a defined population from a health care technology applied for a given medical problem under ideal conditions of use (487).

The question of benefits is perhaps the most important in this area. Traditionally, outcome criteria have been largely restricted to measurement of mortality and morbidity. Less consideration has been given to life expectancy or to psychosocial and functional factors. However, quality of life is becoming more and more of an important factor (see Chapter 9).

In fact, measuring quality of life has become a central part of cost-effectiveness analysis (see Chapters 8 and 9). Furthermore, most valued outcomes have been defined by the health care system itself, but it seems clear that the patient's preferences and values must play a part (439). For example, some patients will choose higher quality of life, but shortened life expectancy.

The range of outcomes can vary a great deal when considering a particular technology. Diagnostic technologies are particularly difficult, where benefit may be examined on five levels (240):

(1) technical capability—does the technology perform reliably and deliver accurate information?

(2) diagnostic accuracy—does use of the device permit accurate diagnoses?

(3) diagnostic impact—does use of the device replace other diagnostic procedures, including surgical exploration and biopsy?

(4) therapeutic impact—do results obtained from the technology affect planning and delivery of therapy?

(5) patient outcomes—does use of the device contribute to improved health for the patient?

In fact, few studies of diagnostic technologies have gone beyond the level of diagnostic impact. Most studies in the medical literature either give diagnostic accuracy or merely report that diagnoses can be made with the technology. If one assumes that the purpose of diagnosis is to improve health, one can readily conclude that this situation is not satisfactory (311).

The specification of benefit is often difficult for other classes of technologies as well. For example, should coronary artery surgery be evaluated for its impact on life expectancy or for its ability to relieve pain? In the case of electronic fetal monitoring, the earliest statements were that it would prevent deaths in the fetus and newborn (47). As that assertion seemed less and less likely, it was then stated that it would prevent neurological damage.

A technology's efficacy can only be evaluated in relation to a particular medical problem. It would be meaningless merely to state that a technology is efficacious. Nevertheless, the specification of medical problems can be complex. Many technologies are efficacious for one indication but not for another. Many technologies are beneficial for dramatic cases, but benefits for less dramatic cases of the same condition have not been demonstrated.

The effect of a technology varies, depending on the population affected or the individual to be treated. A common practice is to carry out clinical trials in severely ill patients, and then to extrapolate the benefits to less severely ill people. Another common practice is to test drugs in adult males and to extrapolate the results to pregnant women and children, where testing is ethically difficult. While such extrapolations may produce correct results, strictly speaking the technology can only be considered to have proven benefit in the specific group in which it was tested.

Conditions of use are critical in a technology's efficacy. The outcome of use of a technology depends on the skills and knowledge of physicians, nurses, and other health personnel (230); by the quality of the drugs, equipment, and institutional settings; and by support systems used by those personnel. In general, for example, institutions that carry out complex procedures more frequently have better outcomes (505). Efficacy is generally estimated from studies done in excellent settings, such as university hospitals. The benefits found from use in average settings will usually be less. For this reason, effectiveness is considered to be of benefit from a technology under average or usual conditions of use. Unfortunately, little information is available on the effectiveness of technology. The effectiveness initiative may produce information that previously was not available.

Safety, like efficacy, is a relative concept relating to several dimensions. No technology is necessarily safe. A statement of safety is a judgement of the acceptability of a risk. Risk can be defined as the probability of an adverse or untoward outcome occurring and the severity of the resultant harm to health of individuals in a defined population, associated with use of a health care technology applied for a given medical problem under specified conditions of use (487). Efficacy and safety can only be evaluated fully in terms of each other.

A technology may provide benefits, but the value of those benefits depends in part on the risk involved in using the technology. Thus, any use of a health care technology involves a compromise between potential benefit and risk.

A difficulty in this balancing is that benefits tend to be rather clear, while risks occur in low rates and harm is often found much later. When a technology is used, some will benefit and some will be harmed. These effects do not divide equally. Some people will be harmed without benefit. Since benefit and risk are both probabilistic, the provider must be careful to be sure that undue risk is not associated with the use of the technology. In general, physicians seem to pay insufficient attention to risk.

7.3 Estimating efficacy and safety

Techniques used for estimating efficacy and safety range from the informal judgements of individual physicians to large complex randomized clinical trials. No technique is universally applicable. In many instances, less complex methods may be more appropriate than more sophisticated approaches. It is not possible to do multiple randomized trials on every technology. A strategy is then needed to determine which method is appropriate in a given case.

7.3.1 *Preclinical*

Many health care technologies are evaluated in laboratories and in animal tests prior to human use. Such tests are usually required by regulatory agencies in the case of drugs, and often in the case of devices. The major function of animal studies is to give an initial idea of toxicity or risk.

The importance of technical studies is often overlooked by clinicians and policy-makers. However, the clinical efficacy of a drug depends on its chemical composition, purity, and dosage. The clinical efficacy of a device depends on such factors as its ruggedness and its reliability.

7.3.2 *Informal clinical assessment*

Despite the increasing visibility of formal studies, informal evaluation is the norm (487). Personal experience by a provider is key to physician attitudes about efficacy. In fact, as described in Chapter 4, physician experience is a key determinant of diffusion of technology.

Peer experience and consensus is more explicit than personal experience. Much of the medical literature is made up of such informal experience, without controls. Peers also interact in such forums as medical society meetings. A community consensus gradually develops concerning any technology (303). Consensus development programmes have the goal of drawing on the experience of clinical providers, as well as the scientific literature, in arriving at conclusions on efficacy and safety.

Informal assessment can seldom give more than preliminary indications on efficacy and safety. The development and course of disease is not understood sufficiently to give much credibility to observations made without control groups. At the same time, the gradual evolution of medicine has probably depended more on individual impressions than on scientific studies.

7.3.3 Epidemiology

Epidemiology is the study of the determinants and distribution of diseases and injuries in human populations. The methods of epidemiology are often used to study the impact of medical interventions. Descriptive studies have often established links between interventions and outcomes. The classic epidemiological investigation was that of Snow in 1855, in which he established that contaminated drinking water was responsible for an outbreak of cholera. Removal of the handle from the pump of the offending water supply ended the outbreak.

While descriptive epidemiology can give evidence of efficacy, it is more often used in determining safety. Controlled studies usually do not include sufficient subjects to find risks or to estimate their frequency. Large descriptive studies, for example of a group taking a certain drug, can reveal such risks.

In recent years, there has been increasing attention to the use of large data sets for assessing technology, especially effectiveness. Methods to use computerized data sets for this purpose are still in development and their results have not been validated (632). None the less, the use of large databases offers attractive possibilities for the future (467,595). Tierney and McDonald (685) have done a useful review of eight large practice databases. The *International Journal of Technology Assessment in Health Care* also examined a number of specific databases and their potentials in two issues in 1990.

7.3.4 Computer modelling

Epidemiological and statistical methods are now used frequently in computer modelling to examine the efficacy of medical interventions. (Computer models are also developed in cost-effectiveness analyses—see Chapter 8.) Modelling is a way to simulate the future, including complicated features of a real-life process to reveal what variables have the greatest effects. Modelling is most useful when based on strong empirical investigations.

The principles of developing a model are simple (350). First, the important factors or variables that influence the benefits of the technology must be identified. Then the relationships between the factors must be specified. A mathematical model uses mathematics to define the relationships between variables. Mathematical models vary greatly in their level of detail and complexity, and therefore in how much time and money is needed to develop them.

An interesting model that has had considerable policy impact in the USA was developed by Eddy to examine the effects and costs of screening for different cancers under different circumstances (207). Eddy's conclusions were generally more conservative than that of the American Cancer Society, but his findings were used in revising the screening recommendations of that organization. In addition, Blue Cross and Blue Shield used his findings in deciding which cancer screening procedures to pay for.

7.3.5 *Controlled clinical trials*

All subjects who agree to participate in a controlled clinical trial are normally assigned to experimental and control groups. In a randomized controlled trial (RCT), considered the 'gold standard' in such evaluations, the determination of a group is done by random assignment (540). In a controlled clinical trial intended to assess efficacy, the experimental group would be treated or diagnosed by the technology under examination; usually the control group would be treated by an established standard technology, although sometimes a placebo control is used.

Randomized controlled trials are most useful when the benefit of a new technology is uncertain or when the relative benefits of existing therapies are disputed (105). There are three major advantages to randomization. First, bias may be eliminated from the assignment of treatment. Secondly, randomization prevents bias with respect to variables that exist in the experiment but are not directly considered in the design (in other words, the control group and the experimental group are comparable in all respects). Third, statistical tests of significance that are used to compare treatments are only valid in such a design.

Ethical objections to randomized trials are often raised. This issue is discussed in Chapter 10.

The method of carrying out a controlled clinical trial and many of its implications have been extensively discussed (22,105,350,607,692).

From the standpoint of technology assessment, the main issue in analysing RCTs is the validity of the evidence presented. All RCTs are not the same. The method must be rigorously applied if the findings are to approximate 'truth'. Methods can be critically assessed by analysing reports and articles presenting trial results. One useful set of criteria for such judgements has been proposed by Meinert (460) (editor of the journal *Controlled Clinical Trials*):

(1) the source of funding for the trial and an indication of whether the reported results are a subgroup of a larger data set;

(2) a list of the treatment groups and the rationale for the choice of treatments;

(3) a description of the method to allocate patients to treatment groups, including reference to the blinding used in each group (i.e., none, single, or double blinded);

(4) the safeguards used in the trial to protect patients' informed consent and privacy;

(5) the criteria used to include patients in the trial;

(6) the rationale for the number of patients studied, including a statement of assumptions used in calculating the sample size;

(7) a statement of the length of time required to complete patient enrolment;

(8) a description of the population from which patients were selected;

(9) a description of the baseline and follow-up examination schedule;

(10) a specification of the key outcome variable(s);

(11) the descriptive information on the baseline comparability of the treatment groups;

(12) the number of patients assigned to each treatment group;

(13) the number of patients followed to the end of the study or to death;

(14) the number of deceased patients;

(15) the number of patients unable or unwilling to return for follow-up examinations, including a count of the number who could not be located at the end of the study;

(16) a description of quality control procedures used in collecting data;

(17) a description of the methods of analysis, including an indication whether the reported p values resulted from a single or repeated evaluation of the data;

(18) a discussion of the power of the study.

7.3.6 *Formal synthesis*

Synthesis of existing scientific information with clinical experience may result in valid estimations of efficacy. This technique is discussed in Chapter 6. Synthesis may be done with the assistance of mathematical models, briefly discussed above.

In synthesizing evidence of efficacy, the quality of the evidence is extremely important. It may be necessary to reach conclusions in the face of poor evidence, and often clinical evidence may be considered to be valid, yet the actual scientific evidence should ideally still be summarized.

One effective method of dealing with this problem is to make explicit the quality of the evidence behind any recommendation. The Canadian Task Force on the Periodic Health Examination graded the quality of the evidence and classified its recommendations accordingly. Quality of evidence was graded as follows (645).

I: Evidence obtained from at least one properly randomized controlled trial.

II-1: Evidence obtained from well-designed cohort or case-control analytic studies, preferably from more than one centre or research group.

II-2: Evidence obtained from comparisons between times or places with or without intervention. Dramatic results in uncontrolled experiments (such as the results of the introduction of penicillin in the 1940s) could also be regarded as this type of evidence.

III: Opinions of respected authorities, based on clinical experience, descriptive studies, or reports of expert committees.

Recommendations were classified as follows.

A: There is good evidence to support the recommendation that the condition be specifically considered in a periodic health examination.

B: There is fair evidence to support the recommendation that the condition be specifically considered in a periodic health examination.

C: There is poor evidence regarding the inclusion of the condition in a periodic health examination, and recommendations may be made on other grounds.

D: There is fair evidence to support the recommendation that the condition be excluded from consideration in a periodic health examination.

E: There is good evidence to support the recommendation that the condition be excluded from consideration in a periodic health examination.

These 'decision rules' were accepted with little modification by the US Preventive Services Task Force, which met in the USA during the period 1984–1988 (743).

7.4 Experiences with assessing efficacy

As indicated in other parts of this book, the assessment of efficacy is not new. What is relatively new is the application of statistical principles, instead of individual judgement, in such assessment. The history of efficacy assessment is discussed in Chapter 2. It can be seen from that discussion that using such methods is relatively recent.

As has been argued at other points in this book, science is not enough in assessing a technology. The scientific base may be perfectly sound. The test, though, is does the technology work? This can only be tested in practice. Learning from controlled experimentation is central to progress in health care (350).

One problem is that physicians often value their own experience more than experimental results (278). Physicians need more training in the importance of prospective evidence on efficacy.

Unfortunately, there are not enough experts in controlled experimentation, nor enough money, to support the careful assessment of all technologies. The present problem for health care is that most technology has never been adequately assessed. The randomized controlled clinical trial began to gain visibility in the 1960s and 1970s. Since that time, more controlled experiments have been done, and the quality of the evidence for many newer technologies is good. An important remaining problem is the lack of evidence on older technologies.

7.5 Conclusions

The limited assessment resources means that optimal studies cannot be done in many cases. This means that decisions must often be made without data from controlled studies. While the methods mentioned above, especially the application of epidemiological principles, can give suggestive evidence, one must always question its validity (756). The lack of good evidence is a serious problem. OTA estimated that only 10–20 per cent of commonly used medical and surgical procedures had been subjected to controlled clinical trials (487). An examination of the syntheses done by the US Office of Health Technology Assessment, which presently gives advice to the Medicare programme, found that evidence of efficacy was insufficient in from 63–76 per cent of the technologies reviewed, depending on the year (403).

One important implication is that more primary research is needed, as well as more research physicians with training in quantitative methods, more epidemiologists and statisticians, and more research teams. Synthesis is of limited value without data, and may be dangerous if its conclusions are not firmly based.

8. Financial costs and their evaluation

A cynic is someone who knows the price of everything and the value of nothing. A sentimentalist is someone who attaches an absurd value to everything and doesn't know the market price.

Oscar Wilde

All progress is based upon a universal innate desire on the part of every organism to live beyond its income.

Samuel Butler

If people know the rules of the game, they can live with tragic decisions, even when the life of a loved one is at stake. Once we accept the principle of differentially valuing life and appropriately interpreting its quality, we are very close to the development of consistent health care policies.

Robert Evans

Increasingly, health care costs are a policy issue. As the percentage of the gross national product spent on health care reaches and exceeds 10 per cent, societies are questioning the value of such care. Economists have long warned that resources are limited. Today, health care systems are truly faced with limited resources.

It is this background that has given health care technology assessment its primary impetus. During the 1970s, most policy-makers expected technology assessment to be helpful in containing costs. Gradually, they have realized that costs must be contained by financial means, such as budgets and prospective payment. The issue for the 1980s has become choice: how does a society determine how to spend its limited resources? Technology assessment seems definitely useful in aiding such choices.

Thus, the basic issue with health care technology is not the absolute amount of resources spent on health care, but how much benefit is obtained from such expenditures in comparison with other possible expenditures.

8.1 The role of technology in health care expenditures

A number of studies have tried to quantify the impact of health care technology on costs. These analyses have been somewhat controversial, in part because of the complexities of the subject. The first complexity is that the definition of health care technology is broad. Using a broad definition, it seems rather obvious that technology must account for a major part of the expenditures. The second is that studies analyse the issue of costs from a number of different perspectives. Most analyses fall into one of four categories:

(1) the aggregate impact of technology;

(2) the impact of particular technologies or classes of technology;

(3) the impact of technology used for a specific age group;

(4) the impact of technology used in a specific disease category.

Total expenditures for health care reflect:

(1) changes in population and health needs;

(2) overall wage and price inflation;

(3) wage and price inflation in health care in excess of general inflation;

(4) changes in service intensity, that is, the quantity of inputs per unit of health care (499).

The last two factors are technology-related and provide a general indication of changes in health care technology and its effects on costs.

Using a 'service intensity' approach, Waldman (708) estimated that labour, supplies, and equipment accounted for about one-half of the daily charge in hospital costs in the USA between 1951 and 1970. Freeland and Schender (255) estimated that from 1971 to 1981, 21 per cent of the rise in costs could be attributed to increased intensity. OTA (499) concluded that in the period between 1977 and 1982, increases in service intensity accounted for 24 per cent of the rise in hospital costs per capita. Considering the total health care sector, the combined effect of increasing intensity and increasing health care prices in excess of the consumer price index is approximately 16 per cent of the increase in per capita health care expenditures during this period.

However, changes in service intensity and excess wage and price inflation are also influenced by forces unrelated to purely technological forces (that is, the introduction of new technology or improvements in existing technology). Examples of such forces include changes in reimbursement methods, attitudes of patients and clinicians towards technology, and the efforts of industry to market drugs and devices. Thus, the division of health care costs in these components does not give a very accurate picture of the contribution of technological change to costs, since it fails to take into account underlying reasons for technological change. It also ignores the patient benefits associated with cost increases or decreases.

In the 'residual approach' expenditures over time are regressed mathematically against a number of variables influencing supply or demand for health services. The unexplained residual is attributed to technological change. Using this approach, Mushkin (472,473) found that between 1930 and 1973, technological change reduced total health care expenditures in the USA at an annual rate of 0.5 per cent. Fuchs (271), on the other hand, found that technological change raised expenditures at an annual rate of 6 per cent between 1947 and 1967. The limitations of the residual approach are related to the sensitivity of any residual estimate to the variables chosen for inclusion, the time period chosen (the difference in the two studies could be due to the two different periods considered, since cost-saving sulfa drugs first were introduced in the earlier period), and the narrow interpretation of technological change embodied in the residual. For example, increased use of technology may to a considerable extent be attributed to demand-related factors such as changes in third-party payment. This means that the factor of technological change is underestimated in the results (499).

Another starting point is to consider particular technologies or classes of technology. Redisch (552) looked at the cost and operating data of seven types of ancillary services (pathology, pharmacy, nuclear medicine, laboratory, diagnostic X-ray, therapeutic X-ray, and blood banks) in approximately 1500 hospitals. He found that about 40 per cent of the increase in operating costs was due to a higher use of these facilities per admission.

The costs of equipment and drugs are a relatively modest part of the overall expenditures for health care, as will be demonstrated in Chapter 23. A typical figure might be that pharmaceuticals account for around 10 per cent of gross national product in industrialized countries, while medical equipment accounts for half of that amount or less.

One of the divisions that can be made when examining types of technology is that between so-called 'big-ticket' and 'small-ticket' technology. Big-ticket technology includes CT scanners, open-heart surgery, and megavolt therapy. An example of small-ticket technology is the auto-analyser in the clinical laboratory. Groot (306,308) estimated that big-ticket technology in The Netherlands accounted for 14.3 per cent of total costs. He concluded that little-ticket technologies might raise costs much more. This is supported by analyses covering the period 1950 to 1970 in the USA (7,237). However, both Showstack et al. (622,623) and Scitovsky (608) found that between 1971 and 1982, little-ticket procedures appear to contribute less than before. Laboratory tests did not contribute to rising costs and new imaging techniques were mostly substituted for older, more invasive procedures in the Showstack analysis. Both studies found that some new and relatively expensive technologies, however, did increase costs. These results are summarized below.

Some studies conclude that increased costs may result more from diagnostic than from therapeutic procedures. In The Netherlands, diagnostic procedures increased from 9.84 to 84.75 per 1000 population between 1960 and 1984 (more than 800 per cent). The number of therapeutic procedures increased in the same period from 50.5 to 146.1 per 1000 population (about 200 per cent) (39).

Considering age groups, it is obvious that the elderly use relatively more health care technology and thus contribute more to costs. A number of analyses have focused on the 'high cost of dying' (611,686). In a review of the studies done, Scitovsky (611) found that medical care costs at the end of life are indeed high. For example, the 5.9 per cent of US Medicare enrolees who died in one year accounted for 27.9 per cent of total Medicare payments. Scitovsky concluded that the high cost of medical care at the end of life is not a recent development, but that the same situation existed 15 or 20 years ago. She also concluded: '. . . the data available at present do not support the frequently voiced or implied assumption that the high medical expenses at the end of life are due largely to aggressive, intensive treatments of patients who are moribund. Given the uncertainty of medical prognosis, it is not at all clear that resources were "wasted" in treating those who died'.

Another group of critically ill are newborns with respiratory distress syndrome. These babies received increasing amounts of surgery during 1971 to 1982, and babies who had surgery received almost twice the resources provided to other infants (608,609).

Finally, technology can be related to its impact on specific disease entities. Beginning with Rice (566), the costs of illness have been investigated by a number of researchers. For example, Mushkin (472,473) did extensive updates of Rice's earlier work, focusing on health expenditures by disease category. Mushkin found that cardiovascular disease was the most expensive disease category for the USA in 1975, costing more than US$13 billion (excluding cerebrovascular disease). Surprisingly, a number of diseases cost US society more than cancer (US$5.3 billion), including mental disorders (US$9.4 billion), diseases of the respiratory system (US$7.6 billion), diseases of the digestive system (US$6.8 billion), diseases of the oral cavity salivary glands (US$7.8 billion), and accidents, poisoning, and violence (US$6.8 billion). Scitovsky (610) subsequently reviewed experience in this field of research.

Studies of the costs of illness are important and interesting, but they do not actually indicate the costs of technology. There have been few attempts to examine this question directly. One exception is renal dialysis, paid for by specific programmes or funds in most countries. In the USA, the cost of the treatment of end-stage renal disease by dialysis in 1987 exceeded US$2 billion.

Scitovsky and McCall (612) traced the change in costs of treating 11 conditions at the Palo Alto Medical Clinic in California. Between 1951 and 1964, the real costs of treating only two of the nine conditions studied fell: otitis media and pregnancy/delivery. From 1964 to 1971 the real costs of treating five of eleven conditions fell: pregnancy/delivery, breast cancer, closed reduction of children's forearm fractures with anaesthesia, non-hospitalized pneumonia, and non-hospitalized duodenal ulcer. Those whose costs rose from 1964 to 1971 were otitis media, simple and perforated appendicitis, children's forearm fractures with cast only and with closed reduction but no anaesthesia, and myocardial infarction.

The increase in diagnostic tests and therapeutic procedures found by Scitovsky and McCall (612) were especially striking. Laboratory tests per case of perforated appendicitis rose from 5.3 in 1951, to 14.5 in 1964, to 31.0 in 1971. Inhalation therapy procedures per myocardial infarction rose from 12.8 in 1964 to 37.5 in 1971.

Scitovsky (610) subsequently updated her work to 1981. She found that the net effects from 1971 to 1981 were cost-saving in eight conditions, cost-raising in seven, and neutral in one. However, in most cases the differences were small. The largest differences were in breast cancer and myocardial infarction, where new 'big-ticket' technologies increased costs considerably. The other large difference was due to increasing use of Caesarean section with its high costs.

Overall, Scitovsky (608) and Showstack *et al.* (622,623) agreed in their findings on primary reasons for rising costs. These were found to be surgery for people admitted for myocardial infarction; delivery of a baby by Caesarean section; respiratory distress syndrome of the newborn; and the provision of other intensive treatments for the critically ill (of course, the clinical laboratory test is an important part of intensive care).

From the standpoint of health care technology, these last findings deserve replication in different countries. If the problem does largely relate to very high cost technologies that diffuse into rather widespread use, the policy problem would be greatly simplified.

One problem with the literature cited is that these are studies of past technology. New and future technology can, in many cases, be cost-reducing. For example, new methods of surgery, including lasers, make shorter lengths of stay in hospitals, and even out-patient surgery, possible. Miniaturization means that complicated diagnostic technology, previously available only in large hospitals, can be made available in peripheral hospitals and clinics. Drug delivery devices make it possible to control drug therapy much more closely, making expensive hospitalization often unnecessary. A variety of technologies make home care more feasible for both medical and functional problems. Future analyses will need to examine such technologies.

8.2 Evaluating specific technologies

The formal techniques of comparing costs and benefits have been applied to health programmes only since the late 1950s. Cost-benefit analysis (CBA) and cost-effectiveness analysis (CEA) are designed for programmes that receive an insufficient evaluation in the marketplace. The marketplace fails to reflect the full effects of using a health care technology for a number of reasons. Unintended side effects occur. Knowledge is incomplete. Technologies such as immunization have broader consequences than those for the individual because of herd immunity. But the most significant reason that market evaluation is insufficient in health care is because of the nature of the health care system. Consumers do not pay directly for health care, or pay only a small part of the cost, in many industrialized countries. They are then unable to make rational choices that take into account all anticipated costs and benefits. Furthermore, many decisions are now made by the policy structure and by the health care system. These decisions also need guidance. Increasingly, cost-benefit analysis, and especially cost-effectiveness analysis, is the tool used to aid these decisions.

The terms cost-effectiveness and cost-benefit analysis refer to formal analytical techniques for comparing the negative and positive consequences of alternative projects. These terms are used in different ways by different people, and they may encompass a range of techniques from large prospective experimental studies that include collection of cost and effectiveness data to partially intuitive, best-guess estimates of costs and benefits done to assist a pressing policy decision. The main point is that some technique of this nature must be part of any rational decision. People use such techniques in their own personal decisions. For public policy purposes, the techniques may be more formal, but the philosophy is similar.

Both CEA and CBA require analysts to identify, measure, and compare all of the relevant costs and consequences of alternative ways of addressing a given problem. Costs are the monetary valuations of resource inputs required to produce a health outcome. Consequences are the monetary and non-monetary results of applying a particular intervention. It is vital to recognize that socio-economic evaluations are grounded in the clinical efficacy of the interventions which they evaluate; the clinical effects of a medication must be clearly understood before the relevant socio-economic hypotheses can be generated. The objective of these evaluations is to structure the information so that it is helpful to the decision- or policy-maker.

Through socio-economic evaluations, it is possible to make better-informed decisions regarding the use, distribution, and financing of health care services and technologies. Although socio-economic evaluations are not a panacea for rising health care costs, they provide information which health care decision-makers can use to optimize their resource allocation decisions.

It is helpful to visualize two streams of events pertaining to each medical intervention (see Fig. 9). The first is the medical stream. In this stream, a patient arrives at a physician's office, receives treatment, and is cured or not. This stream can last a few hours, days or months, years, or a lifetime, depending upon the disease and the intervention. Paralleling this stream is the socio-economic stream of events. Each activity in the medical stream is associated with a particular socio-economic result: medical services and other resources are used, the patient's level of social, personal, or employment functioning is altered, and so on. The task of a socio-economic evaluation is to delineate and value this latter stream of events.

Figure 10 will help to visualize the process of a socio-economic evaluation. The clinical intervention (box (A) in Fig. 10) normally is intended to change the health status (B) of a patient, which is roughly analogous to the safety and efficacy or effectiveness, including quality of life impact of the technology. In turn, the altered health status of the patient is related to three independent economic effects. First, health status change may well alter health services resource use (C). For instance, a cured person is not hospitalized, or fewer or different medications may be consumed. Most economic analyses attempt to value these costs very carefully. These costs are considered to be direct medical care costs. Also, a change in health status has an intrinsic value (D); that is, people are willing to pay, and do pay, for better health. If this box (D) is valued,

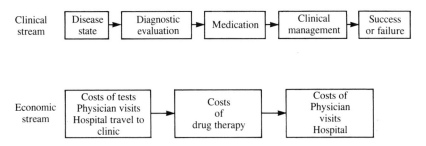

Figure 9. The clinical stream and the economic stream in clinical health care.

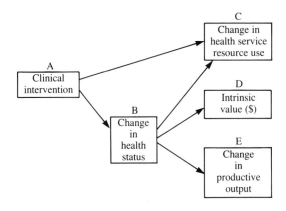

Figure 10. Measuring value in health care (source: 186).

it is considered one expression of indirect costs of the intervention. Third, the change in health status can change productive output (E)—healthier people tend to be more productive in the workforce. Valuing productivity is another expression of indirect costs; specifically it is referred to as human capital. Finally, referring back to box (A), the interventon can directly change the use of health services resources (see vector (A–C)), with no impact on health status. For instance, a new laser technique may permit out-patient instead of in-patient cataract surgery without affecting efficacy, or an oral formula of a medication may replace an intravenous formula of that same medication.

8.3 A brief review of literature volume

The volume of cost-benefit and cost-effectiveness studies in the scientific literature has been increasing at a rapid rate since the mid-1960s (497,498) and the pace shows signs of picking up (Fig. 11). Overall, there has been a trend toward more CEAs (Fig. 12), although a breakdown of the European literature

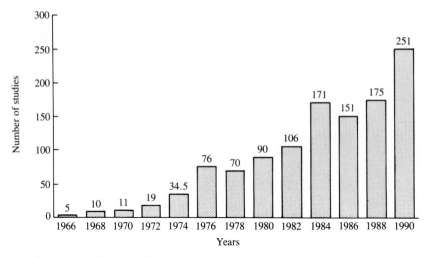

Figure 11. Growth of CBA/CEA literature, 1966–1990 (source: 214).

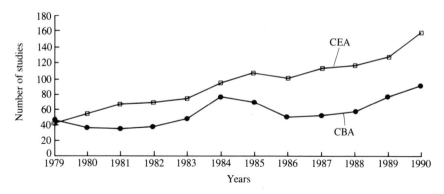

Figure 12. CBA/CEA literature, methods type of publication (source: 214).

indicates a slight preference for CBAs in Europe (214). Whereas the majority of studies from 1979 to 1990 were of US origin (66 per cent), that gap has been decreasing rapidly since 1986 (Fig. 13), probably mainly due to an increase in the volume of the European literature. Table 2 shows the breakdown of non-English language studies by country.

It has commonly been said that CBA/CEA studies are primarily for administrative decision-making, such as decisions to regulate, cover (for insurance purposes), reimburse or set price and purchase amounts. Also, it is common wisdom that physicians are not particularly interested in costs. Yet, the literature reveals that the preponderance of studies continue to be published in clinical

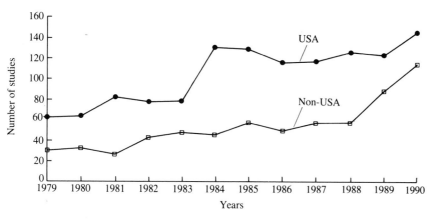

Figure 13. CBA/CEA literature, USA/non-USA (source: 214).

Table 2. Breakdown of non-English published CBA/CEA studies by country during the period 1979–1990.

Country	Per cent
Germany	23
France	15
Italy	12
Spain	10
Denmark	9
Norway	9
Netherlands	7
Sweden	6
Other	5
Unknown	4

Source: ref. (52).

journals rather than in the non-clinical health journals (Fig. 14). Why is there this publication pattern? Physicians are still critical to the acceptance of a technology. Perhaps the clinical literature may be considered to include more influential journals, and also physicians themselves are often the authors or co-authors of CEA/CBA studies.

The literature was also analysed by class of technology. Between 1979 and 1990, 20 per cent of the studies concerned preventive interventions, 36 per cent concerned diagnostic technologies, and 45 per cent concerned medical or surgical procedures (Fig. 15).

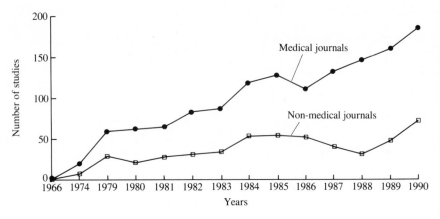

Figure 14. CBA/CEA literature, publication vehicle (source: 214).

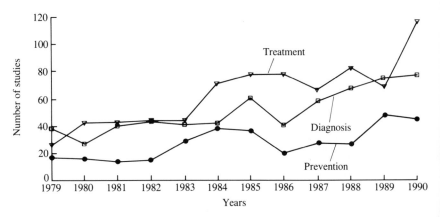

Figure 15. CBA/CEA literature, trends by class of technology (source: 214).

Thus, it is clear from looking at the health care literature that there is a growing demand and interest in cost-benefit and cost-effectiveness studies internationally.

8.4 Types of socio-economic evaluation

There are a number of evaluations that can be used to estimate the socio-economic effects of medical technologies. They are distinguished primarily by whether and how costs and consequences are measured. Three types of studies assess both the costs and consequences of medical interventions: cost-benefit, cost-effectiveness, and cost-utility analyses.

In cost-benefit analysis (CBA), the costs and the consequences of a technology are expressed in monetary terms. This often entails placing a dollar value on health outcomes. Because all consequences are valued in the same way, cost-benefit analyses allow comparisons of disparate types of interventions with widely divergent outcomes. For example, it would be theoretically possible to compare the construction of a hospital to the construction of a dam. One drawback of CBA, however, is that not all consequences are easily estimated in monetary terms, and placing dollar values on human lives can be problematic. Furthermore, consequences that are not easily expressed in monetary terms may be ignored in a CBA, thus potentially misestimating the true consequences of an intervention. In addition, policy-makers and health care professionals may find it distasteful to explicitly place a monetary value on life and limb.

Cost-effectiveness analysis (CEA) was developed to address this limitation of CBA, and it has been used extensively in medical care. In CEA, the values of all resources consumed are measured in monetary units, but health outcomes or consequences are measured in their natural units, such as number of lives saved, years of life saved, cases diagnosed, or cases prevented. The strength of CEA lies in the fact that no dollar value is placed on human life or health outcomes. It is assumed that economic costs are not a valid representation of the entire effects of a treatment, nor should decisions be based solely on economic effects.

Although CEA allows researchers to examine the costs per unit of health outcomes, only interventions whose outcomes are measured in equivalent units can be directly compared. For example, in a CEA, it is assumed that all years of life are equivalent: adding ten years to one person's life has the same value as adding one year of life for ten people. A year in the life of a debilitated cancer victim is considered the same as a year in the life of a patient with simple high blood pressure.

Cost-utility analysis (CUA) addresses this limitation of CEA by measuring the 'utility' or value of years of life rather than just enumerating them. Outcomes are measured in terms of their quality or states of consumer preference. One drawback of this method is that the field of utility analysis is relatively young and the methodology is still developing. Another drawback is that, unlike CEA, which can examine a number of intermediate health outcomes such as cases found or cases prevented, there is only one outcome measure in CUA: quality-adjusted life years (QALYs).

There is another method, termed cost-minimization analysis, which concentrates solely on netting the direct health care costs associated with interventions, and is generally useful only when efficacy is similar or identical for each of the interventions being compared.

Collectively, these types of socio-economic evaluations attempt to measure the social and economic effect of diseases and their treatments. They step beyond an assessment of the clinical efficacy of a treatment and attempt to understand the effects of treatments in a much broader sense. The specific formulation used in a study depends on the problem to be analysed, the data that are available, and the valuation methods that will be used. One type of socio-economic evaluation is not inherently better or worse than another. However in any particular case, one method is likely to be more appropriate than another based on the types of questions asked and the types of data which are available.

Although there is no single 'correct' method of carrying out a CEA, there seems to be an agreement on general principles (497,190,718). OTA (497) has summarized the principles as follows.

1. Define the problem. The problem should be clearly and explicitly defined and the relationship to health outcome or status should be stated.

2. State the objectives. The objectives of the technology being assessed should be explicitly stated, and the analysis should address the degree to which the objectives are (expected to be) met.

3. Identify alternatives. Alternative means (technologies) to accomplish the objectives should be identified and subjected to analysis. When slightly different outcomes are involved, the effect this difference will have on the analysis should be examined.

4. Analyse the benefits/effects. All foreseeable benefits/effects (positive and negative outcomes) should be identified, and when possible, should be measured. Also, when possible, and if agreement can be reached, it may be helpful to value all benefits in common terms in order to make comparisons easier. One scheme for considering costs and consequences is shown in Fig. 16.

5. Analyse costs. All expected costs should be identified, and when possible, should be measured and valued in currency units (dollars, kroner) (see Fig. 16) (231).

6. Differentiate the perspective of the analysis. When private or programme benefits and costs are different from social benefits and costs (and if a private or programme perspective is appropriate for the analysis), the differences should be identified.

7. Perform discounting. All future costs and benefits should be discounted to their present value.

8. Analyse uncertainties. Sensitivity analysis should be conducted. Key variables should be analysed to determine the importance of their uncertainty to the results of the analysis. A range of possible values for each variable should be examined for effects on results.

9. Address ethical issues. Ethical issues should be identified, discussed, and placed in appropriate perspective relative to the rest of the analysis and the objectives of the technology.

10. Discuss the results. The results of the analysis should be discussed in terms of validity, sensitivity to changes in assumptions, and implications for policy- or decision-making.

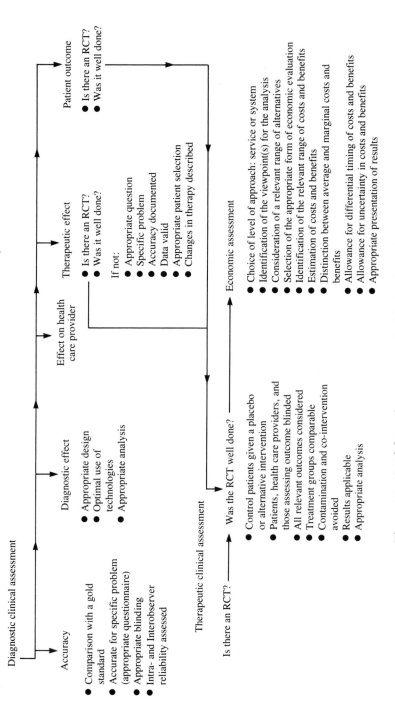

Figure 16. Guidelines for assessment of technology (source: 231).

8.5 The research question

A socio-economic evaluation begins with a clinically-based hypothesis and a research question which states the objective of the study. The research question outlines the alternatives that will be examined, the perspective taken, and the pathway of clinical management that will be considered.

8.5.1 *The socio-economic hypothesis*

To develop relevant socio-economic hypotheses, one must first understand the clinical effects of the technology. For example, hypotheses that are designed to test the costs and consequences of a medication are derived from clinical information on the efficacy and safety of the drug. The clinical efficacy and safety profile is the basis for any socio-economic advantages or disadvantage. A technology with socio-economic advantages, when applied appropriately, may lead to lower costs for outpatient care (fewer concomitant medications, fewer outpatient visits), lower inpatient costs (fewer hospitalizations, shorter lengths of stay), lower costs in the non-medical sector of the economy (fewer days absent from work, longer productive life), and greater quality of life (improved social and emotional functioning, greater sense of well-being). Conversely, a poor safety profile can lower quality of life and increase health care utilization. When applied inappropriately, a technology can increase costs and lower quality of life due to side effects while producing few health and economic benefits.

8.5.2 *Alternatives*

Most socio-economic evaluations compare one treatment with an alternative one, even if the comparison is 'no treatment'. Ideally, socio-economic evaluations should examine those alternatives that are actually available or that would be realistic options in the clinical setting. It is important that the choice of alternatives is not too narrow. For example, there may be a tendency to compare one drug against another drug when a feasible and possibly illustrative option is to compare a drug with a non-drug therapy such as surgery or behavioural/educational approaches.

The choice of alternatives can introduce unacknowledged biases into the study: the cost-effectiveness of a particular technology depends to a large extent on the alternative analysed. Thus, the analyst should justify why specific alternatives were chosen and why others were not.

8.5.3 *Perspective*

Perspective refers to the viewpoint from which the study is performed; in other words, whose interests are considered in the evaluation? Perspective largely defines the types of costs and consequences that will be assessed and is also a powerful determinant of the conclusions that will be drawn from the study results. The most common perspectives are: society, the third party payer (insurance companies or national sickness funds), and the health care provider. Studies are rarely performed from the perspective of patients alone. Generally, the societal perspective is preferred because it considers the general social welfare rather than only the well-being of a specific player in the health care arena. Because studies conducted from the point of view of a specific player will tend to examine only those costs and consequences that are relevant to their budgets, the solutions from these narrower perspectives are almost always sub-optimal and may lead to wasteful decisions when examined in the context of the general social welfare.

For example, a government agency in charge of decisions about reimbursement for a new imaging technology may wish to examine the impact of that device on its own health care expenditures. Such a narrow analysis would ignore a vast array of costs and consequences that should be considered in making a judgement regarding the adoption of imaging technologies. Such costs might include non-reimbursed costs borne by the patient, the costs covered by other third party payers, and the costs absorbed by health care providers.

Inclusion of these costs and consequences provides a much richer base of information for decision-makers, allowing them to understand the varied effects of a technology, those costs that are often hidden, and those consequences which fall outside the limited scope of the agency's perspective. Ignoring these costs and consequences can result in decisions which are not optimal for society in general. One agency's budget may benefit, but overall costs may increase. It is often erroneously assumed that the government's perspective is necessarily societal. Although in some instances this may be the case, when a specific component of the government is concerned with the impact of a new programme or technology on its budget to the exclusion of all other budgets, a definite non-societal perspective has been taken.

8.5.4 *Clinical management and epidemiologic pathways*

The research question also sets the parameters for the pathways of clinical management and epidemiology of disease that will be assessed in the evaluation. These pathways define the clinical stream and epidemiology of events which form the basis for estimating the socio-economic stream. It is at this point that the potential areas of resource use are defined. The results of the study can be altered considerably by the addition or deletion of a particular category of costs or consequences, for example, by including one pathway of clinical management rather than another. Clinical knowledge is absolutely vital at this stage of describing the pathways of clinical management because without it important inputs and outcomes may be neglected. The same is true of the epidemiology of chronic disease such as diabetes or osteoporosis.

8.6 Fundamental concepts of economic analysis

Two fundamental concepts lie at the heart of all economic analyses: opportunity cost and marginal analysis.

8.6.1 *Opportunity cost*

The true economic cost of an intervention is the value of the benefits that would be derived from using the resources required for that intervention in their next best use. This is termed the opportunity cost. The concept of opportunity cost is the basis of the monetary valuation of medical resource use.

In a truly competitive market, prices will equal economic or opportunity costs. The medical care market, however, is not a truly competitive one because of a number of influences such as lack of consumer sensitivity to prices (due to health insurance coverage) and providers' control of demand for services. As a result, the prices or charges affixed to goods and services do not generally reflect their true economic value. In the case of resources in global budgeted systems such as those found in hospitals outside the USA, neither costs nor charges for resources are routinely encountered at all. Because of the difficulty of estimating opportunity cost, many socio-economic evaluations use prices, charges, or *per diem* values as a proxy for costs. To the extent that the purpose of the analysis is to assist in making choices between alternatives rather than to determine true societal value, these substituted values may be an acceptable proxy for costs.

8.6.2 *Marginal analysis*

The second fundamental concept of economic analysis is marginal analysis. Generally, the basic question assessed in socio-economic evaluations is not whether to employ a particular intervention; rather, it is when to employ it, how often, under what clinical conditions, and in what specific circumstances. Thus, the question is, 'what is the additional cost of producing one more unit of that good or service and how much additional benefit will be derived from that level of investment?' This question deals with the marginal or incremental costs of an intervention and the marginal benefits that are expected.

Although socio-economic evaluations should ideally examine marginal costs and consequences, a major limitation faced by these studies is that generally only data on average costs and consequences are available. By using average rather than marginal costs and consequences, it is much more difficult to determine the optimal use of a technology.

8.7 Measuring costs and consequences

Ideally, socio-economic evaluations should include all potentially relevant costs and consequences over all time. However, practical compromises must inevitably be made. Because of limitations in money, time, and data availability, many studies examine only those particular costs and consequences that are expected to be most salient. Researchers must use judgement in simplifying a broadly stated research question into a workable study plan.

8.7.1 Costs

There are two general categories of costs: direct costs and indirect costs. Direct costs include the value of actual changes in resource use that are attributable to the technology. It is important to examine not only those direct medical costs that are associated with the technology, but to look beyond technical-related costs to other sectors of the health care market. Direct non-medical costs include resource expenditures outside the medical care market, such as costs borne by patients in seeking care.

Direct costs are subdivided into fixed and variable costs. Variable costs vary with the volume of services rendered while fixed costs remain constant across the entire range of service volumes. By definition, variable costs such as medical supplies or medications are gained or lost depending on whether they are used and in what volumes. On the other hand, fixed costs are 'fixed', that is, they cannot be 'saved', at least in the short term, regardless of whether or not they are used. From a policy- or decision-maker's standpoint, it is critical that costs be examined carefully to estimate which are truly variable to the programme that is affected by the medical technology under study.

Less obvious but often important to many comprehensive economic evaluations are indirect costs. Indirect costs reflect the value of changes in health status and productivity that result from the health care intervention. These costs are termed 'indirect' because they are not directly expended in the production of health care services or products. These changes in health status may be valued in monetary or non-monetary terms.

There are two main approaches to reaching the monetary value of indirect costs. First, in the human capital approach to measuring indirect costs, changes in productivity are measured as the average earnings of persons in the labour force that will be lost or gained as a result of using a technology. A second approach to placing a monetary value on health and life is the willingness-to-pay method which is preferred conceptually by many economists because it theoretically takes into account a broader array of costs than does the human capital approach.

The willingness-to-pay method elicits values which individuals would spend to stay healthy. Both the human capital and willingness-to-pay methods can be useful in estimating the indirect costs and benefits associated with a medical intervention but both also have several ethical and analytical limitations. One major concern is that people who earn more are valued higher than lower earners.

8.7.2 Consequences

The consequences of medical interventions are the clinical, psychosocial, and economic outcomes of employing that intervention. Clinical consequences include measures of death, disability, and illness. Psychosocial consequences include personal outcomes such as pain and anxiety, and social effects such as work days lost and job changes resulting from illness. Many of these outcomes were considered intangible until methodological advancements such as utility analysis and quality of life assessment were made. Economic consequences are health outcomes which have been valued in monetary terms. Of course, very important economic consequences of a medical intervention are the changes in health care costs themselves: savings or additional expenditures that result from the use of particular interventions. Although the goal of socio-economic evaluation is to assess the full range of consequences that result from the use of a technology, this is often not feasible, practical, or sometimes even necessary.

Measuring consequences is a challenging issue. Many important outcomes are not quantifiable in monetary terms, and thus cost-benefit analysis is not always possible. Clinical consequences such as morbidity and mortality may be appropriate for a given research question. However, these measures often do not capture the full range of outcomes that result from treatment.

Quality of life assessment and utility analysis, discussed more fully in Chapter 9, are means of measuring those effects that have previously been considered intangible. In quality of life studies, patients are asked to respond to a series of questions about their social, psychological, physical, and intellectual well-being in order to identify precisely what aspects of a patient's life are affected by a disease or intervention. Such studies can result in detailed accounts of the impact of interventions and can provide the basis for choosing among interventions which have very similar costs but which can have different effects on patients' personal well-being. These consequences of therapy are not assessed using typical clinical measures.

Utility analysis, on the other hand, seeks to compress these psychological effects into one summary measure in order to compare vastly divergent outcomes in terms of a common metric, usually expressed on a scale that ranges from 1 (perfect health) to 0 (death). Life-years weighted by utility values form the denominator of a cost-utility ratio, a measure that is easily grasped and which effectively summarizes information on health effects.

In general, researchers should begin a study by enumerating the full range of consequences that are based on the clinical evidence that is available. They should evaluate which consequences are most relevant and which are most likely to differ between the alternatives compared. They should examine these consequences to appraise which are measurable in monetary terms, which are measurable in natural units and which can be valued using quality of life or utility measures. Finally, in reporting results, researchers should make explicit which potentially important outcomes are not included in the final results and what the impact of these omissions might be on the interpretation of results. A qualitative description of the consequences that have been excluded from the analysis is often helpful.

8.8 Sensitivity analysis

Researchers face significant challenges in accurately estimating the impact of interventions on costs and on patients' well-being. These challenges often mean that relatively rough estimates must be made and that these estimates are subject to considerable uncertainty. Assumptions must often be made regarding resource use, the costs of resources, or the health effects of an intervention. When such assumptions are made, researchers cannot be certain that their conclusions are tenable, that is, whether the conclusions are 'sensitive' to changes in these assumptions. Sensitivity analysis is an important analytical tool that can be used to test whether the conclusions of a study change as assumptions are altered. It should always be performed whenever there is uncertainty about key variables.

When faced with uncertainty about the true value for some costs or consequences, researchers will generally begin by choosing a value that is a 'best estimate'. They will then vary that estimate, usually suggesting a high value and a low value and then repeat the calculations to see whether their results change under the high and low assumptions. If the conclusions drawn from the study do not change as these values are altered, the results of the analysis are 'insensitive' to changes in this variable and one can be comfortable with the conclusions. However, if the conclusions change with the sensitivity analysis, then one's faith in the analysis is less certain.

8.9 Discounting

When costs or consequences do not occur within a relatively short time frame, or when costs and consequences do not occur at the same time, the results of the socio-economic evaluation should be adjusted to reflect the positive value of time preference. This means that costs and consequences incurred in the present have greater value than those which occur in the future. Basically, discounting reduces future costs and consequences to their present value by a discount rate, commonly between three to five per cent annually.

8.10 Other study design issues

Socio-economic evaluations can be conducted by using prospective or, more commonly, retrospective data. Prospective data might be collected in conjunction with a randomized controlled trial (RCT) of a medication whereas a retrospective study uses data from existing sources, such as the clinical and economic literature or a claims database from a third-party payer (188).

Inclusion of economic measures and quality of life surveys within a clinical trial is a relatively recent phenomenon, but this practice can be expected to increase in the future. Such prospective studies can supply highly valid information because of the strength of the RCT design. However, there may be problems in generalizing the results to other patient groups. Because RCTs are expensive, they are often performed on relatively small and specialized groups of patients, and therefore it is not clear that the results can be generalized to other populations.

On the other hand, retrospective studies often make use of large population-based data sets, or they use 'best estimate' values in conjunction with analytic modelling techniques to simulate general population values. These studies suffer from a different kind of uncertainty. Because the data are seldom derived from well-controlled studies, the precision of values may suffer. Sensitivity analysis as discussed above is particularly helpful in analysing the results and improving the 'believability' of retrospective studies.

8.11 Conclusions

One of the principal reasons that health care technology assessment is an issue today is due to its impact on the cost of medical care. Health care technologies tend not only to be expensive themselves, especially new technologies, but their use is apt to have signficiant economic consequences as well as health consequences.

The history of economic evaluation is too short to draw firm conclusions. In the last 10 years, cost-effectiveness analyses have been increasingly used as an aid to public policy-making. This trend is probably due to the increasingly severe budget constraints and high costs of care in all countries. One can be concerned about this trend. Policy-makers often seek the easy decision. They have more interest in the 'bottom-line' than in the actual framework of the analysis. The methods described in this chapter are not reliable enough to base decisions on them without the input of human judgement, and it seems unlikely that they will ever be. Policy-making can never be—and should not be—a totally rational process.

Although socio-economic evaluations attempt to measure and evaluate the costs and consequences of a medical treatment as accurately as possible, they face restrictions of having to gather data in the real world and having to draw conclusions on the basis of incomplete information. As a result, the costs measured in economic analyses are not true opportunity costs. Rather, they represent either an imperfect price set in a non-competitive marketplace or an arbitrary price set by a government commission or other proxy. And even though marginal analysis is a critical goal of an economic evaluation for optimal decision-making, average costs and consequences are usually the only costs available.

Furthermore, socio-economic evaluations generally collect data on only the most salient costs and consequences on a few alternatives, and do so over a relatively restricted time frame. As a result, some important costs and consequences may be neglected and some important alternatives ignored. The perspective of the analysis also determines, to a large extent, the outcome of a study. Studies conducted from the perspective of society take into account costs and consequences regardless of to whom they accrue. Therefore, they are least likely to result in a shifting of costs from one segment of society to another.

Socio-economic evaluations are important tools for decision-makers in the health care field. Health care decision-makers face increasingly difficult choices between competing alternatives, such as choices between imaging modalities or medications with apparently equivalent efficacy. If these choices are based simply on a comparison of the monetary costs per scan or dose of the drugs, other important costs and consequences may be disregarded: these include costs such as those associated with the utilization of medical resources to treat significant adverse reactions, or consequences such as differences in quality of life.

Socio-economic evaluations can provide balanced and impartial appraisals of the relative costs and efficacy of interventions and are increasingly essential tools for decision-making.

9. Health care technology assessment and health-related quality of life

Dennis A. Revicki

Life is short and Art long; the occasion fleeting; experience fallacious, and judgement difficult.

Hippocrates

One critical question inherent in health care technology assessment is whether patients and society are receiving value in terms of improved health for expenditure on new or existing medical technology (210,216,559,713). Health status outcomes, or health-related quality of life (HRQOL), represents an approach to valuing health that incorporates the patient's and sometimes society's perspective.

HRQOL outcomes are critical for evaluating the impact of medical technology aimed at chronic illness. Medical treatment for chronic disease aims to increase functioning by reducing the severity of disease or by limiting illness progression (559,726). Palliative treatments for cancer and acquired immunodeficiency syndrome (AIDS) have increased interest in ensuring that quantity of life does not compromise quality of life. Therefore, health care providers are increasingly convinced that one of the primary objectives of medical care is the improvement of HRQOL rather than the extension of survival (129,265,414,559). HRQOL outcomes have assumed greater importance over the last ten years in the evaluation of health care technology.

9.1 Definition of health-related quality of life

Although considerable progress has been made in reaching consensus about the conceptualization of HRQOL, differences still exist in how it is operationalized and measured (713,601). The World Health Organization defined health as a state of complete physical, mental, and social well-being and not merely the absence of disease (751). Patrick and Erickson (524) view HRQOL more broadly as the value assigned to the duration of survival as modified by impairments, functional status, perceptions, and social opportunities influenced by disease, injury, or treatment. In many studies, health status is operationalized by measures of physical, role, social, psychological, and cognitive functioning, health perceptions and life satisfaction, and general well-being (60,337,559, 601,713). McDowell and Newell (437), Spilker (643), and Brooks (89) provide good introductions to the definition of HRQOL and various instruments that have been used to evaluate these outcomes. Several special issues of the journal *Medical Care* have also concentrated on various methodological and practical issues of health status assessment (422,423,644).

9.2 Assessment of health-related quality of life

A number of measures have been used to assess health-related quality of life. Two main approaches are used to evaluate health outcomes for health care technology assessments, psychometric health status, and health utility measurement. Over the past 30 years, advances have been made in the methods of health status measurement (523,524,713) and utility assessment (267–270,378,524, 687,688). However, proponents of these methodologies have failed to show any clear superiority with respect to the evaluation of health care technology. There are trade-offs in terms of applications in technology assessment and no single approach can be recommended for all studies. The particular method for measuring HRQOL must be matched to the population, illness, and needs of the technology assessment.

9.2.1 *Psychometric health status measures*

Psychometric approaches to measuring HRQOL require the respondent to indicate the presence, frequency, or intensity of symptoms, behaviours, capabilities, or feelings. Responses to individual questions are aggregated to create individual homogeneous scales (e.g., depression, sleep dysfunction) or global summary scales. Psychometrically sound health status scales have been used successfully to assess the outcomes of medical and surgical treatment and to compare patient outcomes under different systems of care (524,713). Health status measures have been used to discriminate among individuals with different chronic diseases at a single point in time, to predict future health outcomes, and to measure change over time (388).

A number of different health status measures are available including both generic and specific scales (523). Generic health status instruments can be applied across a range of different populations and may be used to examine the impact of medical technology aimed at treating a range of different illnesses and medical conditions. Generic measures cover a broad range of functioning, disability, and distress (312). Health profiles are unified instruments that assess different dimensions of HRQOL and share a common scoring system, and can be aggregated into a number of subscales and often into a single global summary score or index. Examples of health profiles include the Sickness Impact Profile (62), the McMaster Health Index Questionnaire (592), the Nottingham Health Profile (341), and the Medical Outcomes Study short-form 36 (655). The strengths of generic instruments include their established reliability and validity, the possibility of detecting treatment effects across a broad range of HRQOL dimensions, and the fact that they enable the comparison of outcomes across a range of different interventions, conditions and populations (see Table 3). However, generic instruments may not be as responsive to changes in clinical status (compared to specific measures) and they may not always focus on the most critical health outcomes of interest in a medical technology assessment.

Table 3. Characteristics of generic and specific measures of health-related quality of life.

	Generic measures	Specific measures
Application	Across diseases, populations, and HRQOL concepts.	Individual disease, population, or HRQOL concept.
Content validity	May not focus on domains of interest to clinicians and patients.	More acceptable to clinicians and patients.
	May not measure domains relevant to study of specific disease.	Cannot detect unanticipated outcomes.
Construct validity	Well-established for many instruments.	Less well-established for most instruments.
Reliability	Good test – retest and internal consistency reliability.	Variable reliability depending on the individual measure.
Responsiveness	May not be responsive to change.	May be more responsive to change.
	Effects may be difficult to interpret.	Effects are easier to interpret.
Generalizability	Standardized measures provide a common unit of outcome.	Not intended for application beyond specific disease or population.
	Good for comparisons across diseases, treatments and populations.	Can only be narrowly applied across related diseases and populations.
Practical characteristics	Length is a potential problem. Standardized administration procedures.	Often short, easy to administer.

Sources: refs (312),(523),(524).

Specific measures are designed to focus on the aspects of HRQOL that are specific to a particular disease (e.g., arthritis, cancer), specific to an identified population (e.g., children), specific to a particular area of functioning (e.g., depression, sexual function, sleep dysfunction), or specific to a condition or problem that could be caused by any one of a number of underlying diseases (312). Specific measures have increased responsiveness and, because of their content, appear more relevant to physicians and patients. Disease-specific instruments have been developed for a number of illnesses, such as cancer (51,276,600,646), cardiovascular disease (510,725,726), back pain (226,574), diabetes (161), arthritis (266,458), chronic mental illness (410,580), HIV-related disease (759), chronic lung disease (313,443), and other illnesses. The advantages of specific measures are their responsiveness to changes in the target illness due to the application of medical technology and greater acceptance by patients and physicians (see Table 3). There are disadvantages in that specific measures are not comprehensive, and cannot be used to compare across conditions or across different treatment programmes (312).

Clinicians are concerned about the validity and importance of self-rated health, prefer physiological and biomedical outcomes, are uncertain about the responsiveness of these measures to small, clinically meaningful changes, and have difficulty translating changes in scores in clinically meaningful ways (169,560). There are also concerns that most health status scales do not incorporate mortality, duration of survival, or patient preferences for health care or outcomes (378,687,229,688). Health status measures are sensitive to relatively small differences in clinical symptoms and status in groups of patients experiencing mild to severe disability. For example, Revicki *et al.* (561) found that the General Well-Being Adjustment Scale was very sensitive to clinical symptoms, such as chest pain, skin rash, vision problems, nausea, and nightmares, even after controlling for demographic and clinical characteristics in a sample of individuals with hypertension.

9.2.2 *Health utility assessment*

Utility theory and measurement were developed, in part, as a normative model for individual decision-making under conditions of uncertainty. Utility values are numbers that represent the strength of an individual's preferences for different health outcomes under conditions of uncertainty (687,688,229). Sometimes referred to as patient preferences, these values reflect a person's level of subjective satisfaction, distress, or desirability associated with different health conditions (267). The utility approach uses one or more scaling methods to assign numerical values (utilities) on a scale from 0 (anchored as death) to 1 (anchored as complete health). Either the person's current health condition or a hypothetical health state can be evaluated.

Health utility values for a number of health states are summarized in Table 4. Several points can be made based on these data. First, it is possible to have health conditions rated as worse than death (e.g., unconscious or confined to bed with severe pain). Also, clinician judgements of patient health status may differ from that of patients. For example, Revicki *et al.* (565) found that patients with mild to moderate hypertension rated their health state as 0.88 to 0.92, depending on their current antihypertensive regimen, while physicians rated these same health states 0.95 to 0.99 (Table 4). Clearly, an economic evaluation based on clinician ratings may result in very different findings from one using patient ratings of utility.

The utility values reflect preferences for the health states and allow morbidity and mortality improvements to be combined into a single weighted measure, quality-adjusted life years (QALYs) (688) or healthy years equivalent (459). Utility scores can be generated by patients, clinicians, or the general population

Table 4. Health-state utilities for different health outcomes.

Health outcomes	Utility value
Complete health (reference state)	1.00
Life with menopausal symptoms (J)	0.99
Mild to moderate hypertension (J)	0.95–0.99
Maintenance treatment for depression (J, SG)	0.93
Mild angina (J)	0.90
Mild to moderate hypertension (SG)	0.88–0.92
Kidney transplantation (TTO)	0.84
Moderate angina (J)	0.70
Depression episode (J, SG)	0.69–0.73
Some physical and role limitations with occasional pain (TTO)	0.67
Home dialysis (TTO)	0.54–0.64
Chronic renal disease with anaemia (SG)	0.63
Severe angina (J)	0.50
Hospital dialysis (SG)	0.49
Anxious or depressed and lonely much of the time (TTO)	0.45
Blind, deaf, or dumb (TTO)	0.39
Hospitalized for acute schizophrenic episode (RS)	0.30
Dead (reference state)	0.00
Confined to bed with severe pain (RS)	<0.00
Unconscious (RS)	<0.00

J, clinical judgement; SG, standard gamble; TTO, time trade-off; RS, rating scale.
Sources: refs (317),(560),(688), and author's unpublished data.

using visual analogue rating scales, standard gamble, time trade-off, or other scaling methods (267,268,687,688).

Decomposed or holistic approaches can be used to elicit health utilities. In the decomposed approach respondents are asked a series of questions about their functioning. Based on their responses, individuals are assigned to one of several categories and each of these categories has a utility score attached to it. These utilities are developed from previous ratings by samples from the general population, clinicians or some other reference group. For example, the Health Utility Index (687), Disability/Distress Index (577), and the Quality of Well-Being Scale (377,378) use a decomposed approach to generate utilities.

The holistic method uses hypothetical health state scenarios or descriptions as stimuli to get individuals to assign utilities to different health outcomes. These scenarios include several brief statements that describe important aspects of the health condition in terms of physical, psychological and social functioning, pain, and, sometimes, medical treatment. It is also possible to use this approach to get ratings of the person's current health condition. Visual analogue, standard gamble or time trade-off scaling procedures are most often used to obtain utility values using holistic health states, but there is no reason that other methods, such as paired comparisons, could not be used to scale the health states. These scaling methods involve presenting multiple standardized health state descriptions to individuals and eliciting directly or indirectly the relative preferences for each health state.

The utility approach has several advantages. First, it is possible to integrate morbidity and mortality effects into a single score. For economic assessments based on clinical decision models, utility assessment allows for the estimation of values for hypothetical health states. Other advantages include the incorporation of time and risk preferences for different health-state evaluations into the measurement process and its consistency with economic analyses (229). There is, however, some controversy regarding the definition of utility values and the methods used to derive these values (470). Utilities for some health states vary widely among individuals and by the structure and content of health-state descriptions, the way outcomes are framed, and the different scaling methods (560). Other disadvantages include the cognitive complexity of the measurement task, imprecision of individual values, potential population and contextual effects on utility values, and the interpretation of the scores (560,229,269, 470,548). Utility scores may not be sensitive to subtle changes in clinical status.

Utility assessment has been successfuly incorporated into a number of clinical studies and medical technology assessments (74,81,102,104,109,229,317, 378,563,736,737,760,761). For example, Boyle *et al.* (81) examined the cost-effectiveness of neonatal intensive care for low-birthweight infants. They found that the costs per QALY gained, for this technology, was $4500 for neonates that weighed 1000–1499 g. It is likely that the use of patient preference of health utility measurement as outcomes in medical technology assessments will increase as health care systems in both developed and undeveloped countries struggle with resource allocation decisions. Utilities and QALYs are likely to become the common measure of health outcome for comparing the costs and health care benefits associated with different kinds of health care programmes, prevention efforts, and medical treatments (404).

9.3 Health-related quality of life in health care technology assessment

The evaluation of HRQOL requires the collection of primary data from either randomized clinical trials (RCTs) or prospective observational studies. HRQOL measures have been successfully incorporated into studies of medical treatments for hypertension (98,147,675), anaemia associated with end-stage renal disease (109,127,222,406,563), AIDS (562,760), cancer (51), arthritis (74,418,690), low back pain (168), stroke (194), mental disorders (580,634), and the outcomes of surgery (128). HRQOL measures have been used to examine the outcomes of different systems for delivering health services (88,394) and to examine differences in the functioning and well-being of patients treated in primary care practices (564,724).

A number of studies have been performed to evaluate the impact of medical treatment on HRQOL. Most of these studies evaluate the effects of pharmaceutical treatment. For example, Croog *et al.* (147) conducted a randomized clinical trial to examine the impact of antihypertensive treatment on quality of life. They selected a number of different measures of HRQOL dimensions that were thought to be affected by drug treatment for high blood pressure, including measures of general well-being, sleep dysfunction, sexual problems, work performance, social activity participation, physical symptom distress, and cognitive function. The investigators found that there were significant differences between the drug regimens on some of the measures of HRQOL despite comparable efficacy in reducing blood pressure. The captopril group showed improvements on measures of general well-being and physical distress symptoms compared to the propranolol or methyldopa groups.

Several studies have incorporated both psychometric and utility assessments into evaluations of health care technology. Bombardier *et al.* (74) used a number of clinical, health utility, and HRQOL scales in a randomized clinical trial comparing auranofin therapy to placebo in patients with rheumatoid arthritis. Clinical outcome measures were combined with functional health status, pain, depression, health perception, and health utility measures to evaluate the treatment over a six month period. The authors reported that auranofin was superior to placebo on a number of clinical indicators, activities of daily living, Quality of Well-Being scale, range of motion, and pain assessments. No differences were found on measures of depression or general health perceptions. Differences favouring the active treatment were found on the Patient Utility Measurement Set, a measure of the patient's perception of his or her current state of health relative to his or her state of health before treatment and relative to perfect health. Standard and modified time trade-off and lottery procedures were also used to elicit the patient utility values. The evaluation of HRQOL contributed to an understanding of the effect of the therapy on a broad range of outcomes important to the rheumatoid arthritis patient.

A more recent placebo-controlled, randomized clinical trial of r-HuEPO treatment was conducted in Canada. The Canadian Erythropoietin Study Group (109) evaluated 118 patients randomized into a placebo group or one of two r-HuEPO groups (high and low dose) and followed for 6 months. The HRQOL assessment included the Sickness Impact Profile, the Kidney Disease Questionnaire (a disease-specific health status measure), and time trade-off utility. Haemoglobin concentrations in the r-HuEPO group increased. Compared to the placebo group, erythropoietin treated patients demonstrated significant improvements in measures of fatigue, physical symptoms, social relationships and depression on the disease-specific scale. Improvements were also observed on the total physical score of the Sickness Impact Profile and moderate increases in exercise tolerance were observed in the r-HuEPO group. No differences between the treated and placebo groups were detected using the time trade-off utility measure.

Another randomized clinical trial is underway to evaluate the clinical, HRQOL and economic outcomes of r-HuEPO therapy for patients with anaemia associated with chronic renal insufficiency (563). Preliminary data analyses indicate that after 48 weeks of treatment, the r-HuEPO group showed significant improvements compared to the placebo group on energy and vitality, sleep and rest behaviour, and home management. After one month of treatment the r-HuEPO group had higher health utility scores (0.67 versus 0.57), but by 48 weeks this difference largely disappeared (0.69 versus 0.68).

There is also an interest in examining the impact of various treatments for AIDS and HIV disease on HRQOL in clinical trials. Wu *et al.* (761) used the Karnofski Performance Status scale and the Quality of Well-Being scale to evaluate the effect of zidovudine in patients with AIDS related complex over a one year period. This study demonstrated that HRQOL scales were able to detect significant differences between the placebo and zidovudine group. A recently completed observational study found that among a heterogeneous group of 250 AIDS patients with anaemia, r-HuEPO treatment was able to increase energy and vitality, decrease health distress and improve health satisfaction after 24 weeks of treatment (562). More importantly, no significant decline was observed in measures of home management, social functioning, depression, cognitive function, physical or role function, or life satisfaction over this same time period.

9.4 Including health-related quality of life outcomes in health care technology assessments

HRQOL is an important and measurable outcome of health care technology. However, care needs to be taken in including HRQOL measures in evaluations of medical treatment. Several different criteria need to be considered when selecting instruments for either RCTs or observational studies of new or existing medical technology, including appropriateness of the measure, psychometric characteristics, and practical characteristics (61,167,593,711). Each will be briefly discussed, beginning with appropriateness.

9.4.1 *Appropriateness*

The primary consideration in the selection of a HRQOL measure is the correspondence between the study objectives and content of the measure. To ensure such correspondence it is necessary to delineate carefully both the expected outcomes of the study and to carefully review the content of the HRQOL measures. Although not explicitly discussed in many HRQOL studies, the measures should be selected based on existing research evidence, concerning the probable relationship between the medical technology of interest and patient health status outcomes (559). It is often useful to identify the dimensions of HRQOL that might be expected to change as a result of the treatment. These dimensions are identified through a review and synthesis of the medical and health services research literature, and interviews with clinicians and patients.

The evaluation of new health care technologies should avoid restricting the dimensions of HRQOL included in the assessment, since there may be both unanticipated positive and negative consequences associated with a new technology. Scales need to be indentified which best match the purpose of the study, measure positive and negative outcomes of the treatment, and are appropriate for the population of interest. Both disease-specific and generic HRQOL instruments should be considered (524). Comprehensive measurement of HRQOL include traditional clinical measures, disease-specific symptoms and problems, and general health outcomes (713).

Correspondence between the level of health of the target population and that assessed by the HRQOL measure is critical to detecting differences between treatment groups. Lack of congruence will result in a skewed distribution and consequent lack of discrimination, that is, a large proportion of respondents will receive very similar scores, making it difficult to detect meaningful differences between groups or individuals (564). Almost all current HRQOL instruments focus on illness rather than health. However, it is important to consider and assess more positive aspects of health, such as positive well-being. Some scales, however, more clearly focus on higher levels of dysfunction such as those found in a chronically ill, elderly population; for example, the Activities of Daily Living Scale (381). Others, such as the Medical Outcomes Study General Health Survey (655), were designed to measure levels of health status and well-being in a general, primary care population. The level of health assessed by a particular scale may be determined from a review of the content of the scale and findings from previous studies.

A related consideration is the desired level of scale discrimination, that is, the range of scores or the number of categories in which individuals may be placed. In general, scales that provide greater discrimination include more items to assess a particular dimension of HRQOL. Changes in health status over time will be more accurately measured when the HRQOL scales measure the full range of health states (713). Measures that include few items may be adequate for detection of large differences between treatment groups. However, much finer levels of discrimination and responsiveness are usually required to detect differences between patients receiving alternative medications for chronic conditions such as hypertension (564).

Multidimensional measures of HRQOL (e.g., Sickness Impact Profile) are designed to provide an overall score, separate scores for each dimension, or both. The advantage of an aggregated score is that it provides an overall picture of HRQOL. Clearly, this is useful for comparing a profile of the effects, both positive and negative, of a medical technology on HRQOL. A second advantage of a summary index score is that it can be incorporated as the effectiveness outcome for a cost-effectiveness analysis. The major disadvantage of aggregated scores is that they conceal variability of individual dimensions and therefore may obscure valuable information on health outcomes. Conversely, dimension scoring provides a clear picture of the levels of the dimensions of HRQOL, but does not provide a method for combining scores to provide an overall estimate of HRQOL.

The selection of instruments for measuring HRQOL in medical evaluations is normally based on the appropriateness of the instrument for the research question and population, psychometric characteristics (e.g., reliability, validity, responsiveness to change), and practical considerations (e.g., respondent burden, resources available).

9.4.2 *Psychometric characteristics*

Reliability refers to the consistency with which an instrument measures a given trait or behaviour, while validity refers to the extent to which it measures what it is intended to measure (485). Assessment of reliability and validity has received extensive attention in the psychometric and HRQOL literature and thus is not discussed in detail here (see for example, 61,167,485,524,592,711). The types of reliability most frequently reported for HRQOL measures are internal consistency, interrater, and test–retest reliability. Internal consistency reliability assesses the homogeneity of a scale. It measures the extent to which the items in a scale measure the same underlying trait or behaviour. Interrater reliability is important when a scale will be administered by more than one interviewer. This type of reliability evaluates the correspondence or agreement between different raters of the same individual (167). Test–retest reliability, or stability, is applicable for cases where outcomes are assessed on two or more occasions. It evaluates whether scores remain unchanged over time in populations where changes in health status have not occurred. Standards for reliability vary with the type of reliability being assessed and the purpose of the study data.

Validity of HRQOL scales cannot be determined directly because there is no external criteria or standards for evaluating this construct (e.g., health status, mental health). Validity refers to both characteristics of the measure and its application in a particular disease or population. Therefore, evidence for validity is determined by an accumulation of findings from studies addressing such issues as the extent to which the measure discriminates between groups and its responsiveness to clinically important changes. Validity findings must be carefully reviewed since some types of evidence reported in support of validity of a scale may be relevant for an intended application while other types of evidence may not be appropriate (61,485,524,564). The important consideration is that validity must be established for each application and population of interest.

One aspect of validity, responsiveness, is the ability of a measure to detect small yet important clinical changes (167). The changes are those that patients and clinicians view as discernable and important, are detected with a treatment of established efficacy, or are correlated with valid physiologic indicators. Information on an instrument's responsiveness to change is important for planning medical evaluations and to ensure that sample sizes are sufficient to assure acceptable statistical power, and to select among alternative competing measures of a HRQOL domain for a specific study. There are a number of methods for assessing a scale's capability to detect clinically meaningful changes in health status (167,485). For example, Revicki *et al.* (563) determined, using both cross-sectional and longitudinal data on hypertensive patients, that the General Well-Being Adjustment scale was sensitive to the incidence of various physical symptoms (e.g., nausea, chest pain, skin rash) and to the development of these symptoms over time. Again, establishing a HRQOL measure's clinical responsiveness requires the accumulation of experience using the scale in different clinical evaluations for different medical conditions with different populations. Unfortunately, establishing that an instrument can successfully discriminate between individuals with different severity of illness at a single point in time does not ensure that the instrument can detect subtle changes in health status over time.

9.4.3 *Practical characteristics*

For a HRQOL scale to be useful for medical technology assessments it must be shown to be practical for RCTs and other investigations. It is, therefore, critical to determine the practicality of the instruments with respect to administration, respondent burden, and data analysis (714). Practical characteristics to consider when selecting measures of HRQOL include respondent burden, use of proxy respondents, and interviewer training. Respondent burden, which may be due to the length of an HRQOL assessment, complexity of the response task, or frequency of data collection, can directly affect data quality through incomplete or unreliable responses (564). Use of proxy respondents is necessary in some populations such as young children, the very frail elderly, head injured, or severely mentally ill. However, there is considerable evidence that the responses of parents and informal caregivers may be quite different from those given by patients in some dimensions of HRQOL (417,582). Interviewer training and ongoing supervision is especially important in collection of HRQOL data since interviewers can unintentionally influence outcomes resulting in measurement error that may obscure treatment differences. The more complex the instrument, the more time and effort will need to be invested in training and monitoring data collection activities. Issues related to investigator burden are also important when planning RCTs.

The field of HRQOL assessment is complex and many of the issues related to selection of measures represent trade-offs in that improvements in one area may result in problems in another area. Attempts to decrease respondent burden by selecting a shorter measure, for example, may result in a decrease in discrimination and power to detect differences between treatments. Particular attention needs to be focused on planning the HRQOL assessment strategy, selecting various HRQOL measures, and in determining the data collection protocol during the design phase of a medical technology assessment. In this way, the investigator can ensure that important health outcomes are included and that clinicians, health care policy- and other decision-makers, and society will have the necessary findings needed to understand the health benefits of a new technology.

9.5 HRQOL outcomes and economic evaluation

HRQOL outcomes are an integral part of health care technology assessment. Economic evaluations of new or existing medical technology require some measure of health outcome, whether mortality, health status, or QALYs. Incorporating HRQOL into economic analysis was initially proposed by Bush and his colleagues (102,228) in the early 1970s. Their work was based on the notion that quality of life should be included in the concept of life itself in order to express health status as a unifying concept, thus enabling comparison of any two health interventions. Based on their work, the concept of quality-adjusted life years saved (QALYS) was born and today one finds league tables in the literature (190,398,688) comparing interventions in terms of net direct health care costs per QALYS. Weinstein and Stason (721) argued that cost-effectiveness analysis inherently includes quality of life and that health outcomes of an intervention equals the years of life saved, quality of life lost due to adverse effects of treatment and quality of life gained due to decreases in morbidity and symptoms. Table 5 summarizes the costs per QALYS for a number of medical technologies.

In practice, however, researchers have often had difficulty incorporating HRQOL into economic studies for several reasons. This is due in large part because much of the HRQOL research has come out of psychology and sociology, not economics, and the resulting health status measurements (89, 437,643) are simply not compatible with economic concepts. For example, Croog *et al.* (147) examined outcomes across various HRQOL dimensions for different antihypertensive medications. Edelson *et al.* (210) could not directly use this information in a cost-effectiveness analysis of some of those same medications. Croog *et al.* (147) found that captopril was either superior to or comparable with propranolol across a number of HRQOL dimensions; Edelson and colleagues found propranolol to be much more cost-effective than captopril in terms of cost per year of life saved, but not cost per QALYS. The reason HRQOL was not included in the Edelson *et al.* (210) study was because of technical problems of meshing the two concepts.

More recently, the economic profession has been developing practical methods to incorporate utility, or preference, values into cost-effectiveness studies. As mentioned previously, utility assessment is compatible with economic evaluation. The outcomes of different medical technologies or health care interventions can be compared using a common metric, QALYS. In this way, it is possible to compare the medical costs and the health outcomes of such disparate medical technologies as heart transplantation, neonatal intensive care for low-birthweight infants, and antihypertensive treatment for mild to moderate hypertension, in order to make resource allocation judgements. The main problem is that the psychometric health status measures provide a greater richness

Table 5. Cost–utility ratios from selected medical technology assessments.

Medical technology	Cost/QALY gained in US dollars (1990)[1]
PKU screening	<0
Antepartum anti-D	$1970
Maintenance treatment for depression	$6160
Coronary artery bypass surgery	$6800
Neonatal intensive care, 1000–1499 g	$7300
T4 (thyroid) screening	$10 200
Treatment of severe hypertension (diastolic ≥ 105 mmHg) in males age 40	$15 200
Treatment of mild hypertension (diastolic 95–104 mmHg) in males age 40	$30 900
Oestrogen therapy for post-menopausal symptoms in women without prior hysterectomy	$43 700
Neonatal intensive care, 500–999 g	$51 500
Coronary bypass for single vessel disease with moderately severe angina	$58 700
School tuberculin testing programme	$70 700
Continuous ambulatory peritoneal dialysis	$76 200
Hospital haemodialysis	$87 400

Sources: refs (190),(317),(688).
[1]Inflated to 1990 dollars using the US Consumer Price Index for Medical Care.

of detail regarding the impact of medical technology on HRQOL, while the utility assessment methods provide a common, yet less responsive metric for examining health outcomes.

Currently, only a handful of studies have incorporated both psychometric health status and health utility assessments in evaluations of medical interventions (74,109,560,549,760). The Canadian Erythropoietin Study Group (109) found statistically significant differences between the erythropoietin and the placebo groups on haemoglobin, exercise stress test, and disease-specific and generic measures of health status. A time trade-off utility measure was insensitive to these clinical and health status changes. The Quality of Well-Being (QWB) scale has been found to be responsive to changes in clinical status in AIDS, arthritis, cystic fibrosis, and other patient populations (378). However, the QWB did not detect the short-term adverse effect of zidovudine on the health status of patients with early AIDS-related complex that was demonstrated using the MOS general health survey (760). At this time there is conflicting evidence regarding the responsiveness of utility scales, despite their increasing use in cost-effectiveness analyses of new medical technology.

Several investigators are working at merging the measurement approaches of psychometrics and utility assessment to take advantage of the strengths of each method. The psychometric approach is the best method for examining the structure of health outcomes, and for developing and validating scales to measure specific health concepts (713). Psychometric health status instruments do not meet the assumptions of utility theory which are needed for their use in cost-effectiveness analyses. John Ware and others are exploring whether the utility methods for enumerating scale levels and for combining different components of health can be applied to psychometric scales. Other research has demonstrated that utility scores and psychometric health status scores are only moderately correlated and that they measure different aspects of health (560, 562,689). Both psychometric and health utility measures are valuable for assessing medical technology, but the investigator must remain aware of the differences between the two measurement methods.

A second constraining factor associated with the use of HRQOL in economic evaluations is that these types of patient outcomes must be administered in prospective observational or randomized clinical trials. Cost-effectiveness analyses based on retrospective economic assessments or mathematical clinical decision models may not be very amenable to the inclusion of HRQOL measures. There are exceptions to this rule, but only for incorporating utility values. For instance, a number of studies have estimated the utility values of various states of health (see Table 4, p. 118). In some cases the health utility values for these studies were derived from investigator or clinician judgement, or convenience samples of patients or the general population. Clearly, there are problems associated with this approach since there may be systematic differences between patients, clinicians, and the general public in the magnitude of utility values for different health states (269,470). Also, the utility values for different health outcomes included in these economic and clinical simulation models are dependent on the utility scaling method and the objectivity and accuracy of the health-state descriptions. It may also prove possible to estimate utility scores for members of the population with different chronic and other diseases based on national health survey data (217).

Another technique which can be used to incorporate utility in a retrospective cost-effectiveness study is to describe relevant health states and develop utility values empirically. For instance, patients, family members, physicians, or even the general population can be surveyed for their preferences for various health states (688). For example, Hatziandreu *et al.* (317) evaluated the cost-effectiveness of maintenance compared with episodic antidepressant therapy for individuals with recurrent major depression. A clinical decision model was constructed to model the lifetime medical costs and outcomes for the different approaches to depression treatment. Utility values for various health outcomes were generated from expert psychiatrist and general practitioner panels. The study found that the maintenance treatment with a serotonin uptake inhibitor resulted in costs of US$6280 per QALYS and sensitivity analyses suggested that the cost-utility ratios ranged from US$3780 to US$13 460.

It is likely that an increasing number of economic evaluations of new medical technologies will combine health utility assessment techniques with careful collection or estimation of medical care costs. Australia and Ontario are currently experimenting with the use of cost-utility or cost-effectiveness analyses in addition to evaluations of safety and efficacy before approval of new drugs and procedures. Utilities and QALYs may well become the common metric for effectiveness outcomes in economic assessments of new medical technologies (404).

9.6 Use of HRQOL outcomes for health care technology assessments

Health status measures have multiple applications in health services research and medical technology assessment, including monitoring the health of populations, evaluations of new health care technologies, and medical outcome assessment. A number of other uses for HRQOL assessments have been specified by researchers, such as health policy evaluations of new systems of care and financing, medical practice and clinical decision-making, assessing quality of care, and forecasting demand for health care services (61,713).

9.6.1 *Monitoring the health of populations*

Mortality and survival information, morbidity rates, and data on the use of health services are insufficient for describing the health of populations, especially in developed countries. HRQOL measures are needed to describe and monitor the health of the general population in different regions or countries. Before health status outcomes can be used to evaluate the health of a population, it will be necessary to develop norms for the most important health concepts or domains. National health surveys, utilizing standardized generic measures, could then be used to estimate the burden of psychiatric and medical illnesses, describe the health status of the population, examine the changes in health outcomes over time, and possibly estimate the relative health benefits of different medical technologies competing for health care expenditures (713). It would be possible to estimate utility values using national health survey data (217). Clearly, large national or international surveys of health status could provide an important resource for evaluating health care technologies over the entire course of their development and diffusion into medical practice.

9.6.2 *Evaluation of new health care technologies*

HRQOL measures are important for evaluating the impact of pharmaceuticals, and other medical and surgical treatments, beyond biological or clinical outcomes (559,713). Although there are a number of randomized clinical trials of new medical treatments (e.g., 74,109,147,251), the majority of studies concentrate on traditional outcomes of safety and efficacy. Surgical procedures are rarely evaluated in terms of health status outcomes before widespread adoption. Comparisons of alternative health care technologies for the treatments of various diseases and medical conditions should be made based on their impact on patient health status and well-being, as well as clinical and laboratory outcomes (559). In some cases, such as hypertension, medical treatments may actually cause a decrease in health-related quality of life, although the clinical parameter, in this case diastolic blood pressure, improves. In situations where there are multiple effective therapies (in terms of clinical outcomes), it is informative to determine whether there are differences in terms of patient HRQOL among the different treatments. Patients and, increasingly, clinicians and health care policy-makers are interested in understanding the impact of medical technology on physical, psychological and social functioning. In cases where there are treatment options, clinicians and their patients can make informed decisions regarding the regimen which best fits the medical needs and maintains patient functioning and psychological well-being.

Research over the past 30 years has developed multiple generic and specific health status measures and efforts are underway to develop generic and specific measures that can be used in different countries (712). The European Organization for Research on Treatment for Cancer (EORTC) has sponsored the development of multinational health status outcome measures that can be used for the evaluation of new chemotherapy for the treatment of cancer (1). Over the next few years research in HRQOL assessment is concentrating on developing and validating short, comprehensive generic scales for use in RCTs of new medical technologies conducted in different countries in Europe and throughout the world. However, there is some concern whether different domains of HRQOL have the same meaning in different cultures. Comprehensive assessments of HRQOL will include generic health status measures combined with disease-specific and traditional clinical measures. In this way critical issues of safety, clinical efficacy, and HRQOL outcomes will be addressed in controlled clinical trials of new medications and other medical technologies.

9.6.3 *Medical outcome assessments*

Medical outcome assessments are designed to evaluate the impact of existing medical technology and physician practices on health, economic, and social outcomes. It is similar to the previous use of HRQOL assessments, except that the targeted medical technologies are already widespread in practice. Within the USA, the US Agency for Health Care Policy and Research (AHCPR) is supporting a number of Patient Outcome Research Teams (PORTs) to evaluate the medical effectiveness of medical or surgical treatments that impact on a large proportion of the population for which there is some ambiguity in respect of health outcome. The major objective of this effort is to improve the effectiveness and appropriateness of medical practice by developing and disseminating research findings on the effects of existing medical services and procedures on patient survival, health status, functional capacity, and quality of life (524). PORT projects are examining patient outcomes associated with cataract surgery, medical treatment of diabetes, hip replacement and osteoarthritis, knee replacement procedures, medical treatment for acute myocardial infarction, medical and surgical treatment for prostate disease, and other medical technologies.

Standardized HRQOL measures are needed to examine the impact of existing medical treatment on functional status and well-being (129,216). Advantages associated with using generic measures to monitor outcomes relate to their sensitivity to both positive and negative effects of treatment and chronic diseases (713). Health status measures will be used to address ways to reduce rising health care costs. In this way, it may be possible to determine the health benefits, using standardized and systematic assessment of patient outcomes, associated with the introduction or limitations in medical technology. These methods could also be used to evaluate the health impact of changing policies for the financing, organization, or provision of medical services.

Continual assessment of HRQOL outcomes using generic scales is needed to assess the impact of changes to the health care system on health. Baseline assessments are essential in interpreting health oucomes from observational or non-experimental studies of health outcomes across health care delivery systems (713). To adequately evaluate the relationship between changes in medical technology or health care delivery systems, attention needs to be placed on HRQOL outcomes, health care expenditures, and survival. HRQOL assessments may prove invaluable for measuring the health benefits of medical technology after diffusion into clinical practice. As the need for more information on the impact of medical practice increases, cost-efficient methods for monitoring the health of populations may assist in assessing health care technology.

9.7 Conclusions

Concerns about cost containment in health care and interest in the impact of medical treatment on patient functioning and well-being have increased the emphasis on HRQOL research. HRQOL assessment is part of the development and evaluation of health care technology and is likely to increase in the future. The techniques for measuring health status and HRQOL are well accepted and validated over more than 30 years of research (713) and health status assessment is currently applied in a number of clinical research areas (89,643,726). HRQOL assessments provide physicians, patients, and society with more complete information regarding the benefits and risks of medical treatment in terms of patient physical, psychological, and social functioning and well-being. This information helps clinicians in targeting the best treatment for their patients. Finally, HRQOL measures, especially health utility assessments, can contribute to defining health outcomes in cost-effectiveness analyses. Demonstrating that there are significant health benefits associated with a new health care technology may offset some of the differences in health care costs compared to alternative existing medical technology.

The evaluation of the effectiveness of medical treatment and surgical procedures is a reality that developers of new technology need to face. Health care decision-makers, physicians, patients, and society are demanding that the impact of a health care technology on patient functional status and well-being be demonstrated in addition to showing that it is safe and effective. There is a greater emphasis on the cost-effectiveness of new medical technology in the current health care environment. HRQOL studies are invaluable for helping to demonstrate the benefits of innovative medical treatments using outcomes that are important to patients and society. HRQOL outcomes are critical for documenting the expected value of an innovative medical technology. These outcomes can then be combined with information on the costs of the medical treatment to provide government agencies and health care providers with sufficient information to make approval, reimbursement, and adoption decisions. The methods for health status assessment are advanced enough to contribute to understanding the effects of health care technology on health and remain only to be more widely applied in research and clinical practice. It is clear that HRQOL represents an important indicator of the benefit of medical technology.

10. Assessing social implications of health care technology

The very success of science has ended its pleasant isolation.

Robert Sinsheimer

Does the truth reside in the computer printout?

Alan Sheldon

What a man calls moral judgment is merely his desire to generalize, and so make available for others, those values he has come to choose.

C. Wright Mills

The social implications of a new or existing health care technology can be the most challenging and difficult aspects of evaluation. Any decision to develop or use a health care technology inevitably rests on value judgements. Social and cultural factors are completely intertwined in questions concerning the place of technology in health care. At the same time, the methods for assessing social implications of health care technology are relatively undeveloped and few mechanisms exist to take action based on the results of such evaluations. Society does not seem to have enough confidence in social scientists and others dealing with social issues to insure that results of this type of assessment are used in policy-making.

It can be forgotten, in this rational and scientific age, that culture and society underlie all actions in health care (379). Life is obviously an important value in all societies, yet different societies value different lives differently, as indicated by the fact that some countries have had age cut-offs in dialysis programmes, ensuring that some young and some old people with serious kidney disease would die. The attitude towards life is also expressed in the controversy surrounding abortion in some countries. Such social values explain much that occurs in health care that may not appear to be rational.

Technology assessment itself cannot be totally objective or value-free. As an activity carried out by human beings, it too is influenced by social and cultural values.

This chapter gives a brief introduction to what should be a much more active and dynamic field of assessment.

10.1 Some interactions between social values and health care technology

The interaction between technology and the broader environment is very dynamic. Cultural factors such as intellectual curiosity, tolerance for new ideas, and social values favouring efficiency and productivity have obviously greatly influenced the course of technological change (111). Culture has affected the 'ideas, facts, modes of thought and observation, instruments, images, language, values, symbols, and rituals of biomedical science and technology' (253). Technology has also influenced the broader environment. For example, it has led to changes in work and leisure, sexual behaviour, and nutrition.

As the rate of technological change has increased dramatically during the last decades, individuals and social systems show signs of not being able to adapt. Some have accepted any technological change uncritically, and have later seen that technology adoption was associated with unanticipated, and often indirect, implications (346). On the other hand, some have become antitechnology, and have ignored the many benefits that modern technology has brought to humans, including the benefits of health care technology (539).

Some scientists see modern scientific knowledge as totally transforming our ways of being and of seeing ourselves. The discoverer of the structure of DNA, Francis Crick, for example, says, 'we are here because we have evolved from simple chemical compounds by a process of natural selection . . .'. He goes on to conclude that this destroys the 'Christian' and 'literary' 'nonsense' that has guided our lives (quoted in 382). Genetics and brain research seem to be leading to the power to 'reconstruct ourselves'. What kind of human beings would then be good? The discoveries of modern biology '. . . seem to force upon man a transformation . . . of his self-understanding and his view of his place in the whole' (379).

Health care technologies and their patterns of use reflect subtle interactions among various social values, such as the value a society places on health, on innovation, on financial security, and on technological progress itself. Why do societies provide health care or health care insurance, for example? One important factor is clearly the need for a sense of solidarity, in the face of decline in the importance of the family and religion. We need a sense that we are willing to take care of each other.

The definition of health and illness shape a society's conceptions of necessary or desirable technologies (111). The changing view of mental illness is an example. Debates over how to care for those with AIDS is another. Cultural forces have led to a widening of the definition of health, so that the World Health Organization now says that it is a 'state of complete physical, mental and social well-being'. The danger is a redefinition of human problems to make them problems for professionals, the process of 'medicalization' (252,762).

10.2 Social values and the development of health care technology

Social values affect which technologies will be developed, and, through the resources available for that development, the speed with which they will be developed. Social values are one factor determining the questions to be addressed. The special concept of the heart in Western society, for example, delayed research on approaches to heart disease for many years (666).

A common effect of social forces on technology development occurs during the early stages of clinical investigation. Who is to be the first recipient of a possibly dangerous innovation? If potential risks are high, it may not be possible to continue the investigation. This helps explain why investigators have often been the subjects of their earliest experiments. It also helps explain why prisoners have often been subjects of experiments. With increasing concern about such issues, it is often no longer acceptable to use captive populations such as prisoners.

The question of human experimentation, brought to the fore so poignantly by the actions of the Nazis in World War II, has led to increasing protection of subjects of research. For example, the Declaration of Helsinki, a formal code of ethics for the guidance of doctors in clinical research, was adopted by the World Medical Association in 1964 and extended in 1975. Many national organizations have developed their own codes and guidelines, including the National Institutes of Health, the British Medical Research Council, and the Association of American Medical Colleges (631, p. 155). For example, the Helsinki Declaration calls for a specially appointed independent committee to review the protocol in advance of any experimental procedure involving human subjects.

With adequate safeguards, the public in Western countries (at least) supports human experimentation. In the USA, studies have shown that a large majority of those with serious illnesses such as cancer and heart disease, as well as healthy members of the population, believe that patients should serve as research subjects (631, p. 164). One serious issue is how to recruit patients for a human experiment. The burden should ideally be distributed over the entire community. In practice, however, human subjects of research are often the disadvantaged, such as prisoners or the economically deprived.

10.3 Social values and the assessment of health care technology

Technology assessment itself is a social and cultural activity and is a part of social and cultural institutions. This has many implications. Perhaps the most important is that the tools of technology assessment—which can give the illusion of objectivity and rationality—must be applied with great caution. Assessment inevitably selects aspects of a problem to consider. In this process, problems can be reduced to terms that mistake their underlying structure and their fundamental nature (508). The collection of data implies selection of what data to collect; the analysis requires value judgements of which aspects to emphasize. And the limited attention to social values in assessment itself indicates cultural priorities.

The limited place of assessment of health care technology in the past is a reflection of social values: the value that lay people placed on the role of the physician and the conviction of physicians that their success was in large part a personally based art. As the technology of much of health care practice has increased, evaluation itself naturally has a larger place. Publicized failures in health care technology have promoted assessment. Successes have helped ease pressures for assessment.

The ethics of the processes of evaluation have developed rapidly during the past decades. The ethics of controlled clinical trials have been hotly debated (49,631). One frequent statement by some clinicians is that it is not ethical to test an 'established' technology, even if there is no clear evidence of its benefit. Those who believe in assessment answer that clinicians cannot just do as they feel best; their practice must be based on sound scientific evidence (399). Is it ethical to subject a patient to a treatment whose effect is unknown and which may do harm?

Bradford Hill, one of the developers of the method of the randomized controlled trial, wrote:

It must be possible ethically to give every patient admitted to a trial any of the treatments involved. The doctor accepts, in other words, that he really has no knowledge at all that one treatment will be better or worse, safer or more dangerous, than another . . . If the doctor does not believe that, if he thinks even in the absence of any evidence that for the patient's benefit he ought to give one treatment rather than another, then the patient should not be admitted to the trial . . . (quoted in Reference 101).

The problem for clinical trials, as in all human research, is balancing the welfare of the individuals in the trial against the potential benefit to future patients. The Helsinki accords raise a particular problem for clinical trials. The accords state that each subject should be adequately informed about the aims, methods, hazards, and benefits of the study and should grant freely-given consent in writing. However, in a randomized trial, for example one involving a placebo, the benefits and hazards are not predictable for the individual patient. Still, the very justification for a randomized trial is insufficient information to permit a rational informed choice (631, p. 166). Other problems arise when the community or the parents must give approval. Current opinion concerning children is that parents cannot consent, but can give permission; older children should make their own decisions in this case (413).

10.4 Social values and the use of health care technology

Use of a technology depends on the complex interaction of many forces. A sick person visits a physician seeking care. The physician, based on the complaints and an examination, uses knowledge from experience and medical science, to prescribe a diagnostic and therapeutic plan. The care is provided in an institution, and will usually be paid for by a public programme that includes certain constraints. Educational programmes attempt to change physician behaviour toward certain interventions. Patient demands are stimulated by press coverage of certain treatments, and physician responses are conditioned by such public demand. But the entire decision-making process occurs in a social and cultural context that may be very difficult to define. This is indicated by variations in use of technology within a country and from country to country (526,727).

The major test for the medical profession is whether the ends of the profession are so humanitarian that experts may be given autonomy (258). Ideally, actions are based on reliable evidence and patients and physicians define 'good' in the same way. Physicians often choose for patients, however, raising the possible problem that the patient would define good in a different way. McNeil (439), for example, has shown that some patients prefer radiotherapy for larynx cancer even though the outcome in terms of life expectancy is worse than with surgery because radiotherapy preserves the ability to speak normally. In the conflict between value judgements of a health care provider and a patient, the patient's values should ordinarily determine the treatment.

A particular example concerning technology is focusing on the physical symptoms and biological problems a patient has and ignoring the human being. Disease occurs in a human being, and information and knowledge bearing on it also can be psychological and social (250,703).

One obvious reflection of social values is laws and regulations dealing with technology. In Sweden, interventions that can be made available to large subgroups of the population are favoured over those of benefit to few people, for example. Sweden was rather late in accepting brain death as the standard for declaring that a person was dead. For these reasons, Sweden offered heart transplant rather late, compared with other developed countries.

The values of the individual may conflict with the values of society in the case of any technology. For example, vaccines produce 'herd' immunity that protects the entire population from epidemics. From the standpoint of the individual in a society with adequate immunization rates, however, the most rational course is to refuse the vaccine. For this reason, most societies require immunization of children before entering school.

Social values seem to have their greatest effect when the technology deals with processes with deep human meaning. Thus, technologies dealing with birth, death, and reproduction have been most controversial in recent years. Technologies in these areas interfere, or seem to interfere, with natural processes, and may be very disturbing to moral feelings.

10.5 Nature of social implications

Social effects of a health care technology can take place at any time in its life cycle: when a new technology is introduced, when a technology is in general use (especially if it is applied to a different purpose, or when its use for the same purpose is significantly increased), or late in its life cycle.

A social impact or implication can be characterized best by specifying certain aspects of its effects. The most obvious is the nature of the effect itself. For example, a change in societal sex ratios, an increased amount of adolescent sexual activity, or an unresolved legal and moral confusion over the definition of life or death are examples of effects that could have (and have) resulted from widespread use of certain health care technologies. Beyond the effect itself, one can ask, which individuals or groups are affected? Which benefit? Which are harmed? Another issue is the conditions giving rise to the effect. Such conditions could be technical, or they could be social and cultural. The example of Sweden and brain death (previous page) illustrates how social factors can determine conditions necessary for application.

Social implications often are indirect effects, they may occur in the long run, and they are generally unintended. They may also occur as the result of other effects, thus are especially indirect. These have been called 'higher-order' effects. For example, the first-order effect of a contraceptive pill might be considered to be the ability to prevent conception reliably. A second-order effect might be loosening the tie between women and the child-bearing function. A higher-order effect might be increased participation of women in the labour market. Another higher-order effect might be loosening of societal attitudes towards sexual behaviour, the 'sexual revolution'.

A particular type of social effect in today's world of limited resources concerns access to and distribution of health care services. In many countries, new technologies diffuse first into private institutions, meaning that the poor are left with less access. To a significant extent, any technological advance fed into a delivery system that discriminates against some people is likely to heighten such discriminatory practices. Thus, technology can worsen problems of equity and help to break down solidarity patterns.

10.6 Techniques for assessing social implications

The techniques for assessing social implications are varied, but generally fall within the area of social sciences such as sociology. Given the nature and complexity of these effects, such assessments will almost always be multi-disciplinary efforts. The social scientist must clearly understand the technical nature of a technology to assure that an analysis is sound. This means that engineers and physicists, and as well as physicians and nurses, have a part to play in such assessments.

The assessment of social implications has lagged in all countries. In a 1976 report, the Office of Technology Assessment suggested a number of questions that could be asked regarding a specific technology to reveal its effects. The questions were intended to be a guide to thinking about such effects. Social assessments involve more than applying a certain method or tool; they also involve creative thinking and 'brain-storming'.

The list presented here is illustrative and not exhaustive.

1. *What are the medical aims, technical characteristics, and developmental state of the technology in question?*

(a) What medical problems is the technology designed to solve, and how severe are these problems? What contribution will the technology make? Diagnose an early form of disease? Treat a life-threatening condition? Correct a functional problem?

(b) Is the technology a major or minor innovation? Will it radically alter medical practice or will it modify and improve established procedures?

(c) How soon can development and adoption of the new technology be expected? Can development and adoption be speeded or slowed by policy mechanisms?

(d) How effective is the procedure? Has its medical efficacy been assessed? How will efficacy be assessed? Are there reasons to think (animal evidence, for example) that the technology will be efficacious? Are controlled clinical trials possible? Underway? If controlled trials are not possible, what methods will be used to assure effectiveness? What are the potential or proved dangers of the technology to individuals using it?

2. *What are the implications of the technology for the patient's life?*

(a) What will be the quality of life of the patient? Normally active? Moderately restricted? Physically crippled?

(b) What psychological effects can be anticipated? Guilt (because of burdens on the family)? Anxiety? Feelings of dehumanization? Dependency?

3. *What are the implications for the patient's family?*

(a) What will be the costs to the family, both financial and non-financial? How will the technology affect family structure? Will there be any physical dangers to the immediate family? Will the device or procedure be psychologically acceptable to the family? Will active co-operation or assistance of family members be necessary on a continuing basis?

4. *What are the implications for society in general?*

(a) Will the technology affect demographic characteristics of the society? For example, can changes in sex ratios or age distribution in the population be anticipated? Will the technology affect reproductive capability of patients and thus change the genetic pool and the prevalence of genetic disease?

(b) Will use of the technology by an individual create threats to the environment?

(c) Will introduction of the technology challenge important beliefs and values of the society about birth, gender, bodily integrity, personal identify, marriage and procreation, respect for life, right to live, right to die, responsibility for each other? Will introduction of the technology result in changes in any of these values?

(d) Will the technology alter any basic institutions of society (e.g. schools, recreational facilities, prisons)?

5. *What are the implications for legal and political systems?*

(a) Will problems of justice, access, or fairness arise? Will they lead to legal action?

(b) Will the manufacturer be liable for damages resulting from failure of the technology (in the case of devices or drugs)? Will liability extend only to damage to the individual or will it cover environmental effects as well?

(c) Will use of the technology require changes in legal definitions of such concepts as death or suicide?

6. *What are the implications for the economic system?*

(a) What is the projected or present overall monetary cost of adopting the technology?

(b) What are the implications for programmes of disability or life insurance? Pension funds?

(c) Who will pay? Will government support be required for development and/or use of the technology?

(d) How will the technology affect the national economy? Will development and use produce jobs? How will this affect overall productivity? Will productivity in health care be affected by the technology? Will the tax structure and rates be affected? Will imports or exports be affected?

If all of these questions were answered for a new technology, the result might be called a 'comprehensive technology assessment', since technology assessment refers to any policy-oriented study of the implications of technology (492).

10.7 Conclusions

It is difficult to characterize available information on social impacts of technology in health care. Information on social impacts is generally not quantitative, and much of it is not in professionally published sources. Much of the available information has been developed by the lay press, both newspapers and journals. This information seems surely to have heightened consciousness of social impacts in the public mind, yet there is no definitive evidence that it is so. Still, except for economic implications, there is little research-derived, organized knowledge on the social implications of health care technology.

Certainly, consideration of social implications has played a part in policy decisions in the past. Debates on the treatment of end-stage renal disease and the frequent exclusion in early days of elderly people from such programmes is an example of serious ethical issues coming into the public debate. More recently, genetics has been the subject of a great amount of political debate. Still, there is no body of literature that could be characterized as a serious attempt to study the social aspects of health care technology.

Increasingly in the future, as technology interferes more with such processes as life, death, and reproduction, and as resource pressures raise problems of solidarity and equity, systematic considerations of social aspects of technology will be necessary. Such studies seem to deserve much more emphasis in the future than they have received to the present (508).

11. Assuring the quality of health care

. . . the use of critical tests will only be accepted when the public understands the extent to which medical practice rests on custom rather than evidence, and when there is general agreement that the obligation to change this situation must be shared equally.

Leon Eisenberg

The medical profession is puzzled by a strange paradox: as medicine becomes more effective it receives more public criticism. I do not find this at all surprising and it is certainly not anti-scientific; sharp criticism is part and parcel of the scientific method.

William Silverman

The quality of medical and health care is becoming an increasingly visible public issue in a number of countries (17,425,428,469,475,553,642,618). While the overall results of advances in health care seem relatively clear, there is considerable evidence that optimal care is not being given, based on available studies.

This book focuses on technology assessment and the information it provides on benefits, risks, costs, and social implications of health care technology. Focusing on technology assessment has a risk; the risk is implying that examining a situation is enough. In fact, information from assessment must be used. One of the most important purposes of technology assessment is to improve quality of health care (296,428).

The objective of quality assurance is to 'improve the outcome of all health care in terms of health, functional ability, patient well-being and consumer satisfaction' (754). The US Institute of Medicine has made a similar definition (425). The term 'quality' often is used in different ways and may denote characteristics such as effectiveness, efficacy, efficiency, equity, acceptability, accessibility, adequacy, and scientific/technical quality.

Technology assessment should support assessment of the quality of a provider's practice. Using standards to evaluate quality of care requires criteria by which to judge how a health condition or disease has been diagnosed or treated (754). The development of such criteria, if they are to be valid, must be based on knowledge about (at least) the efficacy and safety of the health care technology concerned. As described in Chapter 7 and other parts of this report, such information is often lacking. None the less, a start must be made. Limited knowledge is no excuse for lack of action.

Quality assessment measures and perhaps monitors the quality of health care. Quality assurance seeks to safeguard and improve quality. Most quality assurance activities have dealt with the structure or process of care (see below), and therefore have little relation to technology assessment. This chapter will focus on quality assessment measures using health outcomes and early attempts to assure quality as measured by such variables. The experience with quality assurance using outcomes is limited (296). Thus, most of this chapter will deal with quality assessment.

The intent of this chapter is mainly to describe the relationship between quality assessment and technology assessment. This is obviously a relatively minor part of the large field of quality assessment and assurance. This chapter does not attempt to do justice to the entire field of quality assessment.

11.1 Approaches to quality of care

The term quality implies a degree of excellence. To measure such excellence, a standard of comparison must exist and a method of measurement must be available. The development of broad goals for quality is not a problem. Measurement of quality, however, is a major problem.

The Office of Technology Assessment (505) has defined quality of medical care as 'the degree to which the process of care increases the probability of outcomes desired by patients and reduces the probability of undesired outcomes, given the state of medical knowledge'.

Donabedian (178,179) provided the generally accepted classification of techniques when he used the terms structure, process, and outcome. As he points out, evaluating structure requires the acceptance of two assumptions: that better care is more likely to be provided when better qualified staff, better physical facilities, and so forth, are employed; and that available knowledge allows one to identify what is good in terms of staff, physical structure, and organization. Process is the evaluation of the actual activities of providers, but requires specifying which activities are appropriate, which should mean having specific knowledge about the links between certain health care processes and health outcomes. However, in practice, the assessment of process has generally been limited to evaluating the extent to which the care conforms to accepted norms of care rather than linking them with outcomes. Assessment of outcomes is the evaluation of end results of health care in terms of health and satisfaction. It should be emphasized that health outcome involves more than survival. Donabedian includes recovery and restoration of function as outcomes, for example.

The literature on quality of care is extensive, and gradually a consensus has begun to emerge about how assessment can be done (11,475,553,642). None the less, a confusing array of approaches and philosophies still characterizes the field.

Approaches to quality assessment may be thought of as either general or specific (363). General approaches examine the ability of an individual or institution to meet certain standards. Individuals are usually measured in terms of experience, education, and knowledge. Common approaches are to license physicians and to grant certification to specialists. Institutions are evaluated on the basis of physical structure, administrative and staff organization, minimum services, and personnel qualifications. Standards and guidelines are used for the purpose of accreditation of hospitals and other institutions. Standards and guidelines are also developed for specific services, such as trauma centres and neonatal intensive care units. In many instances, institutions and physicians must be licensed or certified before they will be paid by national health care programmes. A recent trend in the USA has been for hospitals to assure clinical competence of medical staff through granting of clinical privileges to carry out specific procedures. For example, privileges to carry out a procedure may not be granted until the physician can demonstrate that he or she has carried out a minimum number of that procedure (10). In general, quality assurance activities have been focused on hospital care. They are more difficult to develop in the ambulatory care and home care setting (425, p. 2).

Specific approaches to quality measurement and control examine specific interactions of providers and patients. A common method used is to focus on selected diagnoses or activities in hospital care. For example, in northern Europe, attempts have been made to draw up model health care programmes, using the expertise in the health care professions. These attempt to establish the optimal manner of dealing with a specific health problem such as hypertension or lower back pain. Review is carried out by medical staff review committees, and is based on review of patient records. Such a review is generally used as an educational tool in attempts to improve quality. Firmer action is uncommon. Physicians on peer review groups are quite reluctant to discipline colleagues. These activities have traditionally been internal and voluntary. Increasingly, external audits have been necessary.

Europe now shows a mix of voluntary internal and external mechanisms for quality assurance and a range of information coming from providers, consumers, patients, and administrators (754). However, Europe is considerably behind the USA in implementing quality assurance programmes (553). In part, this may be because the quality definition in Europe is often physician-oriented, whereas in Canada and the USA it is more patient-oriented (11).

Evaluating process of care is easier than evaluating outcomes, but it produces less definitive and useful information on quality. The problem is that the relationship between standard health care procedures and health outcomes is often not known (296). There are two problems. One is knowing whether physicians follow currently accepted medical procedures in their practices. In other words, are they using technology effectively? The second is establishing the effect on outcomes under ideal circumstances, that is, efficacy.

In evaluating structure, process, or outcome, criteria are used in the evaluation process. These criteria can be either explicit or implicit. If explicit, they are written down, and can be examined for their relevance and validity. Evaluation of such criteria has led to the conclusion that few in use today are based on good evidence of effectiveness of the intervention (425, p. 290). The development of criteria, or what is often called 'practice guidelines' or 'practice policies' has become a very active endeavour in the USA (206).

Finally, the question of site for quality assurance activities can be considered. As already noted, quality assurance activities have dealt with hospital care. It should be clear, however, that quality in clinics and primary care settings is also important. All types and levels of health service are open to scrutiny and improvement (754).

11.2 Outcome as a focus for quality assurance

Ideally, quality assurance activities review health outcomes and relate them to health services delivered (86,425). Without consideration of health outcome, quality assurance activities seem at best irrelevant and at worst harmful (30). Ellwood (216) has proposed a radical shift to 'outcomes management'. For these reasons, the remainder of this chapter will only consider evaluation of outcome.

Outcome assessment is related to technology assessment, to the extent that the technology assessment is concerned with efficacy and safety. The assessment of outcome is dependent on the results from controlled clinical trials and other attempts to measure outcome scientifically.

Health outcome is the important result of health care, but there are few links between technology assessment and measuring structure or process of care. Outcome evaluation is still undeveloped (425, p. 54). Current measures cannot adequately adjust for patient and environmental factors that may influence patient outcomes independently of quality of care (505). This greatly impedes widespread use of outcome measures. In addition, there is no accepted conceptual framework for the most likely hazards of health care to indicate how care is likely to fail and how to test for each major failure (505).

A review of the literature on quality assurance programmes found little attention to either immediate or long-term outcomes (326).

Outcome information can be developed for use by multiple parties. A recent trend in the USA is to furnish such information directly to the public (505). Such public involvement seems in general to be a good move. However, to the extent that the measures used are invalid, the public may be badly informed. If information is to be released publicly, its weaknesses and limitations must be carefully described. (While the same might be said of efficacy and safety information, the field of efficacy and safety evaluation is considerably further advanced than that of quality assessment.)

Although process and outcomes are often difficult to relate, using the clinical literature in combination with expert opinion can produce useful standards for quality assurance. The RAND Corporation has pioneered such a method (87, 121,328).

The remainder of this chapter will review a few selected methods of quality assessment and assurance that are beginning to come into widespread use and that seem to have considerable promise.

11.3 Hospital mortality rates

The use of patient death rates to compare quality of care delivered by specific health care providers has been expanding. It has also been controversial. Its problems include the fact that mortality can result from many factors other than poor quality care and that techniques to adjust for such factors are generally inadequate.

One of the most challenging questions is how to construct an indicator that takes into account the characteristics of the patients who come to a hospital. Large university-affiliated hospitals generally receive sicker patients with the same diagnoses. Their outcome will thus often be worse.

The experience with hospital mortality and attempts to adjust it to the type of experience in the particular hospital is fairly extensive (505). Dubois and his colleagues have become identified with recent work in this field (192,193). They used insurance claims data to identify hospitals with high and low mortality rates. After adjustment for differences in patients' risk of dying, they found significant differences in preventable deaths between high- and low-mortality hospitals for cerebrovascular accidents (CVAs) and pneumonia. They estimated that 5 per cent of patients with those conditions entering one of the high-mortality hospitals would have a preventable death, compared to a 1 per cent chance in a low-mortality hospital (193). In a more recent study, Dubois and colleagues examined the experience of 12 hospitals and 182 deaths, examining three conditions: cerebrovascular accident, pneumonia, and myocardial infarction. Using a panel of physicians, they attempted to determine the percentages of deaths preventable. Two physicians agreed that 27 per cent of deaths were preventable, while all three agreed that 14 per cent were preventable. The major problems were mismanagement of myocardial infarction, poor diagnostic examination of patients with CVA, and both poor diagnosis and poor treatment in people with pneumonia (192).

There are a considerable number of methodological and conceptual issues that must be resolved before hospital mortality rates can be regarded as a valid indicator of the quality of care. Resolving these issues involves considerable research. In particular, links to health care processes must be identified and valid techniques found to adjust crude mortality rates for patient characteristics.

While such data have problems, their release can initiate a dialogue between different parties, such as consumers and providers. In addition, making such information publicly available is itself a quality assurance programme, since one can expect involved hospitals to examine more carefully the care that they provide.

11.4 Monitoring adverse events

Health care is associated with safety problems, and minimizing these is part of quality assessment and assurance. All technology is associated with possible adverse effects. Unnecessary and unduly prolonged hospitalization results in serious health risks. More than 3 million hospital infections are acquired each year in US hospitals, afflicting almost one patient in every 18 admitted to an acute care facility (315). In one study of 815 consecutive patients on a general medical service of a university hospital, 36 per cent experienced an iatrogenic illness, most arising from drugs or invasive procedures (650). In 9 per cent of all patients admitted, a major untoward event occurred; in 2 per cent, it seemed to be a factor related to the patient's death.

In attempting to control such events, almost all US hospitals have implemented 'occurrence screening' or 'incident reporting' systems. While these systems vary widely from hospital to hospital, their main utility is as a first step to identify poor quality care (505).

This field was pioneered by Rutstein and his colleagues in the early 1970s (588). Working with panels of expert specialists, these researchers developed a list of specific conditions for which adverse outcomes should not be expected to occur, such as a death from tuberculosis. In 1976 the California Medical Insurance Feasibility Study developed screening criteria for 20 'potentially compensable events' for the use in hospital quality assurance activities (505).

Among the most common adverse events used as criteria are deaths, nosocomial (hospital-acquired) infections, unusually long lengths of stay, and unscheduled procedures, readmissions, or transfers.

The largest study in this area was the Study on the Efficacy of Nosocomial Infection Control (SENIC) (315). Incidence rates of nosocomial infections in the urinary tract, surgical wounds, lower respiratory tract, and bloodstream were determined from a random sample of records in 338 hospitals. Using sophisticated statistical methods, changes in infection rates were correlated to changes in infection control programmes. The method described by SENIC was estimated to reduce nosocomial infections by 32 per cent, which would save the USA US$260 000 per 250 beds annually.

Aside from this one programme, none of the systems for reporting adverse events has been validated (505). Perhaps this is not as serious a problem as it seems. Such systems have only recently been developed and implemented. The field is in a rapid state of development because of pressures in the USA to assess quality of care. Most likely, more information on the reliability and validity of the data will be available within the next few years.

11.5 The tracer method

In the early 1970s, Kessner *et al.* described an approach to quality assessment called the tracer method (385). The approach combines the examination of both process and outcome, using a particular disease as a tracer. A tracer is a well-defined disease whose natural history is related to effectiveness of health care. Williamson (738) developed a method similar to tracers, based on health outcomes, called health accounting. The point of the tracer approach is to focus one's evaluation on a representative complex patient management process in order to make inferences on how well the system of care is functioning.

One model for such a system is care for hypertension (high blood pressure). Hypertension is one of the most prevalent and costly medical disorders in Western countries. Approximately 30 per cent of the adult population in industrialized countries is hypertensive. Serious sequelae of uncontrolled hypertension include strokes, renal disease, cardiac dysfunction, and increased risk of premature death. Treatment of hypertension can and should be effective. Finally, an advantage of using hypertension is that most care is given in the ambulatory care setting.

Such studies seem quite feasible, and they generally produce reliable and valid information. One major problem with such studies is the lack of clear criteria based on good prospective studies. This means that studies usually depend on panels of experts to define guidelines for treatment. The validity of these guidelines can be questioned. In fact, little relation between process and outcome has been found in a number of studies. Romm and Hulka (576) concluded that the setting and promotion of standards for the process of care do not guarantee adequate patient outcomes and that peer review groups should recognize the limitations of both process and outcome methods.

11.6 Patients' assessments of their care

The outcome of care is the health of the patient. One possible approach, then, is just to ask the person who has been treated. The key question is the validity of such responses.

What is relatively clear is that patients are more qualified to judge the interpersonal aspects of quality than the technical aspects (505). OTA's review of 23 studies of patients' assessments of care found that 17 contained evidence of the validity of patients' assessments.

Several studies have examined patients' ability to judge technical aspects of their care. Few such studies have been done, however, and have only examined the ambulatory setting. In summary, the findings indicate that consumers generally judge the technical excellence of their care higher than physicians do. Still, consumers seem to have the ability to differentiate between different levels of technical excellence (505). More research is needed in this area.

OTA summarizes its review as follows (505, p. 247):

Finally, it can be argued that routine and careful monitoring of patient-based indicators of the quality of physician and hospital care is important regardless of conclusions about the validity of these indicators in measuring true quality. Instead, the argument is based on strong empirical evidence that patients' perceptions of quality of care influence patients' behavior. Patient behaviors that are affected include doctor-shopping, complaints, disenrollment, compliance, and use of services. Such behaviors have noteworthy consequences to their health and the quality of their care.

11.7 Conclusions

There are many quality assurance activities not discussed in this chapter, including medical audit activities, peer review, hospital tissue committees, and utilization review activities. In all cases, quality assurance attempts to improve the quality of care. Naturally, the important aspect of care is improving patients outcomes, both in terms of 'objective' health measures and in terms of personal satisfaction or quality of life (425). In the future, such concerns will become increasingly visible. The important point is to forge links between the fields of technology assessment and quality assurance to ensure that the best available information is used to improve quality.

Section IV SELECTED CASE STUDIES

The purpose of this section is to present briefly several case studies of technologies in some depth. Each case study has been drawn from much more extensive literature. The interested reader is urged to acquire that literature, which is referenced in the appropriate place.

The cases presented range from preventive measures to computer applications. One important general point in these cases, and in many other examples, is that any technology that falls under the very broad definition presented in Chapter 1 can be assessed using the methods summarized in this book. Health care technology assessment has dealt with psychotherapy (45) and physiotherapy (704). As caring has become more of a respectable subject in the health care literature, it too has been assessed as a technology. In fact, Bryce (95) has argued that 'soft' technology, such as social supports, require the same standards of scientific evaluation that are required for such technologies as *in vitro* fertilization.

12. The assessment of prevention

Historically speaking, assessment of preventive activities is well-established. One of the first assessments on record is that of John Snow, who investigated the origin of a cholera epidemic in London in 1854. One of the first randomized clinical trials was that of pertussis (whooping cough) vaccine, organized by Bradford Hill (454).

As cost-effectiveness analysis began to be used in the health field, many of the earliest analyses were of preventive interventions. In the period preceding 1984, about a quarter of all cost-effectiveness analyses concerned prevention. After 1984, however, there was a shift toward evaluation of treatment activities. In its 1980 report on the methodology of cost-effectiveness analysis, the Office of Technology Assessment (497) noted, 'The shift away from prevention may not be permanent . . . the Federal Government's recent emphasis on prevention, increasing public acceptance of ideas of disease prevention and health promotion, and the conscious linking of prevention to cost containment, may promote renewed interest in prevention-oriented CEA/CBA.'

This prediction may partially have come to pass, with a virtual spate of books and articles assessing prevention. Some prominent examples include assessment of cancer screening tests (207), assessment of general screening (203), assessment of obesity screening (585), and a number of cost-effectiveness analyses of vaccines (31). In the late 1980s the US Preventive Services Task Force carried out assessments of 169 preventive activities, focusing on interventions applied by clinical physicians (697). Cohen and Henderson (135) have reviewed the economics of prevention in some detail. Also, in the USA, the Centers for Disease Control (CDC) has initiated a 'Prevention Effectiveness' initiative designed to develop methods for, and evidence of, prevention effectiveness (676,679). In addition, the US Office of Health Promotion and Disease Prevention of the US Public Health Service released a report in 1992 that is essentially a proposal for a standard method for evaluating costs and benefits of prevention and other programmes (371).

Notwithstanding all the attention which is being paid to assessing prevention, the sheer volume of the cost-effectiveness prevention literature continues to lag behind both treatment and diagnostic technologies (see Fig. 15, p. 102).

This chapter will discuss general issues in assessing preventive activities and then will present an example of measles vaccine to illustrate how an assessment might be done. The chapter is presented with the attitude that prevention should be assessed just as rigorously as any other health care activity.

12.1 The nature of prevention

Due to its very nature, prevention assessment poses special challenges compared to assessing therapeutic technologies. First of all, many prevention activities are outside the health care system arena, for instance programmes to control smoking behaviour, diet, and exercise. Other activities such as environmental efforts, e.g., lead abatement, may be the responsibility of non-health agencies, while public health practices including well-baby clinics, immunization programmes, and health education activities, occur within public health departments which may be organizationally and financially completely separate from the medical care system. Still other prevention activities, such as blood pressure, cholesterol, and diabetes control, occur within the health care system. Thus, prevention activities may compete with very different budgets within society, including individuals' time and budgets, general local, regional, or state budgets, or medical care budgets. Assessments of prevention need to be made with the respective competing priorities in mind.

Societal spending on prevention is considerable (93,94). In the USA prevention-related spending for 1988 was $32.8 billion, amounting to an estimated 0.67 per cent of the gross domestic product. These monies were used for health promotion activities aimed at influencing individual behaviours and developing healthy lifestyles; health protection including environmental measures aimed at protecting large population groups by reducing exposure to disease and risks of injury and disability; and prevention health services, consisting of screening and counselling services generally offered in a clinical setting, sometimes at the worksite. $18.2 billion or 3.4 per cent of US national health expenditures was spent in direct health services-related programmes. Thus, dollar amounts can be large, but the relative proportion of the health care dollar allocated to prevention is quite small, at least in the USA. Assessing prevention scientifically and objectively can help society reach an appropriate balance of investment relative to other uses of its health care funds and, indeed, societal resources in general. Many believe society underfunds prevention activities.

Teutsch (676) presents two complementary frameworks for conceptualizing prevention programmes. The first framework concerns the delivery of prevention technologies and consists of three components:

(1) clinical prevention strategies, which is the traditional medical model. It includes vaccination and early detection of disease through screening, diagnosis, and early treatment;

(2) behavioural prevention strategies, which are more orientated to the individual to encourage healthy lifestyles such as exercise, smoking cessation and healthy diets;

(3) environmental prevention strategies, which are population-based efforts such as fluoridation of water supplies, environmental lead abatement programmes and governmental regulations such as bicycle helmets, public smoking, and seat belt laws.

The second, more familiar framework concerns targeting interventions by stage of disease or injury and also consists of three components:

(1) primary prevention, which is the reduction or control of causative factors for health problems, such as smoking, sex education, and environmental exposures;

(2) secondary prevention, which involves early detection and treatment, such as screening and diagnostic activities;

(3) tertiary prevention, which involves supportive and rehabilitative services to minimize morbidity due to existing disease or injury.

The assessment process itself is greatly affected by the kind of prevention activity involved. In terms of health care technology assessment, prevention strategies within the clinical setting are most often addressed. An assessment would require identifying the population at risk for a disease, for example for breast cancer, women over 40; determining the potential for finding these women and providing mammography; determining the specificity and sensitivity for the diagnostic test itself; identifying the different resulting treatment strategies available; and determining the probability of successful treatment. Note that the chain of events is long, complex, and often uncertain. This chain tends to be both longer and more complex and contains more uncertainty than therapeutic technologies. Much of the assessment process will require data from multiple sources, probability estimations which may or may not be readily available, and will often require sophisticated modelling and possibly expert opinion.

Primary prevention assessment often requires sophisticated epidemiologic modelling of the disease; secondary prevention assessment may require both epidemiologic modelling of the disease and clinical decision modelling of the various treatment options, including the likelihood of success.

Figure 17 presents an idealized depiction of the process of prevention activities and their assessment (676). This ideal process begins with new prevention techniques and technologies being developed by basic and applied researchers. Following testing for efficacy, demonstrations are sponsored to test for effectiveness and preliminary estimates of cost effectiveness. Finally, cost-effective strategies are implemented and evaluated in community settings. This ideal process should be iterative and is rarely achieved. However, it is important for authorities and other responsible individuals to recognize the relational nature of discovery, development, diffusion, and assessment in prevention as in all other areas of health care.

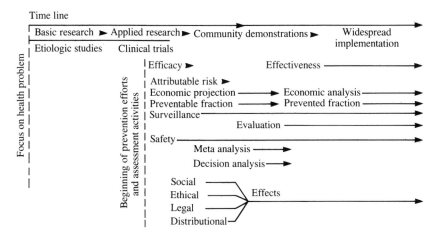

Figure 17. Natural history of the development of an effective prevention strategy and temporal relationship to the types of assessment activities (source: 676).

12.2 Methods for assessing prevention techniques

For a more extensive discussion of the issues covered, the reader is referred to Teutsch (676).

12.3 Efficacy, safety, and effectiveness

Efficacy of prevention techniques is the initial concern as with any new technology. They should be assessed very early in its life cycle. As in the case with therapeutic or diagnostic technologies, the first question is, 'does it work when applied appropriately in ideal circumstances?'. Even efficacy testing may require much antecedent work to be done. Consider the nicotine patch for smoking cessation. Initially, one must have firm evidence of the link between smoking and adverse health consequences as well as the link between smoking-cessation and positive health consequences. Then, randomized clinical trials need to be sponsored to establish the link between the use of the nicotine patch and smoking cessation under carefully controlled clinical conditions. Of course, many prevention interventions, for example lead abatement or health education techniques, are seldom the subject of randomized controlled trials due in part to the high costs of such studies.

Safety may also be a concern and should be assessed. A systemically applied drug has obvious side-effects concerns, but so do other strategies such as lead paint abatement where, for example, sanding produces lead dust that can be inhaled.

Effectiveness assessment concerns the real world. Does the nicotine patch really induce smoking cessation when prescribed by the average physician to the average patient in the community setting? Here, the patch needs to be assessed once it is made available to the general public. Since it is fairly expensive and requires a physician's prescription, will people buy it? Is it covered by insurance? Do some portions of the population have no access due to costs or other reasons? Is it acceptable to users? How effective is the patch compared with other smoking cessation programmes? All these questions should be answered to fully assess the effectiveness of this technology.

12.4 Population-attributable risk and prevented fractions

Besides some of the general characteristics of prevention noted above, including complexity, time, and uncertainty, there are two specific assessment issues which seem to be unique and critical to assessing many prevention technologies. Population-attributable risk (PAR) and prevented fractions (PF) are quantitative techniques to measure the impact of risk factors and preventive interventions.

Population-attributable risk (PAR) is a descriptive term which links the relationship of a risk factor, for example high blood pressure, to the likelihood of disease, for example stroke. It is calculated as follows:

$$\text{PAR} = \frac{P_e \ (RR_e - 1)}{1 + P_e \ (RR_e - 1)}$$

where P_e is the population prevalence of the risk factor, and RR_e is the relative risk associated with the risk factor. Relative risk is the probability that the presence of the risk factor will lead to the adverse event of interest (e.g., the chance that smoking will cause lung cancer).

Whereas the attributable risk is the theoretical limit of the health benefit which could be achieved if the risk factor were to be totally eliminated, the prevented fraction (PF) is an estimate of what can be achieved in actual practice. The prevented fraction is calculated as follows:

$$PF = \frac{P_1 \ (1 - RR)}{RR + P_1 \ (1 - RR)}$$

where P_1 is a measure of the proportion of the population that is both at risk and that accepts the intervention.

The prevented fraction is likely be different when calculated from efficacy studies (where the effect of a prevention intervention might be maximized) than from actual community interventions (effectiveness), where whole populations may be targeted with lesser success.

12.5 Cost-effectiveness and other economic analyses

Cost-effectiveness analysis is applied in prevention as it is with all technologies. Due to the nature of many preventive issues, extensive modelling and simulations may be required. This is partly due to the dearth of well-controlled trials establishing efficacy, in part due to the ever-present uncertainty in applying preventive programmes to whole populations, especially a problem when behaviour change is required, and partly due to the very long lead time which is often present between the intervention and the effect.

In an attempt to develop a standardized method for assessing costs and benefits of prevention activities, Kamlet (371) recommends that all assessments use a utility approach to value benefits.

Interestingly, the prevention literature seems more forgiving of the limitations of cost-benefit analysis (CBA) techniques (44). For instance, many analyses of immunizations use CBA, valuing indirect cost savings using the human capital approach (5,392,740). In such studies, health benefits of immunizations are valued in terms of lifetime earnings gained. Generally such valuation is contrary to policy-makers' own value systems and thus is discouraged. This valuation tends to inflate the perception of benefit, resulting in a perception of large economic payoffs. The point is that, while there may be such benefits, they are quite diffused through society. No one party may be able to recognize benefit. For assessments of prevention programmes, certainly immunization programmes, the concern for lifetime earnings seems to be less present than in other situations.

12.6 Discounting future costs and benefits

Since one of the main characteristics of prevention, which may complicate the assessment, is that the benefits often occur far in the future, the benefits may be uncertain. It also means that an evaluation may have to be continued for years before the value of the activity can be determined. It also means that third parties may be reluctant to pay for it, since they incur the costs but may not accrue the benefits.

From the standpoint of economic analysis, this fact also complicates the analysis. Present benefits do not have the same value as future benefits, as pointed out in Chapter 8. Discounting must be used to put a present value on both costs and benefits. The result may be that costs occur at the present, and therefore are not reduced by discounting, but benefits can be reduced considerably by discounting. Large benefits of prevention occurring far in the future, then, may in fact not be as important as they seem.

Discounting future benefits due to prevention has not gone unchallenged. Many in the prevention community argue that the social rate of discount should be quite low, possibly even zero, and that to use higher discount rates penalizes prevention activities compared to the therapeutic technologies, and devalues potential benefits to future generations, for example in a lead paint abatement programme. However, economists argue that discounting both benefits and costs at the same rate is required. To do otherwise is to face illogical results (718). For instance, by only discounting costs, a rational decision would always be to postpone investing in the prevention programme, waiting for a year when one would have more money and could accrue more benefits.

12.7 Case study: measles vaccination

This section presents an example of an assessment of a primary prevention programme, measles vaccine. The section draws from a recent paper by Thacker and colleagues (679). More details can be found in their paper.

Measles was once a universal childhood disease, causing a large amount of death, permanent disability and discomfort. Measles vaccines were licensed in the USA in the early 1960s and a national campaign to eradicate the disease was launched in 1966 (396). By 1983, fewer than 1500 cases were reported, also resulting in major reductions in measles-related diseases including encephalitis, mental retardation, death, and lesser complications such as pneumonia and otitis media. Substantial costs were also averted.

Assessments of vaccines have extended from safety and efficacy trials themselves to assessments of costs and benefits using modelling studies. Cost-benefit ratios were calculated to be upward from 5:1 (5,392,740). More recently, an analysis of the combination measles—mumps—rubella vaccine estimated a 14:1 ratio. Thus, assessments indicated these immunization policies to be very cost-effective.

Recently, there has been an alarming increase in measles in the USA. By 1989, over 18 000 cases were reported and projected to grow to almost 28 000 in 1990. Although an estimated 97 per cent of all children are vaccinated, clearly a new assessment is needed. There is a suggestion that the vaccine may fail in some cases which has led to a second dose vaccine policy for all school-age children (112). This policy needs to be assessed (679), certainly for cost-effectiveness. In addition, although a high proportion of the general school-aged children population may have received the vaccine, as many as 50 per cent may not receive it in certain poor inner-city areas (112,113,332). Thus, the costs and benefits of making the additional efforts to ensure vaccination of this group should be assessed. There is no doubt that both the two-dose policy for every child and an intensive effort to ensure inner-city children receive at least one dose will prove to be much less cost-effective than the one-dose policy for the general population. The question is whether these new policies are a good use of society's money compared with other public programmes. In addition, some clearly important social and ethical issues are involved in these assessments, including cultural factors, access to care, and possible religious exemptions.

The measles vaccine is an excellent example of a very efficacious preventive technology that is effective and cost-effective in many instances, but clearly ineffective in certain instances. Good assessments can help guide public policy to determine when society should make special efforts to extend benefits to all the populations. With rapid developments in the vaccine area because of new biotechnological techniques, such assessments will continue to be important in the future (40).

12.8 Conclusions

The assessment of prevention is conceptually no different from the assessment of any other technologies. It should be done routinely and should compete on a level playing field for scarce societal resources. There is an old adage that an ounce of prevention is worth a pound of cure. That may be true philosophically, but it does not always hold economically. Most prevention activities, like most diagnostic and therapeutic activities, cost money. Many promote prevention by arguing that it is cost-effective, but they mean that it saves society money. Except for special cases, such as many immunizations, this is seldom true. Russell argues that preventing disease has intrinsic value to society and individuals in society, just as treating and curing disease has value (585). Society is or should be willing to pay for prevention because of that value. The purpose of sound scientific assessments of prevention is to measure this value and to ensure that prevention competes effectively for society's scarce resources.

Notwithstanding the conceptual similarity of assessing prevention compared to other classes of technologies, prevention poses special challenges to the analyst, as noted in this chapter. Besides uncertainty, lack of controlled trials and the long time frames often involved, prevention often involves a degree of compulsion. The intervention may be effective and cost-effective, but an assessment should also pay attention to social factors, such as how much freedom of choice and autonomy may be acceptable. Several countries, for example, allow people to refuse immunizations for their children based on religious objections. The same concern applies to anti-smoking laws, bicycle helmets, and seat belts or air bags in cars. How much freedom of choice is allowed is a social choice, and needs to be considered in an analysis of prevention.

On the whole, however, prevention can be assessed just as any other health care intervention can be. Effectiveness can be determined in terms of mortality and morbidity. Cost-effectiveness can be estimated, and these estimates can be compared to alternative uses of the same resources, such as in treatment programmes.

13. The assessment of medical imaging

Diagnostic imaging has been subjected to intense scrutiny since the introduction of the CT scanner in 1972. At that time, relatively few assessments of diagnostic imaging had been done aside from assessments related to safety, especially in minimizing doses of ionizing radiation. Assessing diagnostic imaging was also seen as difficult from the beginning, because the impact of an image on health cannot be direct. The diagnosis must change therapy, and the therapy must be effective.

13.1 Technology assessment and diagnostic imaging

In 1977, Fineberg *et al.* (240) formulated four (later five) levels of evaluation for the efficacy of diagnostic imaging.

1. Technical evaluation: the technical output gives accurate information concerning the structure of the part of the body imaged.
2. Diagnostic accuracy: this output contains information that potentially improves the clinician's ability to diagnose disease and assess the patient's prognosis.
3. Diagnostic impact: the information can alter plans for additional diagnostic tests.
4. Therapeutic impact: the information can lead to changes in therapeutic plans for patients.
5. Health impact: the end result may be improved patient outcome.

Prior to the mid-1970s, almost all assessments in the field of diagnostic imaging (or radiology) were at the first level. A few studies examined the diagnostic accuracy of specific imaging procedures by collecting data on their specificity and sensitivity. However, the field has developed rapidly since then, partially stimulated by demands from policy-makers and others for evidence of health impact, and a number of studies have been done to assess the impact on diagnostic or therapeutic plans. It is now possible to develop decision rules for the use of diagnostic imaging in specific circumstances. For example, Harvard Medical School has published a useful book of such guidelines (440).

13.2 Technology assessment and CT scanning

After its introduction in 1972, computed tomography (CT) scanning rapidly became the most visible technological advance in health care. As a complex, expensive device, it came to symbolize the problem of health care technology. The CT scanner is a device that uses X-rays, radiation sensors, a computer, and complex software to construct images of cross-sections of the body.

A CT scanner that could be used only on the head was introduced to the international market in 1972 and began to diffuse rapidly into use. The diffusion has been presented in Fig. 2 (p. 25). The Office of Technology Assessment (502) did one of its first health reports on this subject, using the Fineberg framework (240) to review the literature. The basic conclusion of the report (502) was that 'well-designed studies of efficacy of CT scanners were not conducted before widespread diffusion occurred'. By the time of the report it was known that CT scanners performed reliably and provided accurate diagnostic information. In addition, CT scanning was replacing other diagnostic tests, especially pneumo-encephalography and cerebral arteriography. Little was known about how CT scanning affected the planning of therapy or patient health.

The CT scanner was also an issue in Sweden. The first CT scanner was imported in Sweden in 1973. Swedish investigators carried out a cost-effectiveness analysis of CT scanning, based on its ability to replace other expensive diagnostic procedures (274,366). The study suggested that large hospitals could pay for a scanner out of replaced procedures. Subsequently, large regional hospitals did buy CT scanners, but others were prudent. By May 1978, the USA had 4.8 scanners per million population, whereas Sweden had only 1.6 per million. In the USA, which had no effective planning mechanism, the OTA report had relatively little impact on the situation with CT scanners. The scanner diffused very rapidly into practice.

Another early experience with CT scanning was described from the UK (659,661). The Department of Health and Social Security (DHSS) was involved from an early stage in the development of the CT scanner, since it provided prototype funds. The DHSS was quite restrictive towards purchases of the head scanner, and set up an explicit evaluation plan intended to guide policy. By 1978, the UK had 0.9 scanners per million population, compared to the 4.8 scanners in the USA (661). In the case of the body scanner, however, although the DHSS made a policy similar to that for the head scanner, scanners were taken up rapidly out of non-government funds, both endowment funds of institutions and private funds, such as those of donors. There were also explicit fund-raising drives by some hospitals. In the case of the body scanner, the strategy of restriction and assessment failed.

One of the most interesting evaluations of CT scanning was developed by Fineberg *et al.* (240) and extended by Wittenberg and Fineberg (741,742). All physicians requesting a CT head scan were asked to complete a questionnaire at the time of their request (240). The questionnaire asked three questions:

1. What diagnoses were considered, in probabilities?
2. What diagnostic tests would definitely be required and what tests would be required if CT scanners were not available?
3. What would the treatment plan be if the physician had no CT scanner available?

At the time of discharge of the patient, the physician was interviewed to ascertain the diagnostic tests actually performed, treatments undertaken, and final diagnostic understanding of the case. In the first study, cranial CT was found to reduce other neurodiagnostic procedures by up to 73 per cent in the case of pneumoencephalograms, and lead to changes in therapy in 19 per cent of cases. In later studies by Wittenberg and Fineberg (741,742) of body CT scanning, more extensive questionnaires were used. CT improved diagnostic understanding in 52 per cent of patients, reassured the physician about previously planned therapy in 43 per cent, improved precision of previously planned treatment in 23 per cent, and contributed to a change in therapy in 14 per cent.

A number of other European countries developed standards for the number of CT scanners 'needed'. The early standards were often based on information in the OTA report and the Swedish report. For example, in 1979 the French standard called for one CT scanner per million population. The standard in The Netherlands in 1979 called for one head scanner per 500 000 population (43).

The case of the CT scanner has been visible in most countries of the world, including less developed countries. It has been a test of the new field. On the positive side, a number of useful reports and studies were carried out. The CT scanner probably has been studied more than any other health care technology. A number of countries did develop standards for the number of scanners that were effective in their planning programmes. On the negative side, the CT scanner was seen as a prototype technology, whereas in fact it was one of the most expensive technologies in the medical marketplace. Lessons from the CT scanner did not readily transfer to other technologies.

An important aspect of the CT scanner, however, was that it did demonstrate clearly that technology developing in one country, the UK in this case, could rapidly diffuse over the entire world. The result was that technology assessment was seen as having an important international dimension from its beginnings.

Today, CT scanning is fully accepted as a fundamental diagnostic tool for many conditions. Its purchase is no longer regulated in countries that earlier controlled it, such as The Netherlands. Table 6 shows the rates of CT scanners in selected countries in 1986 and 1988.

13.3 Preliminary assessment of magnetic resonance imaging

Magnetic resonance imaging (MRI), sometimes called nuclear magnetic resonance (NMR), is an imaging device that was introduced in the late 1970s and is now rapidly spreading into use as a diagnostic tool (435). MRI is projected

Table 6. Numbers and rate (per million population) of computed tomography (CT) scanners by country and year.

Country	Number scanners		Scanners per million pop.	
	1986	1988	1986	1988
USA	3000	4991	12.8	21.7
Japan	3300	5448	27.5	44.3
France	264	350	4.7	6.3
Belgium	64	118	6.4	12.1
West Germany	423	595	6.9	9.8
Denmark	23		4.6	
Netherlands	45	83	3.2	5.7
England	149	204	2.7	3.6
Italy	201	338	3.5	5.9

Source: ref. (80).

to diffuse at a rapid rate throughout the world, with an increase in the market size of 90 per cent per year, almost a doubling. Numbers and rates of MRI scanners in some selected countries in 1986 and 1988 are shown in Table 7. One reason that this rapid diffusion is a concern is because of the high cost of MRI units, more than US$1 million for the least expensive device. It is striking that the USA has a high rate of both CT and MRI scanners, as well as gamma cameras (an important technology in radionuclide imaging) (Table 8) and ultrasound (Table 9), another imaging device. It seems that the USA puts a high value on this type of diagnostic tool.

Table 7. Numbers and rate (per million population) of magnetic resonance imaging (MRI) devices by country and year.

Country	Number MRIs		MRI per million pop.	
	1986	1988	1986	1988
USA	110	1150	0.5	5.0
Japan	10	256	0.1	2.0
France	29	34	0.5	0.6
Belgium	7	7	0.7	0.7
West Germany	41	91	0.7	1.5
Netherlands	2	7	0.1	0.5
England	14	28	0.3	0.5
Italy	13	29	0.2	0.5

Source: ref. (80).

Table 8. Numbers and rate (per million population) of gamma cameras by country, 1988.

Country	Number cameras	Cameras per million pop.
USA	7639	33.1
Japan	1139	8.9
France	234	4.2
Belgium	197	20.2
West Germany	1167	19.2
Netherlands	137	16.4
England	369	6.5
Italy	451	7.9

Source: ref. (80).

Table 9. Numbers and rate (per million population) of ultrasound scanners by country, 1988.

Country	Number scanners	Scanners per million pop.
USA	50 370	219
Japan	15 744	123
France	9 007	162
Belgium	989	101
West Germany	17 996	296
Netherlands	496	34
England	1 249	22
Italy	4 985	87
Spain	1 978	51

Source: ref. (80).

MRI produces images of cross-sections of the human body similar to those produced by CT scanning. There are importance differences, however. A CT scanner depicts the X-ray opacity of structure of the body. MRI images depict the density or even the chemical environment of hydrogen atoms. These properties of parts of the body are not necessarily correlated.

MRI has several advantages (501,651). It gives a high contrast sensitivity in its images. It does not employ ionizing radiation as CT scanning and other imaging methods do. It is not necessary to inject potentially toxic contrast agents, as is often done with CT scanning (although contrast agents are being used more and more frequently with MRI scanning). MRI allows choice of different imaging planes without moving the patient; CT scanning can only produce an image of one plane at a time, and some planes are not possible. Finally, images can be obtained from areas of the body where CT scanning fails to produce clear images. It may be that an MRI scan can replace many diagnostic laboratory tests in the future.

Despite this great potential, a technology must be assessed in reality. One can ask such questions as these: Is present MRI an advance in imaging technology as compared with (say) CT scanning? Does it produce useful information at a reasonable cost? Does it produce diagnostic information not otherwise available?

13.4 Technology assessment and magnetic resonance imaging

Magnetic resonance imaging has been repeatedly assessed since its introduction. One of the early reports was done by the Dutch Health Council (322). It has been assessed by several groups in the USA (501) and has also been formally assessed in the Nordic countries, in Australia, and in Switzerland by means of a consensus conference.

There is widespread agreement that MRI is a reliable diagnostic device that produces information that can be quite useful at times (501). It has potential advantages over other modalities such as CT scanning: MRI is able to distinguish between various normal and abnormal tissues; blood flow, circulation of the cerebrospinal fluid, and the contraction and relaxation of organs can be assessed; since the compact bone emits no signal, tissues surrounded by bone (e.g., the contents of the posterior cranial fossa and of the vertebral canal) can be represented without disturbance by artefacts; and MRI also has the advantage of easy selection of planes, which is particularly useful when imaging the spine and spinal canal.

Thus, despite the fact that magnetic resonance images contain artifacts that can be confusing and that require expertise to interpret, MRI can be said to produce information that is useful for the diagnostic process. However, this is not sufficient for answering practical questions such as the following: Which patients should be scanned with MRI, and which with other diagnostic modalities (in other words, where does MRI have real advantages in making diagnosis)? Which conditions that can be diagnosed by MRI can also be effectively treated? What is the place of MRI in relation to other diagnostic imaging modalities such as CT, nuclear medicine, ultrasound, and conventional X-ray techniques?

A literature review published in 1988 found that 54 evaluations did poorly when rated by commonly accepted scientific standards such as use of a 'gold standard' comparison of blinded readers of the images (the expert doing the reading did not know the status of the patient). Only one article had a prospective design. Also, over the period examined, there was no improvement in quality of research over time (142). Kent *et al.* (383,384) pointed to a continuing problem in later articles. A recent review done by the author shows no change in this situation.

The most thorough literature review was by Kent *et al.* (384). The literature showed that MRI is probably superior to computed tomography, its main competitor, for detection and characterization of posterior fossa (brain) lesions and spinal cord myelopathies, imaging in multiple sclerosis, detecting lesions in patients with refractory partial seizures, and detailed display for guiding complex therapy, as for brain tumours. In other diseases, the efficacy of MRI was found to be similar to computed tomography. In fact, the best designed study, carried out in a heterogenous group of patients in neuroradiology, studied in a matched pair design, found that sensitivity and specificity of CT scanning were somewhat better than that of MRI. More recent literature does not contain articles refuting these conclusions.

As for diagnostic or therapeutic impact, little information is available. For diagnostic purposes, brain imaging is by far the most frequent use of MRI. For example, Bradley (82) found that more than 65 per cent of scans were of the brain, and between 10 and 20 per cent of the spine. MRI does not appear to have replaced other modalities such as CT scanning in the brain except that it is used preferentially in suspected posterior fossa tumours. In a prospective randomized study in patients with suspected posterior fossa tumours, Teasdale *et al.* (674) found that in groups of about 500 patients each, 93 of those who had CT first were referred subsequently for MRI, whereas only 28 of those who had MRI first were then referred for a CT scan. In the spinal cord, two studies have examined the relative accuracy of MRI in relation to myelography (an X-ray procedure) and computed tomography (464,465). The studies found that MRI and CT were roughly equivalent in terms of true positive results, but that both were superior to myelography. Several studies have indicated that MRI may replace CT scanning and myelography in scanning of the spine (63,464). Peddecord *et al.* (528) found that MRI gradually replaced both CT scanning and myelography. In their study, the percentage of physicians ordering myelography prior to MRI dropped from 15 per cent to zero during the two-year period of their study. This could be significant, since myelography is a risky procedure.

Another area where MRI could be quite useful is in imaging joints. A common problem is torn or damaged menisci (cartilages) of the knee. The standard diagnostic procedure is either arthroscopy by scope or arthrogram, an X-ray procedure. Both are invasive, in that the scope must be inserted into the joint or a contrast material must be injected. MRI is non-invasive. Crues *et al.* (149) found that, for more serious meniscal tears, the false-negative rate of MRI was 6 per cent, a figure comparing favourably with the alternatives. Manco and Berlow (445) reported similar findings. However, the advantage of arthroscopy is that a therapeutic procedure can be done if an abnormality is found.

One study has been carried out in Norway, using the Wittenberg/Fineberg method (538). The investigators found that 33 per cent of patients had their main diagnosis changed by MRI scanning. Plans for surgery changed in 20 per cent of the patients, and plans for radiotherapy changed in 8 per cent of patients.

13.5 Costs of magnetic resonance imaging

The capital cost of an MRI scanner varies greatly, depending particularly on the strength of the magnets. A basic unit costs at least US$1 million.

Evens (223) reported 1983 survey results that found that operating an MRI facility in the USA cost US$840 000 a year. Bradley (82) reported that the costs of operating two MRI facilities varied from US$841 000 to US$1 115 000 per year in 1985. It is worth noting that only about one-third of this operating cost is accounted for by the capital investment in the MRI scanner. Other expenses include space, personnel, equipment, and maintenance. The cost per scan in Bradley's two centres was between US$370 and US$550, and the fee for the scan was US$500 (1986 dollars). The costs apparently do not include the payment to the physician.

Bradley (82) comments on the possibility that costs will be offset by replacement of other diagnostic procedures, particularly myelography. Invasive diagnostic procedures such as myelography must be done with a hospitalization of at least one day, whereas MRI can be done on an out-patient basis.

The author (DB) made rough estimates of the number of cases of specific disease problems in The Netherlands that might be imaged with MRI. Important disease problems and number of cases include:

Brain tumours	850
Tumours of the spinal cord	70
Multiple sclerosis	400
Herniated nucleus palposis	22 000
Torn meniscus	3 735

It can readily be seen that the potential for MRI scanning in terms of numbers is with herniated nucleus palposis ('herniated disc') and torn meniscus. Otherwise, the demand for MRI scanning can readily be met by a relatively small number of units in university hospitals.

13.6 Conclusions

Diagnostic imaging makes up about 5 per cent of the national health expenditure in industrialized countries. This 5 per cent is highly visible, and diagnostic imaging has been perhaps more subject to regulation than any other area of medicine.

This scrutiny will continue. In most industrialized countries, hospital budgets are now tightly constrained. This means that each new purchase must compete

with other alternatives. It is probably a frequent occurrence that imaging departments must choose between several possible purchases. Thus, technology
assessment may become more useful at the hospital level as well as at the
national policy level.

The main problem with the field of technology assessment in diagnostic
imaging remains the poor quality of primary data. Technology assessment
reports are usually based on syntheses of available scientific information, with
an input of judgement and clinical experience (440). Without good data, the
usefulness of the assessment of imaging will be limited.

14. The assessment of surgical practice

The assessment of surgery in a formal sense has been limited. The Office of Technology Assessment (496) concluded in 1983 that 'The impact of RCTs on surgery has been minimal, largely because RCTs in surgery are the exception rather than the rule'.

None the less, the situation seems to be changing slowly. Since the land-mark publication *Costs, risks, and benefits of surgery* in 1977 (99), surgery has been subject to increasing scrutiny. Some specialties of surgery have begun to pay formal attention to the situation with assessment in their particular area. For example, a group in the UK is collecting information on randomized controlled trials (RCTs) in gynaecology and will publish a large review modelled after the Chalmers *et al.* (117) review of obstetric care. Figure 18 shows that cost-effectiveness studies of surgery increased somewhat during the 1980s, although they are still not very frequent.

14.1 The nature of surgery

Surgery has existed as long as written history. The Hippocratic Oath contains an admonition not to 'cut for stone', a particularly life-threatening procedure at that time. Historically, much of the practice of surgery was in setting bones or suturing wounds; these procedures are clearly effective. The sanitary revolution

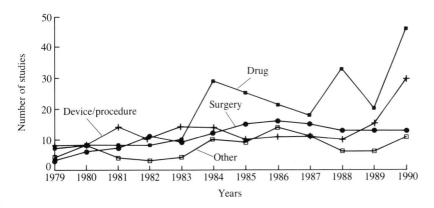

Figure 18. CBA/CEA literature, trends by type of technology (source: 214).

of the late 1800s made more invasive surgery possible with its developments in antisepsis, with associated advances in anaesthesia and nursing care. Much current surgical practice had its beginnings well before RCTs were available as a tool. In many cases, the surgical procedure developed empirically as a response to severe and even life-threatening conditions. If the patient survived or improved, the surgeon had some reason to feel that the procedure was responsible.

The removal of diseased or cancerous organs also seems to make such good sense that the value of such procedures was rarely questioned. The theory behind much cancer surgery, which has been done since the last century, is that long-term survival depends on removing all diseased tissue. Successful surgery, meaning an operation that the patient survived without a following infection, was taken as a successful treatment. Long-term outcomes have not been considered carefully until fairly recently.

14.2 The assessment of surgery

The nature of surgical procedures contributes to the difficulty of testing them through RCTs. Unlike drugs, which are fixed compounds, surgical procedures evolve (76). The efficacy of a drug does not necessarily depend on the skill of the prescriber. In surgery, the skill of the surgeon is vital, and this skill changes over time. Bunker *et al.* (99) attribute the limited use of assessment in surgery to the 'very real conceptual, practical, ethical, and economic difficulties of carrying out in adequate numbers and sizes experiments involving complex surgical procedures in human beings'.

Funding agencies have generally not supported trials of cancer surgery, perhaps because they do not receive proposals for assessments. In 1978, for example, the Office of Technology Assessment (487) carried out an analysis of National Institutes of Health (NIH) expenditures on clinical trials. In that year, of 756 clinical trials supported, 575 were of therapies. Of those, 400 tested drugs in isolation, and only 25 evaluated surgical procedures. This is all the more ironic considering that drugs are reasonably well-evaluated because of regulatory requirements.

Another problem with the assessment of surgery is what control group to use, especially when there was no effective therapy before. Withholding treatment for the purposes of assessing a new therapy is considered unethical by some. Sham procedures also raise ethical problems. For example, in the 1950s, a form of surgery, internal mammary artery ligation, spread for the treatment of coronary artery disease and angina pectoris (542). Because of doubts that the procedure had any effect, trials were carried out in which patients were randomized to two groups (174). One received the procedure. The other had a sham operation, in which an incision was made in the skin, the artery visualized, and the wound then closed without further intervention. The group that received internal mammary artery ligation had significant relief of symptoms. The problem was that the group that received the sham operation had equivalent relief, showing the strong placebo effect of a surgical operation. The procedure has since been totally abandoned.

There have been a number of reviews concerning specific surgical procedures that indicate that inappropriate surgery is common, even considering the lack of assessment information. Perhaps the prototype operation in this regard is the hysterectomy, one of the most frequent surgical operations. Hysterectomy is appropriate when performed in cases of suspected or diagnosed cancer, but it is also frequently done for other purposes. In the USA, studies have indicated that perhaps as many as 30 per cent of hysterectomies were done for sterilization or cancer prophylaxis (496). In The Netherlands, hysterectomy is frequently done as a treatment for excessive menstrual bleeding (menorrhagia) despite the availability of less invasive alternatives (739). A proposal in The Netherlands would carry out a controlled trial of less invasive alternatives versus hysterectomy for this indication.

Still, this example itself indicates one difficulty in assessing surgery. Patients are often referred for a specific surgery for a specific procedure, or they seek that procedure on their own. Entering a randomized trial of drugs generally tests one drug against another. Since the patient has no ability to choose, the choice is equivalent. However, entering a trial of surgery versus another treatment requires the patient to agree to accept an invasive procedure without choice, or alternatively, to forego a procedure that he or she may wish to have done. Many patients will not enter such a trial. For example, as will be described later in this chapter, conventional gall bladder surgery is being replaced by surgery through a laparoscope, which involves only small incisions. Patients choose to go to centres where this procedure is done. It is unlikely that such patients would then agree to enter an RCT where they would have to agree to have open, invasive surgery if the randomization process so indicated.

A final problem in assessing surgery is that the indications for surgery have changed during this century. Originally, surgery was done only under strong imperatives. However, today surgery is often done for reasons related to quality of life (99). When surgery was extremely dangerous, the patient and physician might decide that it was better for the patient to live with the symptoms than take the relatively high risk of death or serious injury. However, even the most invasive surgery, such as open heart surgery, is now associated with rather low mortality rates (around 1 per cent in the case of open heart surgery). This has led to an expansion of indications for surgery, as well as the development of surgical alternatives, such as vasectomy, as a procedure for sterilization. Haemorrhoidectomy is done primarily for the purposes of improving quality of life. With developments in such technologies as lasers, the procedure seems possible with less pain and faster recovery. However, the assessment problem is difficult. One must quantify pain and quality of life to carry out a full assessment.

Cost-effectiveness analysis of surgery is a relatively new development, mainly for the reasons discussed above. Surgery is expensive, both because of the surgeon's time and the intensity of the time in the operating room and hospital. Long-term follow-up is necessary to see if surgery is superior to other alternatives, but such follow-up is seldom done. One can only suspect that in some situations surgery is more cost-effective than other treatments because of its more definitive nature.

14.3 Recent developments in surgery

Surgery has changed rapidly since World War II. The trend has been towards smaller incisions and more rapid operations. One important innovation has been microsurgery, made possible by the development of operative microscopes and associated surgical tools. Anaesthesia has changed correspondingly rapidly. Anaesthesia began in the 1800s with the ability to make the patient unconscious through inhalation of such drugs as chloroform and ether. More recently, however, anaesthesia has focused more on conductive anaesthesia, in which blockage of nerve conduction prevents the patient from feeling pain. Unconsciousness is then not necessary, and the use of drugs that alter consciousness, such as hypnotics, may also not be necessary. Monitoring equipment for anaesthesia has simplified this process (202).

Surgery has gradually become less invasive through these and other developments (734). In urology for example, the substitution of closed instrumental urethral lithotrity for open lateral lithotomy for removing bladder stones reduced operative mortality from 40 to 1 per cent. Urologists have replaced open prostatectomy with transurethral resection. Percutaneous nephrolithotomy and extracorporeal shock-wave lithotripsy (ESWL) now make it possible to treat more than 90 per cent of renal stones without recourse to open surgery (734). (Table 10 shows the diffusion of ESWL in selected countries.) The ureterorenoscope allows removal of stones and tumours of the ureter, and urethral strictures can also be treated endoscopically.

The endoscope has revolutionalized some areas of diagnosis and is now leading to rapid changes in surgery. In combination with other technologies such as the laser (46) and rapidly evolving instrumentation (24,28), the endoscope will allow a wide range of less-invasive procedures, including removal of the appendix, cholecystectomy by laparoscope, repair of inguinal hernias, treatment of joint problems, and so forth. Such procedures have come to be called 'minimally invasive surgery' or 'minimally invasive therapy'. There is now a Society of Minimally Invasive Therapy that supports the publication of a journal on this subject (see later in this chapter for more details).

Chronic coronary artery disease is now treated surgically. The most frequent operation is coronary artery bypass graft (CABG), in which a bypass is made around a blocked coronary artery. Balloon angioplasty, or percutaneous transluminal coronary angioplasty (PTCA), has subsequently been developed as a

Table 10. Numbers and rate (per million population) of extra-corporeal shock-wave lithotripters (ESWL) by country and year.

Country	Number of ESWL			EWSL per million pop.
	1985	1988	1990	1990
France	2	29	36	0.7
Belgium	0	11	12	1.2
West Germany	7	57	72	1.2
Denmark	0	2	3	0.6
Netherlands	1	8	11	0.8
England	0	12	15	0.3
Italy	6	48	69	1.2
Spain	0	34	50	1.3

Source: ref. (80).

partial alternative to CABG. Tables 11 and 12 show the diffusion of CABG and PTCA in a number of countries. It is striking that the countries with high rates of one tend to have high rates of both. This illustrates the problem of expanding indications. PTCA is not in fact replacing CABG. More procedures are being done.

Changes in surgery have stimulated the development of 'ambulatory surgery' or 'day surgery'. In the USA, more than 50 per cent of all surgery was done without a hospitalization by 1990. The outcome for such surgery is excellent. By the year 2000, as much as two-thirds of all surgery could be done without a hospitalization (160). With more serious surgery, interest is growing in early discharge from the hospital and associated home care. People with hip fractures, for example, who in the past have been hospitalized for three weeks or more, are now often discharged after 15 days with excellent results (543). Financial pressures are likely to force continual shortening of the length-of-stay in hospital.

Technology for surgery will continue to evolve. Videos have now been connected to endoscopes, allowing the entire team to follow the course of a procedure and to assist when necessary. Diagnostic endoscopy can be improved in a number of ways, allowing more precise diagnosis. For example, zoom lenses can make it possible to examine a lesion more closely. Modern imaging such as ultrasound and magnetic resonance imaging (MRI) is allowing more precise diagnosis and localization. Therapy will become faster and safer through 'smart systems'. In other words, the role of skill in surgery will decrease as the technology is embodied in the device itself. In the long run, although the endoscope seems destined to become a central part of medical diagnosis and treatment, the present emphasis on cutting, vapourizing, and stitching through the endoscope

Table 11. Numbers and rate (per million population) of coronary artery bypass (CABG) operations by country and year.

Country	Number of CABGs		CABG per million pop.	
	1985	1988	1985	1988
USA	181 600	291 000	780	1265
Belgium	3 300		340	
France	5 900		110	
West Germany	12 600	29 000	206	480
Denmark	414		83	
Netherlands	6 800	8 280	480	583
England	10 840		195	
Spain	.5 230		140	
Italy	8 415		150	
Sweden	2 050		250	
Austria	825		110	

Source: ref. (80).

Table 12. Numbers and rate (per million population) of percutaneous transluminal coronary angioplasty (PTCA) operations by country and year.

Country	Number of PTCAs		PTCA per million pop.	
	1985	1989	1985	1989
USA	98 100	250 000	470	1100
Belgium	1 175	3 400	120	344
France	3 480	18 000	60	324
West Germany	4 490	18 800	90	307
Denmark		350		68
Netherlands	2 556	6 400	190	428
England		6 450		113
Italy		2 500		44
Spain		1 850		48

Source: ref. (80).

may be replaced by other treatment modalities, such as chemical or photochemical techniques.

Future developments in surgery will see the rapid decrease in the rates of open surgery, so that eventually it will almost disappear except in such specialized areas as cancer surgery and transplant surgery.

14.4 The case of laparoscopic cholecystectomy

General surgeons have been significantly slower than other specialists such as gynaecologists to accept laparoscopic treatment. However, the field is now beginning to grow rapidly. The main force seems to be consumer demand, fuelled by information from a few surgical innovators.

Cholecystectomy, removal of the gall bladder, is one of the most frequent surgical procedures in Western societies. The standard treatment for symptomatic gall bladder disease (inflammation, stones) is surgical removal. Cholecystectomy was first done in 1882. The procedure is associated with ileus pain and a slow return to normal functioning (170). The average length of stay in hospital for the procedure is about five days (719).

A number of new methods of treatment for gall bladder disease are now in development or testing. There is a variety of agents that will dissolve gallstones, depending on their types, size, and so forth. However, on the whole, surgeons feel that cholecystectomy has proven to be a more cost-effective procedure so far (672). Another new technology is extracorporeal shock-wave lithotripsy (ESWL) to fragment the stones (493,544). This procedure is often successful, but recurrence of the stones is usually a problem. This method is beneficial, however, when conventional methods have failed to remove a stone lodged in the bile duct or elsewhere. There are other techniques used less frequently. Stents have been used to keep the bile duct open (156,400). A rotary gallstone lithotrite can be used to fragment a stone in the duct, reaching the duct by the percutaneous route (100). Finally, gallstone dissolution with methyl tert-butyl ether is possible, a sort of chemical surgery. These technologies are experimental.

The first successful cholecystectomy via laparoscope was done by P. Mouret in Lyon, France in the spring of 1987. For several years, the procedure spread in France, and in 1988 it began to spread outside, particularly after publication of the experience of the group of F. Dubois (191). This procedure is spreading rapidly into use in a number of countries, but particularly in America (107). The first procedure was done in the USA in 1988 (550), but the most rapid spread has occurred in 1990. A survey of teaching hospitals in Canada in late 1990 showed that more than two thirds of the 29 hospitals that responded were already in the laparoscopic cholecystectomy business (108). Surgeons in the USA and elsewhere have been sceptical initially; the development has been largely consumer-driven (107). In other words, patients are demanding the less invasive procedure.

The literature on laparoscopic cholecystectomy is small, and there have not been controlled studies. Gadacz *et al.* (273) reviewed 5 reports involving about 500 patients (191,244,273,550,765). They found that the usual reason for the procedure was biliary colic. The average operating time was 95–110 minutes. The average hospital stay was 3–7 days in France, but from less than 1 to 2 days in the USA. Return to normal activity occurred in 3–7 days. The complication rate varied between 1 and 5 per cent. Gadacz *et al.* (273) give no figures for comparison with standard cholecystectomy, but they note that the stay in hospital and the recovery time would be considerably longer, and on this basis they feel that the procedure is cost-effective. While these data are impressive, they must be approached sceptically, because they were not collected in careful prospective trials. Van Erp and Bruyninckx (218), Nathanson *et al.* (476), and Perissat *et al.* (530) report similar findings from case series.

The largest study of laparoscopic cholecystectomy was a report on the experience of 20 surgical groups in the Southern USA in 1991 (640). The 20 centres participating in the prospective, uncontrolled study reported on the experience with 1518 patients. Problems included conversion to open cholecystectomy in 72 patients (4.7 per cent) and 82 complications in 78 patients (5.1 per cent). The most common complication was superficial infection at the site of insertion of the laparoscope. The most serious complication was injury to the common bile duct or hepatic duct (see below). The mean hospital stay was 1.2 days, with a range from 67 hours to 30 days, and the average duration of surgery was 90 minutes. Of the entire group, 79 per cent returned to full-time employment within 10 days. Another large series was from 9 clinics in the USA, reporting similar results in 1986 patients (402).

The European experience from 7 centres in France, Germany, and the UK was reported in 1991 (155). Low morbidity was reported with a median hospital stay of 3 days. Only 3.6 per cent of patients needed conversion to an open procedure.

Peters *et al.* (534) report on 100 consecutive laparoscopic cholecystectomies done in 1990. There were no deaths, and there was major morbidity in 4 per cent and minor morbidity in 4 per cent. They developed a comparison group made up of the previous 58 standard cholecystectomies done in their institution. Operating time was an average 122 minutes, with a range of 45 minutes, compared with 78 minutes (range 30 minutes) for standard cholecystectomy. The mean hospital stay for patients was 27.6 hours. The average patient returned to normal activity in 12.8 days. The hospital charges for the laparoscopic group averaged US$3620, with a range of $1005, while the hospital charges for the standard cholecystectomy group were US$4252, with a range of $988. Physician fees were not included in these estimates, and the authors made no attempt to value the early return to work or other activity.

The only significant complication of laparoscopic cholecystectomy reported is damage to the common bile duct, found in about 1 in 100 patients (107). The standard procedure produces such damage in about 1 in 1000 patients. In the study cited above (640), this complication was seen in 7 patients (0.5 per cent); however, four of these were simple lacerations and were repaired through open surgery. There definitely is a 'learning curve' in doing the procedure (170,719). The incidence of this complication fell in the Southern study from 2.2 per cent with the first 13 patients done by one team to 0.1 per cent in the subsequent patients (substantiating the importance of experience and the learning curve). However, the DATTA programme of the American Medical Association has concluded that data on safety are insufficient to reach conclusions concerning either intra-operative or long-term complications (170). This conclusion was reached before publication of the data from the Southern USA.

Cameron and Gadacz have stated that hospitalization is necessary for laparoscopic cholecystectomy. However, Reddick and Olsen, in a later report than that mentioned above (551), stated that they offer the choice of out-patient cholecystectomy to their patients. Out of 83 patients, 37 (45 per cent) chose the out-patient procedure. No serious complications were seen. In the USA, the out-patient procedure is common (640). One series in the USA reported that 63 per cent of patients were discharged from the hospital within 24 hours of admission (402).

A major problem with laparoscopic cholecystectomy is that complications can be quite severe if the surgeon is not skilled. The Society of American Gastro-intestinal Endoscopic Surgeons (637,638) has suggested that the surgeons doing the procedure should be credentialled in hepatobiliary surgery, should have thorough training in the procedure in animals, and should be initially supervised by a surgeon already experienced in doing the procedure in human patients. Hospital privileges for the procedure are then important (170). No European body has developed such standards, and there are no formal controls on physicians who wish to do such a procedure.

14.5 Conclusions

Laparoscopic cholecystectomy shows how rapidly health care can change. Technology assessment has had little to do with this change. Instead, a few surgeons have adopted a procedure that seemed to be sensible, and patients have then insisted on having the less invasive alternative. In the long run, however, developments will not be so easy. Surgeons continue to resist this innovation, despite its attractive nature, especially when procedures can be done by medical specialists, as in the field of gastro-intestinal endoscopy, where the gastro-enterologist is now actively competing with surgeons to treat patients (28). Budget constraints described in Chapter 5 also slow change. Technology assessment has an important role to play in influencing patients, physicians, and policy-makers.

15. The assessment of drugs

Perhaps more information is available on the efficacy and safety of drugs than of any other technology. The main reason that this is true is because of the regulation of pharmaceutical products, which requires manufacturers to test drugs rigorously before they can be marketed. At the same time, organizations that fund technology assessments pay a great deal of attention to drugs. For example, a study by the OTA published in 1978 and based on 1975 data found that of the 755 clinical trials supported by the US National Institutes of Health (NIH) in that year, 400 tested drugs in isolation, while another 135 tested drugs in relation to another possible intervention (487). It should also be noted, however, that more than 300 of the 400 trials of drugs tested cancer chemotherapy. What this may indicate is that information on drugs may vary quite a lot, depending on the type of drug and its possible uses.

As will be discussed further in Chapter 19, the experience with assessment of pharmaceuticals is extensive. In fact, the only relatively complete, organized system for health care technology assessment is that carried out under the supervision of drug regulatory agencies. When a company has a drug that it wishes to test in humans, it must submit laboratory and animal data to the regulatory agency to obtain a license for human testing. The tests are then carried out and the data are submitted to the regulatory programme. The programme synthesizes and assesses this data and reaches a decision as to whether the drug can be approved for marketing or not.

Traditionally, clinical trials of drugs have been randomized controlled trials (RCTs) in which a drug is tested against placebo or, less commonly, an alternative drug. Historically, clinical trials of drugs play an important part in the development of the RCT method. Fibiger (235) used an alternative assignment of patient design to test a serum for diphtheria in an early trial. Ferguson *et al.* (234) studied vaccines for the common cold and used for the first time a blinding method, making the research workers blind as to who received saline or vaccine injection. During the 1930s two major areas for clinical trials were the sulfonamides and antimalarial drugs (540, p. 16). Penicillin was perhaps the most important therapeutic advance in the 20th century. Clinical trials began in 1941 with a few extremely ill patients and no controls, but the results were so dramatic that clear conclusions were possible (540, p. 17). The first clinical trial with a properly randomized control group was for streptomycin in the treatment of pulmonary tuberculosis (455). The trial was very well organized, and showed significantly better patient survival and radiological improvement in the streptomycin group. Another trial sponsored by the British Medical

Research Council (456) used a placebo control in a double-blind manner to test antihistamines in the common cold. There was no benefit from antihistamine.

An important development in this area has been studies of cancer chemotherapy. The first case reports of children with acute leukaemia gaining benefit from chemotherapy appeared in 1948 (540, p. 21). In 1954, the National Institutes of Health organized the first randomized study of this subject comparing two different schedules. In that same year, the US Congress required the creation of a programme of co-operative clinical studies of cancer chemotherapy, which was followed by a large number of trials of chemotherapy in different cancers. In fact, this Congressional action explains the fact that a great deal is known about the efficacy of cancer chemotherapy.

Thus, assessment of pharmaceuticals by RCTs is well-established. The industry itself has an enormous investment in this field and would probably be the first to point to how useful it is. From the standpoint of the industry, of course, such trials are necessary for legal marketing. In addition, the trial results give protection from product liability suits and furnish the basis for drug promotional activities.

A description of the specific drug regulatory process, that is the Phase I–IV testing requirements, is found in the discussions of health care systems of individual countries (see Chapters 17–23).

Notwithstanding the fact that the assessment of drugs is far more regulated and extensive than is true for any other medical technology class, there is much left undone in this area. For instance, drugs are widely used off-label by physicians, and pharmaceutical firms promote such use indirectly by sponsoring post-marketing clinical (Phase IV) studies, many of which find their way into the clinical literature. This literature is often incomplete. In addition, as is true for all medical practice, patient outcome evidence is often lacking even when the drug is used within the indication. Also, physicians in the real world of medical practice misdiagnose and over- or under-prescribe medications which affect patient outcomes (and costs).

15.1 Pharmaco-epidemiology and post-marketing surveillance

For a complete review of this topic, the reader is referred to Strom (664), from which much of the material in this section is drawn.

The field of pharmaco-epidemiology is a new subdiscipline dedicated to the study of the use and effects of drugs in large numbers of people. Pharmaco-epidemiology incorporates what has been known previously as post-marketing surveillance. It is probably appropriate to characterize the new field as a move to legitimize post-marketing surveillance and other related research as a subdiscipline in its own right. As the name implies, it is a blend of clinical pharmacology and epidemiology. Pharmaco-epidemiology is particularly concerned with the study of drug effects and adverse reactions. Adverse reactions consist of two categories: type A reactions, which result from an exaggerated but otherwise usual pharmacologic effects of the drug; and type B reactions, which are aberrant effects (664, p. 3). Type A are common side effects, which tend to be dose-related and can often be dealt with by lowering the dose. Type B, on the other hand, tend to be uncommon and more serious, sometimes lethal. When they occur, the use of the drug is usually considered to be contra-indicated. Type B reactions are often difficult to predict and they may not be apparent as a risk at the time of market approval due to their infrequent occur-rence. The time-honoured approach to studying these adverse drug reactions is the collection of spontaneous reports of drug-related morbidity and mortality. Spontaneous reporting is described in Chapters 9 and 10 (664).

The history of drug regulation throughout the Western world has parallelled society's concerns with major adverse drug reactions events. For instance, the initial 1906 US Pure Food and Drug Act was passed due to reports of excessive adulteration and misbranding of food and drugs. The 1938 US Food, Drug and Cosmetic Act was a result of deaths due to elixir of sulfanilamide dissolved in diethylene glycol (287). The 1962 US Kefauver–Harris Amendments requiring the present three-phase drug testing regulations was a result of the infamous thalidomide tragedy in Europe (412).

Notwithstanding the drug regulatory process, which requires by far the most systematic assessment of safety and efficacy of any class of medical technology, serious and unpredictable adverse drug reactions still occur. This has given rise to a continuing heightened concern for the safety of the public and has spawned many programmes, organizations, and research endeavours as well as the field of pharmaco-epidemiology itself. For instance, today in the USA there is the Sloan Epidemiology Unit (formerly the Drug Epidemiology Unit); the Boston Collaborative Drug Surveillance Program; the Joint Commission on Prescrip-tion Drug Use; and the Computerized Online Medicaid Pharmaceutical Analysis and Surveillance System. In the UK, there is the Drug Safety Research Trust with its innovative system of prescription event monitoring (349).

15.2 Post-marketing studies

The need for post-marketing studies is due to several reasons. First, pre-marketing studies are very limited and cannot answer many questions. They tend to be rather small and of short duration. They are conducted in artificially constrained environments where patients tend to be homogenous in age and sex, and are less likely to have potentially complicating medical conditions. And they often compare the investigational drug to a placebo rather than to another active ingredient. However, pre-marketing studies tend to have high internal validity due to their experimental design. Post-marketing studies tend to be observational rather than experimental and thus are designed to study effectiveness and, especially, safety in the real world of medical practice. They are useful in learning about drug–drug interactions, about effects in previously untested populations such as the elderly, children, and patients with multiple diseases, effects of overdoses, and many other aspects of real patients as well as real practitioners' prescribing patterns.

Pharmaco-epidemiology embraces several study designs (664), in addition to the spontaneous reporting required by law in many countries. Case reports are simply reports of single patients and are commonly published in medical journals. They are helpful in establishing possible hypotheses about drug reactions. Case studies are studies of a collection of patients who have been exposed to a given drug. Analyses of secular trends is another method which is helpful in linking adverse events to drug exposure. In this case, trends of both exposure to a drug and some event or disease are analysed over time to determine whether an association may exist. None of these methods include control groups. The next two methods do.

Case control studies are ones in which patients with a certain disease or who have had an adverse event are compared with similar patients (controls) who do not have the disease/event and both are analysed for the drug exposure. Case control studies are retrospective in nature. Cohort studies are forward looking in nature. Those patients who are exposed to a drug are compared to similar patients not exposed and both groups are followed over time to study whether certain effects may be present. Cohort studies can be thought of as similar to experimental studies without randomization. The determination of whether a given patient was given a drug is due not to study design, but is due rather to normal medical practice.

All of these epidemiological study designs are termed 'observational studies' as opposed to randomized clinical trials, which are termed 'experimental studies'.

15.3 Health-related quality of life assessments

There has been a clear trend towards including health-related quality of life assessments within clinical trial programmes, especially those sponsored by the pharmaceutical industry. One of the first such studies to appear in the clinical literature was the study published in 1986 by Croog et al. (147), in which the effects of various hypertensive medications on patients' quality of life were assessed in a Phase III randomized control trial. The authors were able to show significant differences across a number of quality of life domains, including general well-being, work performance, visual-motor functioning, measures of life satisfaction, and sexual dysfunction. The study by Croog et al. was considered by many to be a landmark, and was closely followed by both FDA and Wall Street. Also in 1986, a study by Bombardier et al. (74) reported on the quality of life impact of an oral gold product (auranofin) compared to placebo for the treatment of rheumatoid arthritis.

Since these pioneering studies, interest in measuring health-related quality of life has grown tremendously throughout the drug industry and at the Food and

Drug Administration (FDA). For instance, FDA requested quality of life data be submitted as part of the erythropoietin clinical trial registration approval process (222). A survey sponsored by the US Institute of Medicine in 1988 and conducted by Luce and colleagues (433) revealed growing involvement and intense interest within industry in routinely incorporating health-related quality of life assessments in their clinical trials. Of the 34 out of 51 (56 per cent) companies who responded to the survey, 21 (62 per cent) reported they had used some type of health-related quality of life (HRQOL) instrument in their clinical trials of drugs. All but one reported they were currently using such instruments. The two most frequently cited reasons for doing quality of life research were marketing reasons and internal management or clinical decision-making. About half of the companies stated they believed that FDA approval would be more likely if such measures were used. Many of the standardized HRQOL instruments (see Chapter 9) were being used in their trials. In the 1990s the percentage of companies conducting HRQOL studies is undoubtedly higher and probably includes most major firms.

15.4 Economic-related assessments

Experience with assessing the economic consequences of drugs is also recent compared with clinical testing. In its 1980 review, OTA commented, 'Drugs have been the subject of hundreds of biochemical and medical studies . . . [but] drugs have not often been the subject of CEA/CBA analysis' (497). Most of the studies that included drug therapy dealt with drugs only implicitly and tangentially. Perhaps the most frequent drug treatment analysed at that time was treatment of hypertension.

However, this situation is changing dramatically. In 1975, a new drug treatment for peptic ulcer disease was first described: cimetidine. Cimetidine was shown to effectively promote healing of active peptic ulcers, particularly of the duodenum (707). After the introduction of cimetidine, Smith, Klein & French, the manufacturer, funded cost-effectiveness analyses in a number of countries to test the effects of the drug. In the USA, for instance, Gewecke and Weisbrod (284), using Michigan Medicaid data in a retrospective analysis, showed that the state health insurance programme for the poor saved considerable monies once cimetidine diffused into medical practice by substituting drug treatment for ulcer operations and hospitalization. More recently, Ciba-Geigy has funded studies in a number of countries concerning cost-effectiveness and quality of life effects of different forms of nitroglycerin treatment for angina pectoris (175,310,342, 364,407,432,486). Other examples are the study by Martens *et al.* (449) of the cost-effectiveness of cholesterol-lowering in The Netherlands and a study by Edelson *et al.* (210) of the cost-effectiveness of antihypertensive medications. The Martens *et al.* study, sponsored by Merck and Co., was presented to Dutch pricing authorities and reportedly was successfully used in price negotiating with governmental authorities (448). The Edelson study was reported in a prominent

Wall Street Journal article. These two examples help illustrate not only the potential significance of economic analyses of drugs, but also the way in which different cultures and systems use them.

A review of the entire cost-effectiveness-related literature reveals that since 1983 the number of studies associated with drugs are far out-stripping studies on other types of technologies (Fig. 18, p. 167) (214). It seems likely that this trend will continue since the pharmaceutical industry is continuing to gear up for such research efforts by creating pharmaco-economic departments within their companies and incorporate prospective socio-economic analyses within their clinical development programmes for virtually all major products. In addition, companies continue to sponsor retrospective studies following FDA approval or the country registration process.

15.5 Incorporating economic studies into the drug development process

Chapter 8 discussed very general classes of economic analyses which are useful in assessing medical technologies, in particular: cost-benefit analysis; cost-effectiveness analysis; cost-utility analysis; and cost-minimization analysis. Regardless of which method is chosen, there are additional study design issues which need to be considered for drug studies, each one having unique sets of advantages and disadvantages. Overall, there are four types of study designs: prospective, retrospective, modelling, and a combination of two or more of the first three designs (Fig. 19).

15.5.1 Prospective designs

There are two ways economic analysis can be studied prospectively: incorporating an economic study into an existing clinical trial (the 'piggy-back' option); and designing a prospective economic clinical trial (PECT) for the expressed purposes of cost-effectiveness analysis. Each choice carries with it advantages and disadvantages.

The 'piggy-back' pharmaco-economic design is one in which an economic analysis is incorporated into an existing clinical trial. Typically, it would mean

Prospective
- 'Piggy back' onto clinical trials
- Stand-alone economic clinical trials

Retrospective
- Existing clinical trials
- Cohort

Modelling
- Clinical decision-analytic based
- Epidemiological based

Combination

Figure 19. Socio-economic study designs for pharmaceuticals.

that health care utilization (e.g., number of hospital admissions and lengths of stay, all tests and procedures, physician visits, drugs prescribed) consumed during the clinical trial would be collected and valued in money. Additionally, patients may be surveyed as to their work/activity participation. If health-related quality of life or patient utility is of interest, it may be collected via a questionnaire as well. In all designs, the way in which health and economic benefits are valued will determine whether the study is a cost-benefit, cost-effectiveness, cost-utility, or cost-minimization analysis.

'Piggy-back' pharmaco-economic studies are becoming much more widely used in clinical trial programmes throughout the world. The advantages of a 'piggy-back' design are:

(1) efficiency, since the clinical trial costs are already being incurred;

(2) timeliness, in that the cost-effectiveness information is generated concurrently with the clinical information and thus is available at the time of regulatory, coverage, and pricing decision-making;

(3) credibility to many, since it has all the classic features of a randomized often blinded, controlled trial;

(4) high internal validity due to randomization and tight protocol control;

(5) low selection bias due to randomization;

(6) health-related quality of life, utility, and work loss can be included using patient questionnaires.

Disadvantages of the 'piggy-back' approach include:

(1) low external validity due to the protocol restrictions, including inclusion and exclusion criteria, specialized setting and patient control;

(2) protocol-induced costs, such as requiring hospitalization, extra physician visits or special tests, all of which distort the economic effects under study;

(3) statistical significance, which may be difficult to achieve even when mean differences are large, due to the fact that study power, and thus sample size, is typically calculated using clinical endpoints which tend to have a much lower variance than economic end points.

The stand-alone prospective economic clinical trial (PECT) design option is one in which the trial itself is specifically designed to study cost-effectiveness. Thus, many of the disadvantages of the 'piggy-back' design can be addressed. There are several advantages of the PECT:

(1) external validity can be maximized in that the trial can be designed to reflect more closely average patients being treated under averaged clinical conditions;

(2) credibility, in that randomization helps ensure against selection bias;

(3) quality of life, utility and work/activity loss data can be included.

Disadvantages include:

(1) PECTs are very expensive, since an entire clinical trial must be funded;

(2) timeliness, since clinical trials take a great deal of time to set up and conduct, plus PECTs are probably not indicated until at least close to the marketing of the drug;

(3) internal validity may be compromised, relative to piggy-back studies, since protocol constraints are relaxed permitting the introduction of potential confounding variables (e.g., compliance, patient cross-over, variations in practice patterns);

(4) statistical significance, which is just as much of a problem as is the piggy-back design.

PECTs are just beginning to be employed and could be as close to a gold standard for economic analyses as is possible.

15.5.2 *Retrospective designs*

There are two types of retrospective studies: an economic analysis of an existing clinical trial, and a cohort design.

The existing clinical trial option consists of reconstructing the economic history of all patients who had participated in a completed clinical trial. The advantages of this option are:

(1) cost-efficiency relative to some prospective designs;

(2) credibility due to low patient selection bias because of randomization;

(3) the economic hypothesis may be stronger since the clinical results are known;

(4) high internal validity due to the RCT design;

(5) best opportunity if a prospective study is not possible.

Disadvantages include:

(1) data quality tends to be very poor, since the utilization data was not planned at the time of the trial;

(2) statistical significance is often difficult to achieve due to lack of power;

(3) external validity is low due to the protocol constraints;

(4) quality of life cannot be included—utility and work/activity loss must be estimated if they are included.

The retrospective analysis of existing clinical trials has been fairly common in recent years. One concern is another kind of selection bias, that is, choosing the most promising of several completed clinical trials to study.

The cohort design is the first of the options discussed so far which consists of a non-experimental approach. In this case, a patient cohort that has experienced a given drug is compared to a cohort that has not been given the drug. The analysis of existing large data sets is often carried out; for example in the cimetidine study by Gewecke and Weisbrod (284) discussed earlier. This design has been fairly common in the USA due to the availability of these large data sets. This cohort design requires careful statistical control for any possible confounding variables such as age, sex, severity of disease, co-morbid conditions, and competing risk factors. There are advantages and disadvantages to this design as well. The main advantages are:

(1) cost-efficiency because no primary data is collected;
(2) maximization of external validity—in fact, it often is a study of the real world and, of all designs discussed so far, most closely approximates the concept of outcomes and medical effectiveness research;
(3) it is possibly the best or only alternative available when large populations are needed and/or prospective clinical studies are not an option.

The cohort design can be a good choice when the effect is believed to be very large.

The disadvantages of the cohort design are:

(1) selection bias of the cohorts being compared—there often are severe confounding variables which make even the most conscientious statistical control problematic;
(2) data quality, which is usually very poor since the data almost never were collected for economic study purposes;
(3) compromising of internal validity due to the observational nature of the study design;
(4) health-related quality of life, utility and work/activity loss are not possible.

15.5.3 Modelling designs

A very popular design method has been the mathematical simulation model. There are two main types of models: clinical decision-analytic models and epidemiologically based models, the choice of which tends to depend upon whether the underlying medical issue is clinical decision-making of present disease or disease prevention/health promotion of future disease. Modelling is useful when extensive primary data (such as clinical trial data) is unavailable and is virtually required when extremely long periods must be studied; for instance, the prevention of heart disease or osteoporosis. Modelling is also both useful and necessary to use in combination with other methods, as will be discussed shortly.

Models take advantage of data from existing literature, often expert opinion and sometimes primary data collection. They are useful for scenario building and hypothesis testing. Extensive sensitivity analysis is always required when models are used.

The advantages of using models are several-fold:

(1) They are often the only option whereby cost-effectiveness can be analysed. When budgets are constrained and data are not immediately available, models can be constructed to estimate cost-effectiveness. They are virtually essential when benefits are incurred way into the future, such as in many prevention programmes.

(2) They are flexible, allowing for testing alternative assumptions concerning the way disease progresses, is treated, and the way different patients respond. Models also can be used to forecast the impact of future scenarios.

(3) They are cost- and time-efficient since they tend to rely on existing literature, knowledge, and belief.

Interestingly, statistical significance testing is not a problem because calculating it is not possible. Thus, the standards are considerably relaxed, relying on often very wide 'confidence intervals' from sensitivity analyses used to test the sensitivity of results to varying assumptions.

The disadvantages of models include:

(1) credibility, since they tend to be built on uncertain foundations;

(2) accuracy due to often wide confidence intervals;

(3) acceptability, because of the uncertainty involved;

(4) health-related quality of life assessment is not possible.

Utility values would have to be simulated, as would work loss.

15.5.4 *Combination option*

The last option is a combination of the various methods discussed above. For instance, it is not uncommon to have sufficient primary data from a clinical trial, either from a prospective or retrospective analysis, to make very narrow inferences on economic consequences, but still need to extend the data and assumptions beyond the clinical trial setting to estimate ultimate patient outcomes and cost-effectiveness. A good example would be a cholesterol-lowering trial. The trial often will be designed to show statistically significant changes in cholesterol, possibly compared to placebo. Yet the cost-effectiveness question will require comparison to other cholesterol-lowering interventions and will optimally require estimates of final health impact which will be decades away for many patients. Therefore, a cost-effectiveness study might include the clinical (and possibly economic) results from the prospective study at hand; results from other (retrospective) clinical studies previously reported; and modelling for future cardiovascular events and their costs.

The obvious advantage of such efforts is to be able to utilize several study designs to address an issue which probably could not be sufficiently addressed using one method alone. The main disadvantage is the complexity of such a multifaceted approach to cost-effectiveness analysis. In addition, health-related quality of life, utility and work/activity loss may or may not be possible, unless explicitly included as a separate module within the study.

15.6 Assessment of pharmaceuticals by providers and purchasers

As will be discussed further in Chapter 19, technology assessment in the USA is becoming widespread throughout the medical care system. In particular, individual hospitals, hospital systems, health maintenance organizations (HMOs), insurers, and government agencies are each organizing for conducting assessments. Among the hospitals and some state Medicaid agencies, the more sophisticated of the assessors tend to be members of the formulary committees (90). These committees screen drugs for relative efficacy, effectiveness and cost-effectiveness mainly by reviewing literature, but also sometimes conducting technology assessment studies, including economic analyses, in their own institutions. In general, they are increasingly better trained to evaluate the costs and benefits of new additions to their formularies, and are very sceptical of cost-effectiveness claims of manufacturers without sufficient scientific data.

15.7 Regulations and cost-effectiveness

At the beginning of the 1990s, attempts are developing in different parts of the world to regulate the cost-effectiveness of pharmaceuticals. Until recently, the growing interest by the pharmaceutical industry in sponsoring economic analyses of their products, although voluntary, was due to either market pressure, formulary restrictions, or reimbursement and pricing decisions by authorities. In the USA, the main catalyst has been market-generated, fuelled by the concerns for budget control. There has been no attempt in the USA to regulate or to require cost-effectiveness studies of pharmaceuticals. In fact, the recently proposed Medicare regulations permitting—even encouraging—cost-effectiveness considerations during the coverage process, explicitly omits pharmaceuticals (695). In Europe, there is clear evidence that cost-effectiveness of pharmaceuticals is highly encouraged, and even expected, by many national pricing and reimbursement authorities, but no countries formally require cost-effectiveness today nor are they expected to in the near future (318). However, Australia does require that cost-effectiveness data be generated by a prescribed methodology and submitted to authorities at the time of registration of the drugs (140). Ontario, Canada is proposing similar regulations (511,512). One of the reasons why both Canada and Australia have seen fit to prescribe the methods by which cost-effectiveness data are to be generated is that methods are not very standardized, allowing considerable discretion and possibly bias in selecting the methodological approach for a given study (329). The concern for potential bias and for the ability to compare findings across studies has led to calls for a consensus of methods (189), and a voluntary effort by interested parties to develop research and reporting guidelines in this area (330).

15.8 Conclusions

Pharmaceuticals are by far more highly regulated and rigorously tested before market entry than any other medical technology. This is particularly true for basic safety and efficacy. Yet, even in this important technology class, much is not known about their ultimate impact on patient health outcomes and health system economics. There is continuing interest in fostering better post-market surveillance information, especially to protect the public's safety associated with infrequent but important side effects. Today, there is also increasing interest and activity aimed at providing and, in some cases, requiring broader scientifically-derived measures of value, including health-related quality of life assessments, utility or patient preference assessments, and cost-effectiveness analyses.

In all these newer 'outcomes' research areas, pharmaceuticals will likely continue to far outpace all other medical technologies.

16. Picture archiving and communications systems (PACS): an example of the computer revolution

The computer is an extremely important development in health care technology in the 20th century (250). The computer finds applications throughout the health care system. At the level of the individual patient, administrative records are generally computerized. Increasingly, clinical records are also computerized. In practice, computers are part of an increasing number of devices and practices, including the CT scanner and MRI scanner, discussed in Chapter 13. At the level of the hospital or the health care system, organization, evaluation, and feedback would not be possible without the computer. And a very important function has to do with research. Aside from the fact that it is hardly conceivable to do biomedical research these days without the data storage, analytical, and communicative dimensions of computers, large data sets also give clues and in some cases definitive information on disease aetiology or efficacy and safety of specific procedures.

The experience with technology assessment in medical informatics is quite limited, but interest is growing (345). Informatics groups such as the International Society for Optical Engineering (SPIE) frequently hold sessions on this subject (344). In 1990, a conference was held in Montpellier, France, on the subject of 'medical technology assessment, with special emphasis on informatics applied to medicine and health' (245).

A number of publications have dealt with the assessment of Picture Archiving and Communications Systems (PACS), focusing especially on financial costs and benefits of such systems (33). From 1986 to 1989, the BAZIS organization in The Netherlands carried out an assessment of PACS (55), and in 1991 BAZIS sponsored an international workshop on technology assessment of PACS. A number of papers from that conference are referenced in this chapter.

16.1 Assessment of medical informatics

Assessment of medical informatics is difficult for both practical and methodological reasons. Practically, because the range and number of applications is so large. Methodologically, because informatics is a very technical area whose goals and aims vary quite a lot, and are often not clear.

Medical informatics can be divided into several subgroups. The easiest to assess are those applications that are directly a part of clinical care. For example, expert systems are rapidly being developed to support both diagnostic and therapeutic activities (546,691). A computer programme to improve diagnosis or treatment of diabetes can be assessed in the same way as a clinical technology. The most appropriate design seems to be an RCT. If the implementation of a new program in a clinical situation where nothing else is changed does not lead to improved outcomes, its value is questionable, to say the least.

At the highest level are extremely large and complex systems of data collection, analysis, storage, and transfer. One example might be a system of universal medical record-keeping for all Europeans. A minimum data set for this purpose is being developed. Another example might be a network of programmes to improve quality of care in the hospitals of European countries. Evaluating such systems is extremely difficult, even conceptually. What shall be the outcomes? What can be measured? Do all parties agree on important aspects? Who are 'all parties'?

Furthermore, large systems often are intended to meet higher value goals, such as the integration of Europe. This seems a worthy goal, but it seems impossible to conceive of an evaluation in which the contribution of medical informatics to this goal could be quantified.

In between these two extremes is the level of applications aimed largely at efficiency. These applications are also difficult to assess. Informatics systems can have many benefits, including such intangibles as changed morale of health care workers, improved quality of care, and improved patient satisfaction. At the same time, these systems are expensive and generally must justify themselves economically. This means that they can be assessed economically. In other words, although such a system may have a number of benefits, if it is visibly expensive, it is not likely that it will diffuse far into health care unless it can pay for itself or come close to paying for itself. For this reason, assessment of such systems as PACS has focused primarily on economic costs and benefits.

16.2 Computer-assisted medical imaging

The case of computer-assisted medical imaging will be used to illustrate how innovations can be assessed economically.

A quiet revolution began in 1972, as already described in Chapter 13, with the introduction of the computed tomography (CT) scanner. The CT scanner was one of the early clinical applications of computers, which were not of practical use until the 1960s and 1970s. The CT scanner used digital (numeric) data for the first time to construct images of the inside of the human body. Chapter 13 has already described some of the clinical consequences of this new technology. However, assessments from that time made no mention of what is probably a more significant aspect of this and related technologies: that they use digital data.

Imaging methods that have come into widespread use since 1972 have all been based on digital data. These include digital subtraction imaging (including angiography), ultrasound imaging, nuclear medicine (including positron emission tomography), and magnetic resonance imaging.

These innovations have dramatically changed the field of radiology. Many departments of radiology have even changed their name to 'department of medical imaging' or something similar. It was estimated that 50 per cent of images would be digital by the year 1990 (484).

The implication of this change is that digital data can be produced, manipulated, transferred, and stored without production of a hard-copy image.

16.3 The present system in radiology

Conventional radiology continues to be the predominant form of imaging, with the chest X-ray the most frequent procedure. Images are stored in analogue form on film. The physician responsible for interpreting the studies examines a series of films. He or she reviews the images, mentally discards non-useful information, and concentrates on important features of the image. He or she may request further studies to produce additional information. An interpretation or diagnosis is then reached. The film is then stored in a film jacket in an archive until it is needed again. The physician's written report is sent to the clinician ordering the film. If that physician wishes to see the film, he or she can borrow it or visit the radiology department, to review it with the radiologist if required.

This system has problems. Digital imaging has led to an increased number of tests, complicating physical handling and storage. Film jackets cannot be used for several purposes simultaneously, which may make certain films temporarily non-accessible. Transfer of the film jacket from individual to individual takes time, and film jackets are sometimes lost or misplaced. One study found that the retrieval of 25 per cent of requested films was delayed (314). Surveys of physicians have found evidence that delayed access to films increases length of stay of patients in hospital (663). Vanden Brink and Cywinski (698) calculated that radiologists spend 7−11 per cent of their time on film management. A particular problem with patients who are acutely ill is that several different physicians may need to see an image within a short period of time.

Digital imaging modalities can improve this process in certain ways. The supervising physician can alter the diagnostic procedure during its course. Prior images can be called back for examination while the patient is still available. The data collected can be processed and manipulated to emphasize certain possibly abnormal features. This can make the diagnostic process more efficient, saving resources and avoiding excessive radiation dose to the patient. For example, De Simone *et al.* (166) found that picture archiving and communications (PAC) systems decreased the period of time between an examination and the start of the treatment in an intensive care unit.

These advantages have led to proposals for a fully digitized system of imaging, what has been called a 'film-less X-ray department' or a picture archiving and communications system.

16.4 A picture archiving and communications (PAC) system

In a department based entirely on digital systems, all imaging technologies would be integrated by one computer system, with video consoles in the main department, consoles in other parts of the hospital or remote sites, transmission lines connecting sites, and computerized storage of the data both for short-term recall and long-term archiving (340). No complete PAC system is in operation, but several are in fairly advanced development. Literature in this field is accumulating rapidly (602).

One technological change necessary for a PAC system is to replace analogue systems with digital systems. This would require either collecting regular X-ray examinations in digital form or transforming conventional X-rays to digital form for storage purposes. Both are feasible, but the second would always be laborious and expensive. In the long run, a technology that does not use film at all seems the most likely solution.

The other technological changes necessary concern the PAC system itself. A PAC system is a system of stations connected by a network. The stations carry out key functions in medical imaging: acquisition, where the images are created by a diagnostic device in contact with a patient; display, where the images can be selected, displayed, manipulated, and annotated; and archives, where images can be stored for later use. Such a system is extremely complicated, especially if it is integrated with the hospital information system, which it should be for maximum utility (66).

A full PAC system has large mass storage requirements, and developments are needed in display set-up, imaging processing, and data compression. Many hardware components are either not available in reasonable form or are too expensive. One key problem is access to certain images very quickly. Images contain large amounts of data. A chest X-ray contains more than 50 million bytes of data (358). A high-quality telephone line will only transmit 1200 bytes per second. This means that it would take 3.5 hours to transmit the data in a single chest X-ray. Another problem is that physicians are not accustomed to reading images from a video display device, which does not always make satisfactory images.

In the remainder of this chapter, it will be assumed that the technical and personal challenges can be solved. A sample evaluation will be carried out of benefits and costs.

16.5 Effects of a PAC system

To an extent, a PAC system can be assessed as is an imaging device (33). Does it improve diagnosis? Does it improve therapy? Does it improve outcome?

While a PAC system may make diagnosis more efficient, this may be difficult to prove. It seems unlikely that a PAC system can be demonstrated to have an important effect on health except in situations where improved access to images could save lives, as in intensive care or remote sites where an emergency procedure was needed.

From the standpoint of the organization of care, a PAC system has important implications. Instead of visiting the radiology department, clinical physicians can see the image in their own site, and discuss it with the radiologist by phone or other communication device. This might improve efficiency. More importantly, a central location could supervise image collection and interpretation, improving quality. Automation of much of this process could be done. Ultimately, a PAC system stimulates the transformation of a number of health care sites into one system. With such a system, other kinds of information could be transferred: laboratory results, clinical consultations, patient record information, and so forth. Most observers feel that improved access to images for clinicians will be the main benefits of PACS (282,547).

A PAC system has important potential implications for administrative efficiency. In Utrecht, The Netherlands, it was found that a prototype PAC system reduced the number of interactions between people involved in ordering, making, and interpreting an ordinary X-ray by about 50 per cent (13).

A PACS prototype in Utrecht, The Netherlands, was evaluated positively by clinicians. They found that it delivered information about more examinations, and delivered information on present examinations on the same day. PACS allowed faster consultation with more experts. The information in PACS was available at all hours of the day and night. And the information was complete; that is, no images were missing due to being borrowed or lost. In addition, information could be used in more than one place at the same time (55).

Another aspect of efficiency is the storage of data. Conventional X-rays take space. They are often lost. People must keep track of them. A PAC system is hypothesized to reduce the need for space and people in this process.

16.6 A framework for evaluating PAC systems

As indicated in the previous section, evaluating the benefits of a PAC system is difficult (148). At the present time, the cost of a PAC system is very large, probably more than US$3 million for a moderate-sized hospital. The annual cost for operating a PAC system, including amortized capital cost, is more than $1 million.

The policy-maker wishes to know how much benefit has been achieved for how much cost. In this case, the answer cannot be given, because there is no complete PAC system. Furthermore, many of the benefits cannot be quantified and many of the costs are unknown or are high because the technology is not yet well-developed.

Because of the uncertainties, and because of the centrality of economics in this case, those involved with technology assessment of this application of medical informatics have concentrated on detailing the financial costs of a system, the possible financial benefits of a system, and the critical points where costs might be reduced (331).

The capital cost of a PAC system might be US$3.6 million (33). Capital costs are made up of work stations, display stations, archiving equipment, interfaces, and the communication system. All aspects are under development, and costs will surely be reduced over time, with improved performance at the same time.

Financial savings from a PAC system include such factors as savings in capital costs for cameras, darkroom and storage space, savings in consumables associated with film, and savings in staff time because of fewer archiving personnel and better efficiency in general. An important possible financial saving is from shorter lengths of stay, but there is limited evidence at this time that such a result is possible.

Drew (1985) estimated direct annual savings from a PAC system. He estimated savings of $40 000 in capital costs, $20 000 in maintenance costs, $80 000 in consumables (especially X-ray film), and $60 000 in staff savings. The total direct cost is estimated at $200 000. A number of other analyses done since 1985 generally confirm Drew's results (13,148,331,430,710).

The conclusion is that a PAC system is not economic at this time. In other words, a fully comprehensive PAC system would not pay for itself at this moment. According to a simulation model developed by the BAZIS organization, the costs of a PACS will equal the costs of a film system around the year 2000 (55).

16.7 Conclusions

A PACS certainly has the potential to improve communication between and within institutes of health care, and it may improve the quality of patient care. As indicated above, prototype PACS have improved access to medical images. In some circumstances, such access could be quite important. Improved access might lead to reduced length of stay in the hospital. De Simone *et al.* (166) found that films were viewed earlier when a PACS was in use; the authors assumed a shortened length of stay but did not document it. In the evaluation of the Utrecht prototype system, a reduction was found (13).

Such systems also have negative implications. In particular, confidentiality of patient data is harder to protect. If patients are concerned about this issue, they might seek legal or other means to prevent the diffusion of PACS.

Improvements in health care through computer systems will be difficult to classify, much less document. For this reason, economic analysis will continue to be the major assessment method with such systems.

Section V AN INTERNATIONAL
              PERSPECTIVE

Technology and society interact in many ways. This section examines formal policies that make up the health policy structure or framework in different countries.

Because of the importance of health care technology, every society has developed policies that guide the different stages of its life cycle. Policies have a great potential effect at the stage of basic research, because almost the whole of the funding comes from the public. Governments attempt to steer applied research in industry as well; for instance, when they share costs. Governments regulate experimentation and testing in human beings, and require proof of efficacy and safety of drugs, and increasingly of medical devices, before they can be marketed. Planners attempt to rationalize the placement or adoption of health care technology, through licensing laws and other types of regulation. Use of technology is affected by different policies, especially payment for services and budgets for institutions.

In the chapters that follow, policies in several countries are described. These countries have health systems that range widely in their underlying philosophy. The US system of health care is based on a *laissez-faire* philosophy, in which the tendency is to assume that each citizen is responsible for his or her own problems. European systems generally are based on the idea of solidarity, in which the assumption is that citizens of a country have a degree of responsibility for each other. Developing countries have less well-developed policies to control health care technology, although countries such as Mexico are beginning to change this situation.

Systems also differ in their organization. In Eastern Europe and Sweden, policies have developed within the context of a socialization and regionalization that is rather unique in the world. Other countries struggle with problems such as private ownership of hospitals, private practice of physicians, inappropriate financial incentives to hospitals and physicians, placement of expensive, high-technology equipment in small hospitals, and overuse of technological services, in part because of financial incentives. It is because of these problems that most Western countries have a complex of policies and programmes to control technology.

Pluralistic services, such as those found in the USA and The Netherlands, do not encourage efficiency. In those countries, private services and inappropriate incentives are common. Attempts at planning and rationalization have not been too successful, in the face of these fundamental system problems. In Sweden, on the other hand, these problems just do not exist. Nevertheless, all the countries described face the same problems of limited resources and large demand for health services. All countries have seen a rapid technological change in their health care systems, and they realize that they will have to make similar difficult choices in the future. Therefore, the experience with health care technology assessment is very relevant internationally. In particular, the results of such assessments, to the extent that the information can be used in another country, are highly relevant. This fact underlines the importance of international collaboration.

Developing countries have problems that are common to an extent, but they develop less of their own technology, meaning that they must import it. In addition, problems of limited resources are more severe, meaning that choice is more difficult.

In this section, the first chapters (Chapters 17–22) describe the situation in a few selected countries. Chapter 23 uses material from these chapters and discusses international developments in health care technology assessment, including activities in countries not described in specific chapters. The final chapter (Chapter 24) presents overall conclusions and suggestions for future policy changes, focusing on further developments in a system for health care technology assessment.

17. Health care technology in Sweden

Lars Werkö

17.1 The health system

Sweden has a population of about eight million people. Largely urban and highly industrialized, Sweden has one of the world's highest per capita incomes. The country's economy is a mixture of capitalism and socialism.

Sweden has a government-owned and operated health care system. The system is highly regionalized, with four levels: health centres, district hospitals, central general hospitals, and regional hospitals (274).

Responsibility for health care in Sweden rests almost completely with the county councils. The 24 county councils have the right to levy local taxes, most of which are channelled into health care. During the last decades, the central government has successively transferred responsibility for certain sectors of health care to these councils, starting with local district doctors in the 1960s, mental hospitals in the 1970s, and university hospitals during the following years. Each of these moves was coupled to a promise from the state to transfer monies for the costs of the activities to the local councils.

This development was finalized in the Health Act of 1988, when the councils were officially given total responsibility for the health of their inhabitants, including not only medical care but also preventive care and rehabilitation. The money transferred from the central budget to the councils became a lump sum, the size of which is negotiated between the state and the councils each year. These negotiations are almost the only way the central government can influence the policies of the counties regarding the delivery of health care. This subsidy from the state to the councils for the delivery of health care constitutes about 20 per cent of the health budget in Sweden (out of a total of about 10 billion Swedish crowns).

Each county has an elected steering body, but in negotiations with the central government, as well as with the employee's organizations, they are organized within the Federation of County Councils (FCC). The FCC has a powerful board, politically elected, and a well-staffed central office, the director of which is one of the most powerful individuals within the Swedish health care system. During the development of the present system for health care administration, it has always been the understanding that the central government is responsible for research and development as well as for the education of doctors. For historical reasons, most of the education of other health care personnel rests with local authorities, counties, or communities.

To complicate matters further, Sweden is divided into seven regions for specialized health care, with one large hospital in each region defined as the specialty hospital for that region. In six of these regions, the university hospital, partly staffed by the local medical faculty of the university, is the hospital responsible for highly specialized care in the region. The seventh region (Orebro) has no university, but its regional hospital is almost as well-equipped for high technology as the university hospitals. Up to now, there has been an agreement between the county with a regional hospital and the other counties within the region concerning the economic and administrative details for the delivery of highly specialized care.

This whole system of well-defined responsibilities, with agreements of how money should flow within the system and how patients are taken care of, is now under debate. To some extent this debate is due to lack of balance between costs and resources, to some extent it is due to decreased confidence in the system. Many new ideas are being tested, most of them originating in the USA or the UK. It is impossible to state how this experimental period will end. Changes are certainly going to be introduced, but different counties are likely to have different goals and implement different changes.

17.2 Policies towards research

Some counties are richer than others, but all are interested in demonstrating their ability to deliver high-quality health care. While the FCC—partly for political reasons—is totally opposed to counties being involved in research, some counties, especially those connected with regional hospitals or those with a stronger economy, have an unofficial policy of engaging in research activities. They may thus have special research funds, administered by the county council, or personnel paid from the health budget for the purpose of assisting in research projects, in some instances in primary care, in others in high-technology medicine.

With the central state government explicitly responsible for all research and academic education, the state budget contains special resources for education and research in the universities, where the medical faculties have been relatively well-funded. The pre-clinical institutions particularly are well-staffed, with well-trained employees, and these pre-clinical research activities in Sweden are generally considered to be excellent. The clinical institutions are not as well-supported from the state budget, partly because of the dual responsibility for the running of the university hospitals, which have a small academic staff responsible for research and education of both medical students and some paramedical personnel and a large non-academic staff employed by the county for the care of patients. For a long time all academic activity was concentrated in the university hospital with its many specialized beds and large out-patient departments. During the last decade all universities have created specialist departments of primary care—sometimes called family care—headed by a professor and other staff similar to other clinical departments. All academic personnel have a responsibility to take part in research, with an unwritten rule that such activities should comprise about 20–25 per cent of the time, the rest being divided between teaching and medical service.

The other important support for research in Sweden is the organization of research councils. The Medical Research Council (MRC) is the most important source of resources for medical research and for initiatives regarding the research policies of the government. Most of the research funding from the MRC goes to the pre-clinical departments of the universities, but some is also destined for clinical departments, primary care, or social medicine. During the last ten years, the MRC has had a special committee for health services research (HSR) to stimulate such activities. It was partly through the initiative of the MRC and its HSR committee that the Swedish Council for Health Care Technology Assessment was created.

Even though the MRC may be the most important voice regarding medical research in Sweden, other government research bodies certainly have a role in formulating government policy regarding biomedical research, such as the Council for Research (FRN), in which members of parliament take part, and the 'Forskningsberedningen', chaired by the secretary for education and reporting directly to the government. Clinical research is also supported by several large private foundations. Since Sweden is a small country, it has comparatively few individuals competent and interested in the administration of research. It is thus not unusual that the same person may influence both private and public funding policy, as well as both university and research councils, concerning important research questions. This may be good or bad. The relatively high recognition of the quality of Swedish biomedical research indicates, however, that so far these individuals have been able to stimulate scientific activities in a positive way.

17.3 Assessment and control of pharmaceuticals

Sweden has for a long time had a well-organized central agency for the control of pharmaceuticals. This agency was part of the Board of Health and Welfare, but became an independent institution in 1990. It has a reputation for scientific competence and integrity as high as that of the American Food and Drug Administration (FDA) or similar bodies in the UK or Australia. When new medicines are registered—after thorough scrutiny of efficacy and safety—the price of the new medicine is agreed upon between the Medicinal Agency and the provider of the medicine. The drug is then sold through the State Monopoly—Apoteksbolaget—mostly following a prescription from a physician.

Swedish patients have had an unusually favourable subsidy regarding prescription medicines. The patient only pays a nominal amount—slowly increasing from 15 to 90 Swedish crowns (US$2.5–US$15)—for all prescriptions written at the same time by the same physician. This situation has led to the patient requesting the doctor to write many prescriptions at the same time, increasing the amount paid by the government. In recent years some restrictions have been introduced, both regarding the amount that can be prescribed—only three months' supply—and regarding the type of pharmaceutical—vitamins and cough medicines are no longer part of the scheme.

A new bill is being discussed in parliament to decrease the subsidies on medicines, whereby the patient will have to pay a certain sum for each drug on a prescription and that only the cheapest drug of the same kind will be subsidized. This would increase the amount that the patient had to pay, as well as reducing government costs for drugs—now more than 10 billion crowns. This bill is being resisted by both patients' organizations and the pharmaceutical industry.

There are only a few pharmaceutical enterprises in Sweden. Most medicines used are imported through subsidiaries of the large international companies. The few Swedish companies—ASTRA, KABI-PHARMACIA and FERRING—are, however, quite successful and have considerable presence in the international pharmaceutical market. Part of this success is due to unusually good co-operation between universities and industrial research companies. In some respects, this co-operation has been specially designed. University research departments are free to advise companies, for example. Companies can support university research without losing the possibility of retaining patent rights. Of still greater importance has been the personal co-operation between certain individuals in the pharmaceutical companies and some prominent academics. The creation of special posts in academic institutions as adjunct professors for highly qualified industrial researchers has stimulated scientific activities both in the industry and in the medical and pharmacological faculties, including the pre-clinical faculties such as biochemistry and physiology. This co-operation, which used to be questioned as tainting the academic purity of institutional research, has now become essential both for universities, as government support for research tends to fall, and for the companies, which are able to attract highly qualified research leaders, needed in these days of stiff international competition. No-one now questions the intense exchange of ideas and results that goes on.

The Swedish system of registration of the population and the keen interest in clinical research on new therapeutic possibilities has stimulated the international pharmaceutical companies to conduct early clinical trials in Sweden. With the negative attitude of the Federation of County Councils towards research, there was little support for such activities. Physicians interested in this type of research had difficulties in convincing health care personnel, hospital administrators, and patients about the need for such research. In the early 1980s, after rather long negotiations between the organizations of the pharmaceutical industry and the FCC, an agreement was reached concerning rules for conducting clinical studies with new drugs, including advice about how the economic agreement between the hospital administration and the company might be written. This agreement has dealt with most of the earlier criticism. Although the agreement is applied differently in different hospitals, most parties involved in this activity have been satisfied. This agreement has also been of importance for patient safety and has helped the monitors from the company producing the new medicine to gain trust.

17.4 Control of medical devices

In contrast to pharmaceuticals, medical devices are almost entirely unregulated. Since the drug agency became independent, the government has indicated that regulation of devices will become the responsibility of this new agency. The details of this regulation will probably be part of the changes necessary as Sweden harmonizes its rules with those within the European Common Market.

17.5 Academic education

Sweden has a long tradition of university education in Lund and Uppsala. During a time immediately after World War II, the central government had a keen interest in increasing academic education, at first mostly in medicine, but then in other fields. New universities were created, beginning in Stockholm, Goteborg, and Umea, and certain faculties in the older universities were enlarged. One result was a marked increase in central administration of the universities through the office of the Chancellor for Universities in Stockholm, which became a large governmental agency for the administration of academic affairs. This removed some decision-making from universities and academic personnel to the office of the Chancellor and politically appointed administrators. This first wave of development was followed by the creation of 'High Schools' offering all kinds of education, placed in several cities around the country, but all controlled from Stockholm.

The result of these changes has been questioned, in terms of both quality and efficacy. The central administration is now being dismantled. The present government has announced that it wishes to decentralize the administration of both the older and the newer universities and schools for higher education. Instead of having to listen to dictates from Stockholm, it is envisaged that the local governing board of the universities will decide most of its activities by itself, as long as certain measures of quality are adhered to.

A discussion is underway concerning the creation of local foundations to run the universities. The proposal implies more freedom, but also more responsibility for those accepting the challenge. Some academicians would like to accept the challenge, while others who are more cautious question their ability to widen their responsibilities outside their own research field. The parties involved in the discussion include politicians, local administrators, and organizations of employees, including the labour unions of the professors. This bold proposal for change could lead to marked alterations in the administration of education and research in Sweden.

17.6 Assessment of health care technology

Sweden was one of the first countries to become involved in health care technology assessment (365,366). Studies of the computed tomography (CT) scanner done at the Swedish Planning and Rationalization Institute (SPRI) were some of the first studies done in this field in the world (366). During the last 15 years, health care technology assessment has become more and more accepted in Sweden, and is now carried out by the SPRI and in several universities (85,597).

Through the combined efforts of the MRC, some politicians in government and in the parliament, and with assistance from the Board of Health and the SPRI, the government created the Swedish Council for Health Care Technology Assessment (SBU) in 1987. The Council both assesses important technologies and serves as a focus and co-ordinating body for activities in Sweden. The idea was to give the new Council three years to work in order to see whether the results were such that a more permanent organization should be created. The philosophy was consistent with that of this book: assessments should be done to change policy and health care practice in constructive directions. For this reason, the Board of the Council consists of representatives of all important organizations in health care. It was envisaged that this Board should have enough competence to select suitable fields for assessment, as well as suitable methods for working.

The Council created a small central office with a few people working full-time and a project organization heavily dependent on specialists working in the health services, mostly those outside university centres, to assure contact with the problems encountered in the daily routine of medical services. Through its expert committee, a large number of possible projects have been discussed and several have been carried out and published (667–671). Each report contains a recommendation from the Board about how the problem in question might be solved.

The first report concerned pre-operative investigations in elective surgery (669). The report recommended restrictions on certain investigations. An evaluation demonstrated that these recommendations were followed to a certain extent. Another problem concerned the problem of back pain and led to renewed discussion of this disorder in many contexts (671).

The trial period was completed and a special evaluation of the activities of the council was positive. The government then decided that the organization should be permanent. A bill was presented to parliament suggesting the creation of an institution for technology assessment in health care with the same general organization as the council. Since all political parties agree on the bill, the institute should begin to function within the next budget year (1993).

Two large projects are presently underway in the council. One is a thorough evaluation of the treatment of mild to moderate hypertension, where some patients are overtreated and others undertreated. Although many expert committees have made recommendations concerning this condition, there has never been the critical examination of the literature necessary to evaluate results in relation to resources needed in different types of patients. The other large project concerns the rationale for radiation treatment of solid tumours. A large Swedish working group of oncological specialists, economists, and experts in critical assessment is working to evaluate the voluminous literature. Since this is a sensitive field for recommendations, an international expert group has also been appointed in order to assist in the final recommendations.

17.7 Conclusions

In Sweden, it is recognized that even a rich country cannot do everything possible in health care. This means that technology must be controlled and that choices must be made. The regionalized Swedish system for health care and the budgeting system gives great potentials for controlling health care technology. However, the basis for choice—for action—is not fully developed. Health care technology assessment is seen as an important mechanism for helping policy-makers, politicians, and clinicians make these choices. While technology assessment activities are still relatively small in Sweden, they are of growing visibility and importance.

18. Medical technology in the UK

Jackie Spiby and Barbara Stocking

18.1 The health system

The UK consists of four countries: England, Wales, Scotland, and Northern Ireland. There are some differences in the administrative arrangements for health service provision among the countries, but none that has a major impact on policies concerning the introduction and use of medical technology. The UK has a population of 55 million people and currently spends about 6.1 per cent of its gross national product on health care. The 1989 government expenditure on the National Health Service (NHS) was £23.25 billion.

Before World War II, a national insurance system existed through which contributions were made for health care. The provisions were, however, established which entitled all people to free health care with access based on need rather than ability to pay. The NHS is now financed almost entirely out of central taxation with a small percentage coming from national insurance contributions and from other sources (for example from the charges which are made for prescriptions and ophthalmic and dental services).

The overall responsibility for the NHS lies with the Secretary of State for Health in England, and the Secretaries of State for Scotland, Wales, and Northern Ireland. The Secretary of State is a member of the government in power, and is accountable to Parliament for the NHS. He or she exercises responsibility, in England, through the Department of Health (DH). Although the department sets general policy and allocates resources to regions, there is an expressed philosophy of devolution of power to local Health Authorities and care providers.

In 1974, the NHS was reorganized to bring together community and school health services with existing hospital and primary health care services. In 1982, further restructuring took place, organizing health care through 14 Regional Authorities with 191 District Authorities. The Authorities were the statutory bodies for the management of the NHS. In 1984, each District and Region appointed a general manager who became the final person accountable for the service, rather than the previous system of consensus management. This was mirrored by the establishment of a National Policy Board and Management Executive with a Chief Executive of the NHS.

The most recent changes, potentially of major importance for technology assessment, are those changes embodied in the NHS Act of 1989. Following a ministerial review, district health authorities have become responsible for identifying the needs of their local population, determining what services are required to meet those needs, and purchasing those services from the providers of health services (acute, community, and mental health services) who are becoming independent units, called trusts. Thus the management of health provision is separated from those charged with the responsibility of achieving the optimum improvement in the health of the population. This division, along with major developments in primary care where some general practitioners (GPs) have been given their own budgets to purchase secondary care, constitutes a major change in philosophy on the provision of health care in the UK. Its impact on the rational use of technology will need to be monitored.

18.2 Research and development

In 1988 the House of Lords Select Committee on Science and Technology in their document *Priorities in medical research*, stated that there was a lack of coherent arrangements for the NHS to articulate its research needs and to ensure that the benefits of research were systematically and effectively transferred into service. They were particularly critical of the way in which public health research and operational research (i.e., research into the organization and management of health services) have been relatively neglected, and suggested a marked increase in funding for this area. In response to this, in 1990, the Government created a new senior post of Director of Research and Development, to head the Research and Development Division (527). A Research and Development Strategy was launched as the first stage in the creation of an R&D programme and infrastructure in the NHS (477). The prime objective was to see that R&D becomes an integral part of health care so that clinicians, managers, and other staff find it natural to rely on the results of research in their day-to-day decision-making and longer-term strategic planning.

The NHS R&D programme will place emphasis on evaluation of the quality, effectiveness, and cost of methods of disease prevention and treatment, and on research into the delivery and content of health care (165). It will also seek to influence biomedical research by expecting NHS priorities to be taken into account when planning future programmes and expecting the practical implication of major research discoveries to be anticipated at an early stage.

The Government has shown its commitment by including increased funding for R&D in the Secretary of State's objectives, and stating an intention to move over a five-year period to a target of expenditure of 1.5 per cent of the NHS budget rather than the present 0.9 per cent. The development of the R&D strategy is also high on the list of objectives for the Management Executive in 1992/1993. The regions are expected to have a crucial role in the R&D programme by directing, commissioning and managing R&D programmes and helping to ensure that the results of good research are used to full effect. They will also be expected to ensure that there is a dialogue between the local research community and the purchasers (the district health authorities). To date regions are developing their own R&D plans and appointing staff to oversee their programmes. The actual impact of the national and regional R&D initiative has yet to be felt.

At the heart of the strategy is the task of setting priorities and co-ordinating activity for NHS R&D. A Central Research and Development Committee (CRDC) has been set to review R&D of relevance to the work of the NHS, and to identify areas where further work would be of value to the NHS. The committee brings together senior NHS managers, leading research workers from universities and elsewhere, lay members, and others with experience in industry. The membership covers the whole country and a wide range of backgrounds but is not based on formal representation. The work identified as a priority by the committee will either be funded centrally or the regional health authorities and postgraduate hospitals will take a lead (163,336).

The R&D Strategy for the NHS is part of a wider R&D strategy for the Department of Health (DH) as a whole, which includes developing liaison committees between the DH and major funding bodies and ensuring a more coherent strategic approach to medical research in the UK.

18.3 Technology assessment

Until recently, technology assessment in the UK has been characterized by considerable work but limited co-ordination or systematic methods of dissemination and implementation (359,656,661,662). There is a long tradition in the UK of supporting clinical trials, especially randomized controlled trials, following the lead of the likes of Cochrane (132) and Doll. These trials have mainly been initiated within the universities and funded primarily by the Medical Research Council (MRC). The UK is also a leader in the development of health economics as a specialty, both as an observational science (186,187), and also more recently as part of large-scale trials such as the study of coronary heart transplantation (103,104).

The UK has also a strong tradition in equipment evaluation, mainly centred on technical quality, reliability, mechanical and electrical safety, and costs. This task is carried out at 18 centres designated by the DH. Questions of clinical value of the equipment and whether it was in fact required by the Health Service are rarely tackled.

Soon after taking up his post, the DH Director of Research and Development set up a Health Technology Group. (A similar group was set up in Scotland.) This group marks the acknowledgement of the importance of technology assessment and the need to co-ordinate and promote a systematic approach to activities in the field. The group was convened 'to prepare a paper discussing methods for assessing the effects of health technologies; to identify matters requiring action; and to make recommendations'. Amongst the main points and recommendations are the following (4).

1. The range of possible outcome measures by which the effects of health technology might be assessed should always be considered explicitly.

2. Existing evidence about the effects of health technologies should be reviewed systematically and the results disseminated in forms that a wide variety of decision-makers, including patients can understand. Where evidence is strong, means would be used to ensure that it influences practice.

3. There should be a systematic information system for disseminating the results of technology assessments.

4. Every effort should be made to assess the effects of new technologies before it is decided whether or not they should be used within the health service.

5. Multidisciplinary research centres, each focusing on a priority area of health care, should be established to assess the effects of health technologies.

6. There should be training and a career structure for those who wish to specialize in technology assessment.

The report has been considered by the CRDC, which is very positive in its aim to ensure that its recommendations are taken forward.

18.4 The Medical Research Council

The Medical Research Council (MRC) plays a key role in the UK in medical research activities. Although the Council has been moving towards change for some time, it has been mainly dominated by biomedical research and been less interested in health services research or consideration of the wider issues related to the medical technology in practice. Following the House of Lords report, the appointment of the DH Director of Research and Development and a new Secretary at the MRC, change has been accelerated and there appears to be a more positive attitude towards health services research and applied clinical research as evidenced by the new board structure which includes a fourth Board for health services research, public health, and epidemiology. Relations between the MRC and DH are governed by a concordat which now acknowledges the strong role of the DH in health services research. A report is also being considered by the MRC Board which proposes that the MRC take a far more proactive role in evaluating procedures including consideration of economic, quality of life, and psychosocial issues.

18.5 Introduction and use of technology

18.5.1 *Clinical equipment*

As previously described, there has been a strong tradition of technical equipment evaluation in the UK, although clinical value has been largely ignored. The division previously responsible for this work has now been integrated into the

R&D Directorate, and it is expected that in time this work will be combined into the central priorities of the Division and broaden to cover the wider topics of technology assessment.

18.5.2 NHS Supplies Authority

In 1991 the Department of Health reversed its previous policy of devolving purchasing of medical supplies (ranging from catering to expensive scientific equipment), and established a central NHS Supplies Authority. The change of heart resulted from a report by the National Audit Office, a body charged with auditing the public sector, which was critical of NHS buying. The report said that the considerable buying power of the NHS was not being fully utilized due to lack of co-ordination and that there were many missed possibilities for more cost-effective purchasing of supplies. The main thrust of the report was on more cost-efficient purchasing. The new Authority will provide a central co-ordinated policy on the buying of supplies. For organizational efficiency, it will be divided up into six divisions with the national headquarters concentrating on key commodities such as food contracts, medical and surgical items, and X-ray equipment. The Authority will also undertake research into market requirements and will have a small R&D programme. Two early areas of review will be superabsorbent materials and magnetic resonance imaging. However, this new development is rather at odds with the establishment of trusts and the independence of providers. At present, it is expected that trusts will be encouraged to use the purchasing power of the Authority but will not be required to.

18.5.3 *Role of regions*

In the past, regions have held a capital equipment budget from which replacement and new equipment have been purchased. Regions differed in the amount of that budget that was immediately devolved down to districts, but all kept some control of purchasing of large pieces of equipment through a complex and often unclear mix of bidding and rational planning. With the NHS reforms the majority of this direct control is slowly devolving to health care providers, although regions will maintain an advisory role (569).

18.5.4 *Role of health care providers*

As discussed previously, the NHS reforms split the buying of services from the management of them. Since April 1991, providers (hospitals, community service units, mental health services) have been able to apply for Trust status. This in effect means that they are independent units responsible only to the DH for their overall performance, tied to district health authorities by contracts which specify not only how much service is to be provided but what quality is expected. The development of these Trusts signals the development of the UK health care market, so the units are increasingly becoming aware of the need to provide an effective and efficient service. Thus they are looking more critically at the results of technology assessments.

The reforms have also meant that capital charges (i.e., cost of land, buildings, and equipment) are included in the price of services. The aim is promote the efficient use of capital, including more considered buying and use of new and old technology (569). At present the main emphasis is on ensuring better use of capital stock invested in land and buildings, but the larger hospitals are already realizing that their higher prices include the cost of expensive equipment. Units that have been given trust status are not bound by the previous rules for obtaining new equipment but are able, within certain limits, to purchase the new equipment they require, as long as its cost is included in the overall price of the service. Again the true impact of this system has yet to be seen but it should promote the demand for better evidence on the effectiveness and costs of equipment and hence better purchasing policies.

18.5.5 *Medical audit*

The NHS reforms include the promotion of medical audit, the systematic, critical analysis of the quality of medical care. This should include the procedures used for diagnosis and treatment, the use of resources, and the resulting outcome and quality of life for the patient.

New monies have been released by the Department of Health for the development of medical audit. In the third year of this initiative a large number of clinicians are involved in medical audit at some level. At present, much of the activity is centred around collecting data, but in some centres clinicians are now looking more critically at their work and appraising themselves of best practice and judging their work against agreed standards. Again the initiative, along with management changes which are encouraging doctors to be more involved in management issues, is forcing the profession to consider evidence on cost and effectiveness of clinical procedures.

18.5.6 *Clinical Standards Advisory Committee*

The Clinical Standards Advisory Group (CSAG) was established in 1991 as part of the NHS Act to advise the UK Health Ministers or health service bodies, as requested, on standards of clinical care for, as well as access and availability of, services to NHS patients. Most of the members are nominated by the Royal colleges and faculties relating to medicine, nursing, and dentistry although it is funded by the DH. Its initial work will cover:

(1) access to, and availability of, selected NHS specialist services;

(2) clinical standards for women in normal labour;

(3) standards of clinical care for patients admitted to hospital urgently or as emergencies;

(4) standards of care for people with diabetes.

This body is a very new venture into developing and assessing clinical standards and its success is still not assured, especially as it is advisory rather than mandatory.

18.5.7 *Other influences on the use of technology*

18.5.7.1 *Regions*

Apart from their role in the direct purchasing of equipment, regions can also influence the use of medical technology and clinical practice as part of their responsibility to monitor the health and health service provision, both primary and secondary, within the region. This is done both by direct measurement and by monitoring district's purchasing intentions and decisions about priorities. At present this role is in its infancy but ideally it can be expected that by monitoring health care outcomes, regions will become a rich source of effectiveness data.

As discussed earlier, regions also have a key role in spear-heading the development of R&D. A key factor in this will be the appointment of regional directors of R&D who will have to be the local product champions.

18.5.7.2 *Districts*

The role of districts in purchasing health care based on the needs of the population provides a major impetus for technology assessment. Needs assessment, or the population's ability to benefit from health care, clearly encompasses the concept of securing proven effective services. Thus, for the first time managers and public health physicians are working together to assess the literature on effectiveness of health care procedures including cost-effectiveness. The DH has responded by commissioning a series of bulletins on the effectiveness of health service interventions for decision-makers, the first edition being published in January 1992. These bulletins are specifically orientated towards health authorities rather than clinicians.

The need to purchase effective health care packages is also promoting interest in service evaluation and local health services research is increasing rapidly.

18.5.7.3 *Primary care*

The NHS reforms have also put a greater emphasis on the role of the general practitioner (GP). Two initiatives are of particular importance in relation to medical technology assessment. GP fund-holding has given some of the larger GP practices their own budgets to purchase secondary care and to organize and manage their own services. Although it is early days, there is some evidence that this is making those GPs involved consider more carefully their practice and there is a slow shift of inappropriate work away from the hospital back to primary care. The second initiative is the setting of indicative budgets for GP prescribing. In the UK some £6 billion is spent by GPs on drugs. The wide variations in spending between different GPs and practices suggests that not all prescribing is as cost-effective as it could be. As yet the budgets are not fixed, but even an indicative budget is promoting a better focus on the appropriateness of prescribing. The initiative has also meant that most Family Health Services Authorities (FHSAs) have employed medical and pharmaceutical advisers who are charged with the task of promoting the enhancement of the quality of prescribing in primary care.

18.5.7.4 *The role of consumers*

A major part of the NHS reforms was a commitment to the importance of the consumer in decision-making in the NHS. The main part of this policy has been the publication in 1991 of a Patient's Charter. This sets out clearly for the first time the public's right to care in the NHS and National and Local Charter Standards which the Government intends to see achieved. The Charter rights include the right to request a second opinion, a clear explanation of any treatment proposed, including any risks and any alternatives before deciding whether to agree to treatment, access to health records, the choice whether or not to take part in medical research, and to have all complaints investigated and to receive a full and prompt written reply. This increased emphasis on the role of the consumer will no doubt increase actual patient questioning of medical practice and interest in gathering and researching the consumer's view.

The increasing role of the consumer in technology assessment can be seen in the acceptance of the importance of including consumers in the planning of major randomized controlled trials such as the trial of chorionic villus sampling. At present this involvement is primarily in medical specialties relating to women's health, but it can be expected that consumers' expectations will increase generally.

18.5.7.5 *The Audit Commission*

The Audit Commission is an independent body which audits the public sector. More recently it has developed its work in health matters and reviewed services such as those for day surgery, AIDS and HIV prevention, and bed utilization. As a body that has access to all health authorities, it potentially could have a considerable impact on the use of medical technology.

18.5.7.6 *The King's Fund and Consensus Development Conferences*

One of the main proponents of technology assessment in the UK during the 1980s has been the King's Fund, both behind the scenes and in the development of the UK Consensus Development Programme. The latter has now ceased but as district and regional health authorities have come to realize their need for assessment data the method has been adapted to local circumstances.

18.6 Conclusions

The UK has been a leader in developing methods of assessing health care technologies, but until recently it has not acted to ensure active use of research findings in provision of health care services. That situation is now rapidly changing. Health care technology assessment is now a visible activity in the policy environment in the UK and seems certain to become more important in the years to come.

19. Assessment of health care technology in The Netherlands

Henk Rigter

Technology assessment in The Netherlands is based on decision cycles, which have in common four major steps (see Chapter 6): (1) identifying and selecting the existing and emerging technologies that need to be addressed; (2) collecting the necessary information; (3) decision-making; and (4) providing follow-up by disseminating the results and monitoring what happens with the technology in practice. These steps will return later in this chapter in the discussion of pharmaceuticals, medical devices, and other health care technologies.

19.1 The health care system of The Netherlands

The health care system of The Netherlands is pluralistic (589,590). Diagnosis and treatment are primarily provided privately, but are subject to government control, reflecting the tendency of the Dutch to settle things through a strong 'public–private' interface. Health care institutions are mostly private, non-profit foundations, although academic and municipal hospitals are public. Doctors and other professionals generally work either in these institutions or in private practice or both. The government has the primary responsibility for providing preventive care services and for giving general guidance, mainly through the Ministry of Welfare, Health, and Cultural Affairs (WVC). In clinical health care, the government sees its role in the creation of proper conditions for the exercise of private actions (307).

The goverment's role in health care mainly takes shape through the Health Care Charges Act (Wet Ziekenhuistarieven) of 1965, which regulates price setting for intramural institutions, and the Hospital Provisions Act (Wet Ziekenhuisvoorzieningen) of 1971, which regulates the building and renovation of institutions.

The insurance system can be divided into three parts. The first is sick fund insurance, which is a compulsory, public scheme covering about 60 per cent of the population. Members of the scheme include employees whose total wages fall below a certain level. The second part is private insurance, which covers everyone else in the population. The third part is public insurance, for all residents of The Netherlands, under the Exceptional Medical Expenses Act (AWBZ), covering *inter alia* facilities for the disabled, mentally handicapped, and the elderly. Under the Health Care Charges Act, all charges and fees in the health care sector are controlled, as well as the overall budget of each institution. The Central Health Care Charges Agency (Centraal Orgaan Tarieven Gezondheidszorg, COTG), made up of representatives of employers, employees, institutions, doctors' organizations, funding bodies, and independent experts, has the responsibility of drawing up guidelines for the setting of charges and fees. Each hospital is now under a global budget, i.e., a ceiling for the incomes generated from charges. The actual amount of the budget is determined by historical experience and negotiation.

Academic specialists are paid by salary, but other specialists by fee-for-service, thus offering incentives for over-utilization of medical procedures (321). General practitioners are paid mostly per capita.

The major explicit control that the government has over technology is authorized by Article 18 of the Hospital Provisions Act, which gives it the authority to license high-technology services (120,306,308). The purpose of this Article is to limit the number of facilities for reasons of efficiency and quality. Although the Dutch feel that some high-technology services have diffused too widely, this anomaly is small compared to what has happened in many other countries. In fact, the concentration of high-technology services in The Netherlands has been quite successful (78). About ten services are licensed, and thereby centralized, including various transplantations, neurosurgery, heart surgery and invasive cardiological interventions, radiotherapy, intensive care for neonates, *in-vitro* fertilization, clinical genetics, and renal dialysis. This control mechanism has, more than anything else, prompted the development of health care technology assessment in The Netherlands.

Despite the successes attained, the present government is disappointed with the possibilities of the State to control health care technologies. Therefore, it has decided to change policies. This is bound to occur within the framework of a more general change in the health care system in The Netherlands. The idea is that government control creates suffocating bureaucracy and that the health care 'field' should exercise more self-regulation and assume more responsibilities. The AWBZ will be transformed into a national health insurance, to be executed by private insurance companies, including the former sick funds. In 1992, the pharmaceutical services were transferred to the sphere of operation of the AWBZ. The next step may be the transfer of extramural services (463). However, this process of change has been slowed down by political and societal opposition. The lessening of control by the government, and the associated increase in 'free-market' competition in health care, has resulted in a cost explosion, which has jeopardized the plans of the government. As a result, the government has announced that, contrary to earlier ideas, it will continue to regulate high-technology medicine, perhaps even in a stricter and more general way than previously (649). It is hard to predict, at the present time, how things will work out, but this is clear: the government expects technology assessment to play a decisive role in decision-making in the present and in new health care systems.

19.2 Policies towards research and development

Medical research in The Netherlands is mainly funded by the government, especially through the Department of Education and Science, and is carried out in the eight universities that have a medical faculty, in the associated hospitals, and in special research institutes. In addition, research groups may secure funds from other sources, such as charities and industry. This diversity of funding also applies to research in technology assessment. A particularly important source for funding of technology assessment studies is the Investigational Medicine Fund (fonds ontwikkelingsgeneeskunde), which is discussed below.

There have been some attempts to set priorities in the allocation of funds from the Department of Education and Science, through procedures separating excellent research groups from less gifted ones, but in general academic freedom is still the rule in spending research funds. This may change, however. The Dutch government has decided to create research centres of excellence, which will enjoy priority status in the allocation of research funds. The centres of excellence (onderzoeksscholen) will be selected using indicators for high-quality scientific performance. Among the eight centres from all disciplines selected in the first round, there were two medical research groups. Even more gratifying is that one of these groups was an alliance of the Departments of Epidemiology, Social Medicine, Medical Informatics, Health Care Policy and Management, and Medical Technology Assessment, the Institute of Medical Technology Assessment (IMTA) of the Erasmus University in Rotterdam. Thus, health care technology assessment in The Netherlands is not just fashionable; it has achieved the status of academic excellence.

The government will continue to develop methods for priority setting in the allocation of research funds. The Department of Education and Science provides the university hospitals with a fund to develop a 'platform' for doing medical research together with the medical faculty. The government is expected to change its non-discriminative policy in granting this so-called State contribution (rijksbijdrage). Possibly, a national authority will assess the scientific status of university hospital departments, using scientific criteria. Only departments meeting certain standards will receive a share from the State contribution.

In priority setting in the allocation of research funds, not only measures of scientific excellence will be used. The government has also identified areas of research it would like to stimulate because of policy relevance. Among these areas is health care technology assessment. Thus, the government gave the above-mentioned Institute of Medical Technology Assessment some 'seed money' to get started. In addition, nuclei of health care technology assessment research can be found in the hospital of the University of Amsterdam (Department of Clinical Epidemiology and Medical Technology Assessment), the University of Limburg (Maastricht), the Department of Law of the Erasmus University, the State University of Groningen (Department of Medical

Sociology), the various departments of epidemiology, and—outside the university—in the Centre for Medical Technology of TNO (The Netherlands Organization for Applied Scientific Research). Most of these groups perform literature and empirical studies (steps 2 and 4 described in Section 18.1: collection of information and monitoring (follow-up), respectively). The government has assigned step 1 (identification) to the Health Council (Gezondheidsraad) of The Netherlands.

Also of relevance is the recent decision of the government to establish a School of Public Health. This School will be a joint effort of the State University of Utrecht, the Erasmus University, and the State Institute for Public Health and Environmental Protection (RIVM). The School will provide opportunities for education and research. It is likely that health care technology assessment will be part of the curriculum.

The importance attached by the Dutch government to policy research is also apparent from its decision to foster the establishment of the EAC, the European—American Centre for Policy Analysis. The Centre began operations on March 26, 1992 in Delft, The Netherlands, and at RAND in Santa Monica, USA. At both locations the Centre will bring together multidisciplinary teams of European and American researchers to collaborate on projects, including technology assessment, and to exchange data and research methods.

Health care technology assessment has an international dimension in The Netherlands. In October 1992, the Council of European Ministers of Health adopted a resolution, drawn up by the Chair (The Netherlands), in which the value of technology assessment for European health policy was stressed. Health care technology assessment studies already receive support from European research programmes. Health care technology assessment researchers from European countries already collaborate on certain issues. An example is the EuroQoL project, with the objective to develop a common European instrument for valuing health states (219).

19.3 Policies towards pharmaceuticals

Expenditure on medicines in The Netherlands increased over a period of four years to 1990 by almost one-third. Growth in 1990 was over 11 per cent. The increased expenditure can be ascribed to a shift away from cheaper drugs to more expensive ones, and to a far lesser extent to an increase in volume.

Compared to neighbouring countries, consumption of medicines in The Netherlands is low, but prices are high. Of a group of 13 European countries studied in 1989, France scored highest with 49 packets of medicine per head of population, whereas The Netherlands was at the bottom of the list with 8 packets per head (195). In order to ensure better cost control, the government decided to introduce, as of 1 July 1991, the Cost of Medicines Refund System (geneesmiddelen-vergoedingssysteem). Under this system reimbursement for

medicines is subject to limitation for groups of medicines which are inter-
changeable: the price of the cheaper products will determine the reimbursement
level.

19.3.1 *Identification*

The Health Council of The Netherlands is an advisory body that, by law, is
commissioned to advise the government on the scientific state of the art with
respect to health care and environmental protection. This ninety-year-old
Council has approximately 170 members, drawn from universities and other
research institutes, and a further 500 scientists contribute to the 60-odd committees working for the Council. In 1985 the government asked the Health
Council to investigate the possibility of establishing an 'early warning system'
to identify emerging drugs with a potentially great effect on health care, in
terms of quality and cost. It was hoped that appropriate policy measures could
be prepared well in advance of the moment these drugs would enter the Dutch
market. This could only be done if the Dutch Medicines Evaluation Board, the
Dutch version of the Food and Drug Administration in the USA, would reveal
information on drugs submitted for pre-marketing evaluation. Legal prohibi-
tions sealed the lips of the Board and an 'early warning system' has not yet
materialized.

19.3.2 *Collection of information*

Assessment of new drugs is still limited in scope in The Netherlands, as in most
countries, and does not involve fully fledged technology assessment. A company
submitting a drug for marketing approval by the Dutch Medicines Evaluation
Board needs only to submit evidence of safety and effectiveness. Unlike
Australia and probably Canada in the future, the Dutch authorities do not yet
require proof of cost-effectiveness. However, pharmaceutical companies themselves may increasingly decide to generate data on cost-effectiveness, if that
could improve their chances under the above-mentioned Refund System.

19.3.3 *Decision-making*

The decision to approve a drug for marketing is taken by the Dutch Medicines
Evaluation Board at the behest of the State Secretary of Health. Giving this
'green light' does not imply that the cost of the drug will be reimbursed by the
health insurance companies. As far as reimbursement by the sick funds is
concerned, reimbursement depends on an additional decision by the State
Secretary of Health, to be taken on the advice of the National Health Insurance
Board (Ziekenfondsraad). Usually, the private insurance companies follow suit.

As yet, vaccines, sera, and blood products are assessed under a regulatory
scheme different from the one for drugs, with the Health Council and the
National Institute of Public Health (RIVM) being the main actors in the evaluation process (280). This will change shortly, as the law has been altered to

include vaccines, sera and blood products under the definition of 'pharmaceutical'. The Dutch Medicines Evaluation Board will take over the task of pre-marketing evaluation of these products.

19.3.4 *Follow-up*

Commonly, once a drug has been approved for marketing, the indications for its use are expanded beyond the indications accepted by the Dutch Medicines Evaluation Board. The Health Council regularly identifies important cases of expanding use. The National Health Insurance Board may then advise the State Secretary of Health to change the reimbursement rules. For instance, the government has decided to curtail reimbursement of biotechnologically-produced growth hormone to cases where the hormone has been prescribed by a paediatrician for use in a child with an undisputable growth disorder.

Follow-up includes post-marketing surveillance (PMS), intended to detect unexpected positive or negative effects of drugs used in practice. PMS is quite fragmentary and deficient in The Netherlands. In 1991, a committee of the Health Council published a unifying 'concept', which is likely to be adopted by all parties as part of the commitment of The Netherlands to contribute to the establishment of a European network of PMS activities.

The RIVM and the Health Council monitor the national immunization programme. The RIVM collects reports of possible adverse reactions to vaccinations, whereas a committee of the Health Council evaluates the soundness of these reports and advises the government annually on steps to be taken, if any.

19.4 **Policies towards medical devices**

Throughout the years, the Dutch goverment has not shown a strong interest in making a coherent policy for medical devices. Although the Health Council identifies innovations in medical equipment and draws attention to the implications of the use of certain new and old devices, such as the lithotriptor, the MRI, the PET scanner, and lasers, the government rarely takes action. Consequently, there is an overcapacity of some devices (e.g., lithotriptors, lasers) and an undercapacity of others (PET). Perhaps the sharply rising expenditure on medical devices—in part due to the change being brought about in the health care system—will force the government to reconsider its position on this issue. Expenditure increased by almost 20 per cent in 1990 (463).

In general, the Dutch government refrains from controlling the effectiveness and safety of medical devices. While a law was enacted in 1970 to render such control possible, in reality it has never been applied except for condoms and mechanical heart valves. This is not to say that there are no policies at all. The RIVM and the TNO Centre for Medical Technology monitor problems in the use of medical devices, each institute from its own perspective. Unfortunately, the Health Council's advice to turn this into a joint effort, so that a real national PMS system for medical devices would emerge, has not been implemented by the government. The RIVM is specialized in sterilization issues. This institute draws up sterilization guidelines for hospitals and good manufacturing standards for companies making sterilization equipment. TNO addresses the technical safety and the proper use of medical devices.

A special topic is equipment involving the use of ionizing radiation. European guidelines have been translated in Dutch law. The government has established standards for the technical performance of the devices concerned, and has defined requirements for personnel and the sites of installation. These standards are based on reports of the Health Council.

19.5 Policies towards other health care technologies

In a pluralistic health care system such as the one in The Netherlands it is extremely difficult to control the influx of new health care technologies. Furthermore, The Netherlands is a small country. Most technologies are imported and the country does not have sufficient resources to assess all technologies itself. Thus, it comes as no surprise that the present policies in The Netherlands to evaluate new technologies have serious flaws. Nevertheless, important progress in designing better policies has been made the past ten years and further improvements are to be expected.

19.5.1 *Identification*

The government has given the Health Council the responsibility of identifying important emerging and new technologies. However, the Council has not received the permanent resources needed to fulfil this task adequately. The Council signals technologies in its Annual Reports, special case studies and in its bulletins, but this effort certainly is not all-encompassing. Recently, the State Commission 'Choices in Health Care' stressed again the necessity of providing the Health Council with the opportunity to gear up its 'early warning' activities (195).

These activities formally began with a future-oriented study supported by the Steering Committee on Future Health Scenarios (Stuurgroep Toekomst-scenario's Gezondheidszorg) in 1985–1987. The project group, headed by Dr David Banta, was housed by the Council (39).

Late in 1991, the government published a white paper on the advisory bodies within the Dutch health care system. Some of these bodies will be disbanded or given new assignments, but the Health Council was reaffirmed in its central position as scientific advisor of the government. The Steering Committee on Future Health Scenarios will cease to exist and its functions will be transferred to the Health Council (identification) and the RIVM (modelling studies).

The 'signals' published by the Health Council serve various policy functions. The Annual Report contains a chapter on new technologies possibly qualifying for application of Article 18 of the Hospital Provisions Act (see Section 19.1) and on technologies presently under control of Article 18 which may be released from this central regulation. Another chapter lists suggestions for technologies, new and old, to be studied within the framework of the Investigational Medicine Fund. These suggestions are not binding, but they are used by the government for the purpose of formulating research priorities. This priority setting mechanism is still rudimentary, but improvements are likely to be made in the near future.

19.5.2 *Collection of information*

A distinction is to be made between synthesis of the scientific literature and expert (group) judgement on the one hand, and empirical studies on the other. The Health Council is in the first category. At any given time, this organization has some 60-odd committees preparing advisory reports on 'the state of the art' of all sorts of medical technologies and environmental issues, using synthesis of the literature, including meta-analysis and workshops. The reports are public. Belonging to the same category, but with another mission (aimed at members of medical professional societies rather than the government), is the National Organization for Quality Assurance in Hospitals (CBO), which prepares documents for consensus development conferences. Consensus development conferences in The Netherlands follow a process somewhat different from those in other countries. In The Netherlands, opinion-making professionals are brought together, and they prepare a consensus statement in advance of the meeting. This statement is then distributed to all conference participants and discussed at the meeting. The final text is prepared by the experts some time after the meeting and is submitted for publication in a Dutch medical journal and sent to the participants (280).

Empirical health care technology assessment is relatively well-developed in The Netherlands. It began in 1985, when the National Health Insurance Board decided to sponsor three major technology assessment studies, i.e., on liver transplantation, heart transplantation, and *in-vitro* fertilization, respectively (77). These studies were directly linked to decisions to be taken by the government and by insurance companies.

The next step was the creation of the Investigational Medicine Fund, supported by monies from the National Health Insurance Board and the Ministries of Health (WVC) and of Education and Science. More than 30 million guilders a year is available, quite a large sum for research by Dutch standards. The aim of the Fund is to study medical technologies, old and new, the central question being which technologies should be rejected, because of insufficient (cost-)effectiveness, and which ones accepted, and therefore reimbursed. Clinical research groups seek grants from this Fund. Often, technology assessment is part of the grant proposal.

19.5.3 *Decision-making*

The Dutch technology assessment studies, such as those performed by the Health Council or those paid from the Investigational Medicine Fund, usually are commissioned with a specific question in mind; for example, a question posed by the government (should the technology have a place in the health care system and, if so, unlimited or licensed using Article 18?), or one posed by, or on behalf of, the insurance companies (should the technology be reimbursed?). A common problem is that the decision-maker phrases his questions in too loose a manner, thus creating confusion and reducing the efficiency of the technology assessment approach (77).

The government is considering changes in decision strategies, in order to be able to control more technologies with a minimal effort. Presently, the following scenario is being discussed:

(1) put more money into the Investigational Medicine Fund;

(2) limit funding of clinical studies of new technologies, with few exceptions, to the university hospitals and medical faculties;

(3) protect the university hospitals against competition by other hospitals;

(4) while a new technology is being examined, forbid non-university hospitals to use the technology;

(5) concentrate high-technology in university hospitals as long as there is a significant evaluation component.

19.5.4 *Follow-up*

If resources for primary health care technology assessment studies are scarce, so are resources for follow-up. The Health Council regularly revises reports on high technology. So does CBO for its consensus statements. However, an infrastructure for systematic follow-up is not available. The government has announced that it would like to transfer 5 per cent from the high-technology budget (hospital provisions regulated by Article 18) to facilities for continuous monitoring of the services concerned. This would mean an important change, but the necessary steps have not yet been taken, with one exception.

19.6 Conclusions

The Netherlands was one of the first countries to acknowledge technology assessment as a useful tool in health care policy. Various people involved in the health care field have expressed an interest in health care technology assessment, most notably the government, advisory bodies (experts, or representatives of health care organizations advising the government), health insurance companies, universities and other research organizations, industry, and—cautiously—medical professions. The past ten years have witnessed quite a number of actions and initiatives to stimulate health care technology assessment in The Netherlands, although important deficiencies in the technology assessment infrastructure can still be identified (197,280). Plans have been drafted to create a more systematic approach in the evaluation of new and existing medical technologies (77,195), but they have not yet been implemented fully.

20. Medical technology assessment in the USA[1]

The USA has an open, private health care system that does not do well at controlling technological change (587). None the less, the system is innovative and dynamic. Because of the lack of controls on technology, this chapter will concentrate on technology assessment programmes.

Today a number of organizations in government and the private sector have assumed responsibilities for assessing health care technologies in the USA. As a rule, these organizations have been created over time as a response to the perceived needs of society.

20.1 Regulation: an historical overview

In 1906, the Food, Drug and Cosmetic Act established the new Food and Drug Administration (FDA) to regulate the marketing of drugs and foods for safety. It was passed in response to unsafe and falsely advertised products, primarily of the home remedy or 'patent medicine' type. In 1938 an amendment requiring safety of drugs to be demonstrated through more rigorous and sophisticated testing was enacted, largely as a result of public catastrophes such as Elixir of Sulfanilamide deaths (399). In 1962 further drug amendments extended regulatory authority of the FDA to require that drugs be tested for efficacy as well as safety prior to marketing. Passage of this legislation was due, in large part, to the thalidomide tragedy (408).

FDA authority over the marketing of medical devices has lagged behind that of drugs. The 1938 amendments sought truth in labelling and provided some marketing control, but only if devices were 'adulterated' or 'misbranded'. By the 1970s, adverse affects of unsafe medical devices had been documented (36), leading to further amendments to the Food, Drug and Cosmetic Act in 1976 empowering the FDA to regulate the marketing of medical devices for safety and efficacy.

In the period following the 1965 Medicare and Medicaid Amendments to the Social Security Act, there arose a number of other legislative attempts to regulate the adoption and use of medical technologies due mainly to concerns about the ever-increasing cost of medical care. (Medicare is a national health

[1]Reprinted in part with permission from Williams and Torrens, Introduction to Health Services, Third Edition, Copyright 1988 by Detmar Publishers, Inc., Albany, New York.

insurance system mainly for the aged; Medicaid is a state-administered federal-state funded insurance programme for the poor.) In the late 1960s health planning legislation was passed that helped to spur state certificate-of-need (CON) legislation around the country. These laws were intended to guide the diffusion of capital-intensive technologies as well as to guide hospital bed capacity. In 1974, the federal planning legislation was greatly strengthened with the passage of the law establishing a network of health systems agencies (HSAs) around the country.

Other legislative routes were followed to regulate hospital utilization such as the requirement of Medicare that hospitals have utilization review committees and the enactment in 1973 of the national Professional Standards Review Organizations (PSRO) programme which was designed to conduct utilization review for Medicare beneficiaries.

Also during this period, Congress created the Office of Technology Assessment (OTA) to guide itself in the increasingly technological world in which it was operating. OTA's Health Program issued its first major report in 1976 outlining opportunities and needs for assessing medical technologies (492). Two years later, Congress established the National Center for Health Care Technology (NCHCT), whose mission was to 'set priorities' for technology assessment, and encourage, conduct, and support assessments, research demonstrations, and evaluations concerning health care technology (694). NCHCT was also to advise the Health Care Financing Administration (HCFA) on Medicare specific coverage policy issues. Before the Center could mature, it was defunded in 1981 largely as a result of the medical professions' and the medical device and pharmaceutical industries' belief that such co-ordinated government-controlled technology assessment activities unduly threatened the innovation process (532).

Following the demise of the NCHCT, there has been some efforts towards public–private partnerships to develop, guide, and carry out technology assessment policies as well as assessments themselves (352). In the late 1980s, the Institute of Medicine (IOM) of the National Academy of Sciences was given a federal charter to establish a Council of Health Technology Assessment. The federal government appropriated limited funding and required private matching monies. The Council was made up of senior officials from the various private parties of interest, such as insurers, hospitals, physicians, and health maintenance organizations, as well as academics. Federal ex officio members were also appointed. The IOM Council operated for several years, but ultimately failed to generate the requisite private funding support and no longer exists.

More recently, in 1991, there has been a move by the private insurance industry to be a catalyst for a similar co-ordinating mechanism for an assessment effort which is national in scope. Again, that effort appears to be failing to attract support from the medical products industry, without which the federal government seems reluctant to participate.

Today, there continues to be concern that technologies are not adequately and fully assessed prior to their diffusion and use in medical practice as discussed earlier in this chapter. The more prominent organizations whose mission includes the control or assessment of medical technologies are discussed below. Figure 20 shows the relationships of the principal organizations engaged in technology assessment in the USA. Each of these organizations will be discussed in turn.

20.2 The Food and Drug Administration (FDA)

The FDA can be considered the backbone of the government's medical technology assessment activities. It regulates entry into the US market of all drugs and relevant medical devices, requiring manufacturing firms to demonstrate that their products are safe and efficacious. Thus the FDA requires rather than conducts assessments (248). Specifically, it develops product standards, regulates testing, develops and/or approves clinical protocols, evaluates technical and clinical evidence given to it by manufacturers, and carefully regulates product labelling and advertising claims. It does no clinical testing itself.

The FDA generally requires that companies demonstrate safety and efficacy only as claimed in their labelling, not relative to other products or procedures. Thus, testing is usually done compared to a placebo.

20.2.1 Drug regulation

In order for drugs to enter the US market, the manufacturer must proceed through two major steps established by the FDA: (1) the investigational new drug (IND) application process, and (2) the new drug application (NDA) process (248). The IND process normally precedes testing in humans in the USA. The manufacturer describes the proposed clinical studies, the qualifications of the investigators, the chemical properties of the drugs, and the results of all pharmacologic and toxicity testing gained from laboratory animals as well as results from any available human studies, usually from other countries. If the FDA approves the IND application, the manufacturer may proceed with the NDA step, which consists of a three-phase clinical testing programme in humans, culminating in relatively large (usually 700–3000 patients) multisite randomized controlled trials. The results of these studies are then presented to the FDA for market approval. In some instances, additional 'Phase 4' post-marketing surveillance studies are required (248).

The entire drug development process leading to FDA approval reportedly takes as long as 7–10 years and is extremely expensive. When one includes the development costs of unsuccessful efforts, as much as $231 million is needed for each new chemical entity that reaches the US market (173).

20.2.2 Device regulation

The 1976 Medical Device Amendments to the Food, Drug and Cosmetic Act require that all medical devices be classified into one of three groups: Class I,

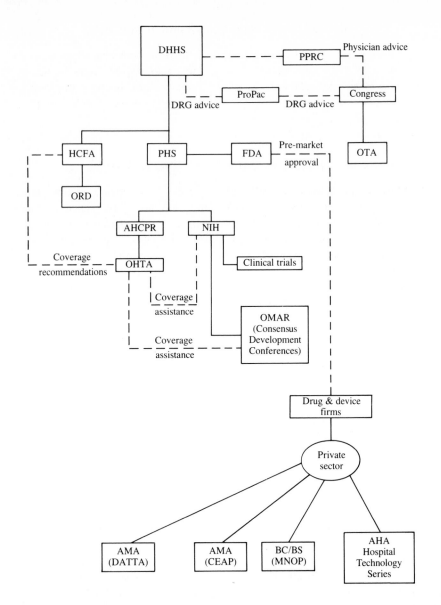

Figure 20. Relationships of technology assessment organizations in the USA, 1992.

(ACP, American College of Physicians; AHA, American Hospital Association; AHCPR, Agency for Health Care Policy and Research; AMA, American Medical Association; BC/BS, Blue Cross and Blue Shield; CEAP, Clinical Efficacy Assessment Project; DATTA, Diagnostic and Therapeutic Technology Assessment; DHHS, Department of Health and Human Services; FDA, Food and Drug Administration; HCFA, Health Care Financing Administration; IOM, Institute of Medicine; MNP, Medical Necessity Program; NIH, National Institutes of Health; OHTA, Office of Health Technology Assessment; OMAR, Office of Medical Applications of Research; ORD, Office of Research and Demonstrations; OTA, Office of Technology Assessment; PHS, Public Health Service; ProPAC, Prospective Payment Assessment Commission.)

general controls; Class II, performance standards; and Class III, pre-market approval.

In general, the approval process for medical devices is less onerous than that for drugs. Class I devices (e.g., medical and surgical supplies) essentially require only FDA notification of intention to market and are not closely regulated; Class II devices (e.g., non-invasive diagnostic test equipment) must pass general performance standards; however, Class III devices (e.g., pacemakers, total hip prostheses) are regulated for safety and efficacy and must pass through a clinical testing phase closer to those mandated for drugs (although much less demanding).

A manufacturer of a Class III device is required to file an investigational device exemption (IDE) application (which is similar to the IND drug process). The IDE permits the manufacturer to test the device in controlled settings on humans in order to establish its safety and efficacy. The resulting evidence is then submitted to the FDA in the form of a pre-market approval application (495,536).

20.3 The National Institutes of Health

The National Institutes of Health contribute to medical technology assessment by sponsoring clinical trials and by conducting consensus development conferences on specific medical practice issues.

The NIH's principal mission is to support basic and applied biomedical research in the USA. Although only 8 per cent of the total budget is spent on clinical trials, this amounted to nearly $610 million in 1990. The National Cancer Institute is the largest sponsor of such research, accounting for 40 per cent of all NIH monies spent on clinical trials, down from 59 per cent in 1985. The decrease is due to additional funding for AIDS research ($146 million, or 24 per cent) (480). While funded by the NIH, most trials are investigator-initiated by research clinicians from medical centres all over the USA.

20.3.1 *The Office of Medical Applications of Research*

Another major technology assessment activity of the NIH is the consensus development programme organized by the Office of Medical Application of Research (OMAR). Whereas the NIH-sponsored clinical trials are typically conducted on medical and surgical procedures in a very early phase of development, the consensus development conferences generally concern medical practice that is in a much more advanced stage of diffusion. Some topics (e.g., magnetic resonance imaging) are chosen because they are important or controversial new technologies; others (e.g., screening for cervical cancer) are chosen because they are widespread yet unresolved issues.

These conferences are meetings of experts to arrive at consensus regarding the appropriate use of a given medical technology. The experts are brought together in an open forum to review evidence of safety and efficacy/effectiveness of the

Table 13. NIH consensus development conferences.

Date	Conference title
1977	Breast cancer screening
1979	Intraocular lens implantation
1981	CT scan of the brain
1983	Critical care medicine
	Liver transplantation
1984	Lowering blood cholesterol to prevent heart disease
1986	Smokeless tobacco
	Magnetic resonance imaging
1991	Treatment of panic disorder

Source: ref. (481).

technology under study. The panel then secludes itself for a short period in order to reach consensus on a statement of what is known about the application of the technology and what it agrees is appropriate state-of-the-art practice.

NIH's objective in sponsoring these conferences is to transfer knowledge to the medical community rather than to create knowledge. The latter is the purpose of the clinical trials. Thus special attention is paid to disseminating the results of the conferences, first by holding a news conference, then by publishing the results in the *Journal of the American Medical Association* (*JAMA*) and by wide distribution of booklets summarizing the findings.

As of the end of 1991, 87 conferences had been held. Table 13 contains a selection of topics chosen to emphasize the diversity of subjects addressed.

20.4 The Office of Technology Assessment

The Office of Technology Assessment (OTA) is Congress' technology research and advisory body. Established by Congress in the early 1970s to assist in a better understanding of complex technological issues, OTA is divided into a number of programmes, including the Health Program within the Health and Life Sciences Division.

The main thrust of the OTA Health Program is to assist Congress in developing policies concerning medical technologies and their assessment. Its reports tend to be general in nature, drawing conclusions from evidence and expert opinion rather than specific assessments of individual technologies. For instance, OTA was instrumental in educating Congress and the country concerning the lack of safety, efficacy, and cost-effectiveness information of medical technologies.

Although general in scope, OTA's reports are often accompanied by one or many case studies of individual technologies. Even these case studies, however, are often syntheses of information rather than evaluations of primary data. Many assessments include not only cost, efficacy/effectiveness, and cost-effectiveness, but legal and ethical implications as well. By 1991 the OTA Health Program had generated 33 main reports of technology assessment issues plus over 60 case studies and other background papers and technical memoranda. Its 1992 budget is approximately $2 million.

Following a specific request from a major standing Congressional Committee, OTA typically conducts its studies by forming an advisory panel for each major topic, gathering evidence from the literature and expert opinion, writing a report on its findings, and circulating drafts of the report to a wide audience for criticism. It then releases its published report to the requesting committee.

OTA is credited with having guided Congress in a number of major technology issues, including legislation establishing the National Center for Health Care Technology in 1978 (which was defunded in 1981). OTA appoints both the Prospective Payment Assessment Commission (ProPAC) and the Physician Payment Review Commission (PPRC), both of which advise the Secretary of Health and Human Services on Medicare hospital technology policy (ProPAC) and physician policy (PPRC). It was also instrumental in passage of the law establishing the Institute of Medicine's Council on Health Care Technology (no longer in existence).

20.5 The Health Care Financing Administration

The Health Care Financing Administration (HCFA) is responsible for administering Medicare and the federal aspect of state Medicaid programmes. Its medical technology activities are mainly associated with coverage and reimbursement policies and, to a lesser extent, research and demonstrations.

New procedures are evaluated for coverage determination at as local a level as possible, and generally must pass a rather loosely defined test to determine whether they are reasonable and necessary (416). When coverage cannot be resolved at the local or regional level, HCFA's central office initiates a more formal process, first by referring the issue to its internal physician panel and then, if still unresolved, referring it to the Office of Health Technology Assessment (OHTA) within the Public Health Service (PHS) for an assessment and recommendation. A more structured coverage process which includes the assessment of cost-effectiveness is presently being proposed by HCFA (457).

The HCFA Office of Research and Demonstrations (ORD) conducts and sponsors some studies associated with medical technology and its assessments, but these studies are generally aimed at more general delivery and reimbursement of services than at individual technologies. An exception was the National Heart Transplant study in which the HCFA sponsored a study to help to determine its coverage policy. The ORD devotes a relatively small portion of its

$36 million research and development budget to technology assessment. A selection of previous ORD topics includes heart transplantation, kidney dialysis and transplantations, cyclosporin, magnetic resonance imaging, and implantable devices.

20.6 The Agency for Health Care Policy and Research

The Agency for Health Care Policy and Research (AHCPR) both sponsors extramural research for the study of technologies and their assessment and conducts assessments intramurally mainly through its Office of Health Technology Assessment (OHTA) in support of HCFA coverage policy.

The extramural programme consists of investigator-initiated research across all areas of health services research including especially medical outcomes research (the 'effectiveness initiative'), as well as topics in health care financing, organization, quality, and utilization; health information systems; the role of market forces in health care delivery; and health promotion and disease prevention and research related more directly to medical technology issues. AHCPR's budget in 1992 was $120.2 million.

20.6.1 *The Office of Health Technology Assessment*

Located within the AHCPR, the Office of Health Technology Assessment (OHTA) is primarily responsible for advising HCFA on coverage policy, assuming this role from the now defunct National Center for Health Care Technology (NCHCT). The Public Health Service (PHS) had previously assisted the Medicare programme in guiding coverage policy; however, when the NCHCT was created, the process became more formalized. In 1981, when NCHCT was deactivated, the then National Center for Health Services Research (NCHSR)—now called the Agency for Health Care Policy and Research—created the OHTA to continue that coverage advisory function for the HCFA.

As stated earlier, when the HCFA cannot resolve a coverage issue within its own system, it formally requests the Public Health Service to advise it. The PHS refers that request to the OHTA, which then publishes a notice to that effect in the Federal Register, requesting information and advice from interested and knowledgeable parties.

Traditionally, OHTA assessments have been concerned with safety and efficacy/effectiveness, not cost-effectiveness, and generally have addressed the acceptability and appropriateness of a procedure. In the past, PHS advice was to either cover or not cover a procedure without explicitly providing guidance as to the appropriate conditions of recommended use. More recently, however, OHTA is addressing the conditions under which a technology should be covered. For instance, in 1986, OHTA recommended to HCFA that heart transplants be covered, but only for persons aged 55 and under and only when performed in facilities meeting certain criteria (e.g., high volume, high success rate). In addition, HCFA has proposed coverage rules which include the assessment of cost-effectiveness of new technologies. Presumably, the OHTA will have a role in assessing cost-effectiveness.

The OHTA reviews and synthesizes existing data, literature, clinical trial evidence, and expert opinion, rather than collecting primary data. It also relies heavily on consultation with the relevant medical specialty societies and federal agencies such as the FDA and the NIH. Between 1981 and 1991, OHTA prepared over 160 coverage recommendations, nearly all of which were accepted by HCFA in its coverage policy determinations.

OHTA technology assessment efforts are guided by its National Advisory Council on Health Care Technology Assessment.

20.7 Prospective Payment Assessment Commission

As part of the 1983 Amendments to the Social Security Act, Congress established the Prospective Payment Assessment Commission (ProPAC) to advise and assist both Congress and the Secretary of The Department of Health and Human Services (DHHS) in maintaining and updating Medicare's Prospective Payment System (PPS). Appointed by the OTA, ProPAC has two primary responsibilities: (1) recommending to the Secretary the annual economic update factor for the entire system that includes an adjustment for changes in technology, and (2) recommending changes in the relative weights to the diagnosis-related groups (DRGs). (Medicare pays hospitals on a per admission basis. Admissions are divided into 367 groups called diagnosis-related groups, or DRGs). The latter responsibility requires ProPAC to study individual technologies as they apply to hospital in-patient care.

When a new technology begins to diffuse into the hospital environment, it must fit within some DRG that has been calibrated based on costs of previous practice patterns. If the new technology either decreases or raises costs of providing care, the DRG may no longer reflect the relative resource intensity of providing care and thus may inappropriately compensate the hospital for that cost. ProPAC's responsibility is to assist in determining whether and when a DRG needs to be created or recalibrated and what that change should be. Two examples illustrate the issues involved and the potential impact of the diffusion of important new technologies.

Magnetic resonance imaging was introduced in the 1980s. MRI is an expensive technology that can apply to a growing number of types of hospitalized cases (i.e., DRGs). The question becomes whether—and,if so, how—the Medicare prospective payment system (PPS) should be modified to reflect the additional costs of providing care. If no change is made, hospitals that adopt MRI are likely to lose money on such cases (126). If all relevant DRGs are increased to reflect the additional costs to the entire system, hospitals that are slow to adopt MRI will be overcompensated and hospitals that adopt MRI will be undercompensated (since the additional payment is spread across all cases). If an additional DRG 'add-on' is made for only those hospitals that adopt MRI or for only those cases where MRI is used, payment may be more equitable on a case-by-case basis, but such a method begins to resemble the previous inflationary cost-based system that the PPS was designed to reform. ProPAC's recommendation was to pay an add-on to the DRG for each scan. However, the HCFA has been reluctant to adopt such a policy, and did not take ProPAC's advice.

Extracorporeal shock-wave lithotripsy (ESWL) provides another example of the new technology-related DRG dilemma. Prior to the lithotripsy technology, the treatment of kidney stones in a hospital could be managed either medically or surgically, depending on clinical indications, with the surgical DRGs being roughly three times more expensive than the medical DRGs. Although the lithotripter is an expensive machine to buy and install, it crushes kidney stones non-invasively and thus tends to be more expensive per case than medical management but considerably less expensive than surgery. Fitting the lithotripsy into either category could either under- or overpay a hospital for adopting the technology. After studying hospital cost data, ProPAC recommended that the HCFA temporarily utilize the higher of the two medical DRGs that it calculated would just cover costs if the machine were used efficiently. The HCFA decided to simply pay ESWL within the existing medical DRGs (493).

Both MRI and ESWL are examples of the importance of ProPAC's role and the potential far-reaching effects of reimbursement policies on the adoption, diffusion, and ultimately, innovation and development of new technologies.

20.8 Other government agencies

A number of other governmental agencies in the USA conduct activities related to medical technology assessment. For instance, the Physician Payment Review Commission (PPRC) has a similar charter to ProPAC in terms of physician payment issues as well as technology-related concerns such as the development of practice guidelines. The new Medicare resource-based relative value scale (RBRVS) fee schedule is designed in part to lower procedure-based services relative to cognitive-based services. This results in lowering financial incentives for physicians to provide technologically-based services. PPRC advises on the new fee schedule system. The National Center for Health Statistics of the Public Health Service collects and disseminates information on health services utilization and health status of the US population and sponsors some relevant methodologic work such as the measurement of health-related quality of life. The Veterans Administration (VA) funds clinical and health services research, much of it related to technology, throughout the system. The Centers for Disease Control (CDC) supports assessments of technologies related to clinical laboratories and disease prevention and health promotion. The Department of Defense conducts some clinical trials, but most of its other medical technology assessment activities are limited to military applications.

20.9 Private sector technology assessment activities

Although public policies and agencies tend to dominate discussion of medical technology assessment issues, the private sector is also very active in this area by contributing funding and generating information.

20.9.1 *Pharmaceutical and device industries*

The pharmaceutical industry devotes enormous resources to the assessment of its products, as mentioned earlier in the discussion of FDA's job in regulating drug entry into the marketplace. The industry reports that 15.9 per cent ($6.8 billion) of its 1990 sales was devoted to research and development (535). As noted earlier, each new chemical entity requires 7–10 years and an average investment of $231 million (173,536). This investment includes all the pre-clinical and clinical trial research required for FDA pre-market approval.

The medical device industry also spends large amounts of money on assessments of its products, although on a much smaller scale than the pharmaceutical industry. A very rough estimate is that 6 per cent of sales in the major firms are devoted to research and development, which total almost $2 billion annually (323). In addition, the medical device industry probably devotes only about 4 per cent of its research and development (R&D) expenditures to clinical trials, in part because it takes less time to bring devices to the market and because FDA evidence of performance standards, safety, and efficacy is usually less rigorous than that required for drugs.

Recently, due to increased pressures from the more competitive marketplace exhibiting greater price sensitivity to costly new technologies, drug and device firms are increasingly investing in cost-effectiveness analysis (CEA) of their products (214). In some cases, firms are integrating economic analysis into pre-market clinical trials as well as sponsoring retrospective CEAs using existing literature and data sources such as claims files. These cost-effectiveness studies also differ from more traditional clinical studies by being comparative studies. That is, rather than being compared to placebo, the technologies are being examined for cost-effectiveness compared to competing choices of therapy; for example, coronary artery bypass surgery compared to percutaneous trans-luminal coronary arteriography (PTCA), a procedure that uses a balloon catheter to open restricted coronary arteries. A new phenomenon is the appearance of prospective economic clinical trials which are set up for the express purpose of examining cost-effectiveness in the real world but using a rigorous randomized design.

20.9.2 *Insurers, medical associations, and providers*

Most of the remaining technology assessment activities sponsored by private sector organizations rely on synthesizing existing information in order to assist technology policy-making. Very seldom are new data collected. In addition, most of these activities assess safety and efficacy issues rather than broader socio-economic concerns such as cost-effectiveness and legal and ethical implications. Sponsoring such activities are several of the more prominent health care organizations, including the Blue Cross and Blue Shield Association, the American Hospital Association, the American Medical Association, and the American College of Physicians.

All insurers must have some system to determine their coverage policy, just as Medicare must, although private insurers often take a 'follow the leader' approach. The leader may be the HCFA (for Medicare), or possibly the Blue Cross and Blue Shield (BCBS) Association. Blue Cross/Blue Shield consists of affiliated non-profit insurance firms throughout the USA. In other cases, such as in organ transplantation issues, the HCFA has been slower than commercial insurers in making coverage decision. Just as the HCFA relies on the Public Health Service, many insurers rely on the appropriate medical societies for guidance as well as having their own internal medical advisory panels.

A prominent and well-defined private insurer assessment activity is the Blue Cross and Blue Shield Association's Medical Necessity Program (MNP). Established in 1977, MNP attempts to assist in formulating coverage policy by selectively reviewing existing technologies in order to eliminate or reduce coverage for outmoded, ineffectual, and/or misused medical and surgical procedures. By 1985, the programme had identified over 90 procedures that were classified as outmoded, had called for the elimination of routine laboratory and X-ray testing, and developed guidelines for respiratory therapy. MNP uses the BCBS' Medical Advisory Panel and requests the co-operation from such medical societies as the American College of Physicians and the American College of Radiology to guide its assessments.

The American College of Physicians (ACP) sponsors the Clinical Efficacy Assessment Project (CEAP), an expansion of MNP (732). This programme relies on literature review and expert opinion from among its membership to review the appropriate application of established technologies used in the practice of internal medicine. The ACP distributes its reports to its membership and publishes its findings in *Annals of Internal Medicine*.

Other medical specialty societies also engage in activities which are at least related to technology assessment. For instance, physician groups such as the American College of Surgeons, American College of Cardiology and many others publish guidelines for the appropriate utilization of selected procedures and technologies relating to their respective fields of interest.

The American Medical Association (AMA) sponsors the Diagnostic and Therapeutic Technology Assessment (DATTA) programme, which is similarly designed to educate its membership of the value and appropriate use of technologies. DATTA tends to concentrate more on new and emerging diagnostic and therapeutic technologies. For each topic, the DATTA programme reviews existing evidence, formulates relevant questions, and surveys a panel of experts within the AMA's membership ranks. Findings are published in the *Journal of the American Medical Association*.

The American Hospital Association's (AHA) Hospital Technology Series is a programme that focuses on hospital devices and equipment from the hospital administrator's point of view. The evaluations are concerned primarily with the cost and service implications of technologies that are entering clinical practice. Evaluations are based on synthesis of technical reports and the professional literature as well as selected and focused interviews with technical and hospital experts. Findings are distributed to its membership as well.

There are also numerous less formalized technology assessment activities that are conducted throughout the USA by the providers of care, and the payers. Luce and Brown (431) recently conducted in-depth interviews with key individuals from hospitals, health maintenance organizations (HMOs), third-party payers, self-insured employers, and government health programmes to determine:

(1) how the organizations make purchase, coverage, and utilization decisions;

(2) what information is sought about medical technologies;

(3) what difficulties are experienced in using available technology assessment information;

(4) what the future holds for technology assessment.

All of the organizations interviewed were actively engaged in some level of assessment activities and use technology assessment in their decision-making. Their interest in technology assessment is based on the perceived need to be cost-conscious in purchase decisions and to determine treatment effectiveness before making coverage policy decisions. All respondents expected that technology assessment will continue to increase in importance and become one of the several *required* pieces of information used in the decision-making process.

They found that most institutions and organizations have committees responsible for assessing new technology before purchase or coverage policy decisions are made. The level of training and experience of committee members varied widely. Hospital staffs generally were less sophisticated and have other duties in addition to their assessment activities. HMO and third-party payer committees are likely to have more training in assessment methods and concentrate on assessment activities.

Most providers identify a threshold cost such as $100 000 to $250 000, above which formal assessments are required. Those technologies not meeting the threshold are typically assessed more informally at the department level in hospitals or HMOs. The assessments conducted by providers are primarily financial analyses of costs and 'pay-back' to make prudent purchaser decisions or a hunt for new technologies that might promote the hospital. Pharmacy formulary committees are separate from other assessment committees; all generally conduct more sophisticated assessments, including outcomes assessment and even cost-effectiveness analysis.

By contrast, third-party payers and the HMOs conduct assessments on both costly and controversial technologies and procedures. Patient outcomes are included when possible for HMO purchase and coverage assessments and are usually considered in insurers' coverage decisions. Long-term outcomes (e.g., survival over a year, rather than immediate outcome of the procedure) are considered by insurers if appropriate data are available.

The primary sources of technology assessment information used by providers and payers are peer-reviewed journals and information from manufacturers. HMO and third-party payers are more likely to include sources such as the Office of Health Technology Assessment (OHTA), the Office of Technology Assessment (OTA), medical specialty organizations and professional organizations such as the Health Insurance Association of America (HIAA) as sources of information. Occasionally providers or payers conduct or commission technology assessment research.

20.10 Conclusions

As this overview of several of the major organizations included in medical technology assessment in the USA indicates, the predominant activity is that of assessing existing information. The principal exceptions are the pharmaceutical and medical device firms who must generate primary data for FDA pre-market approval, clinical trials sponsored by the NIH, and to a much lesser degree other federal agencies. Institutions at all levels in the USA are intensely interested in medical technology assessment, and numerous assessment activities take place. Each class of institution, whether it be government, insurer, or provider, is assessing technology for its own consistency. Although there have been attempts to develop a co-ordinated policy, these efforts to date have failed.

21. The development and assessment of health care technology in Mexico

Carlos Cruz, Julio Frenk, Jaime Martuscelli, and Gladys Faba

21.1 The health care system

Mexico is a federal republic covering an area of almost 2000 square kilometers. The 1990 census reported a total population of 81.1 million inhabitants, 72 per cent of whom reside in urban areas (354). In 1989, the country had a gross domestic product (GDP) of 200 730 million dollars, with a GDP per capita of US$ 2010. The average annual growth rate was 3 per cent during 1965–1989. Mexico is a country with a heavy external debt of US$95 642 million.

The Mexican health care organization is characterized by segmentation of the health care system into three major components: the private sector, social security, and public assistance (260). The private sector is complex, with philanthropy, indigenous medicine, and growth of private health insurance and prepayment schemes. The major form, however, is represented by networks of solo or group practices with admitting privileges to modern hospitals. The private sector covers about 10 per cent of the population and has a disproportionate share of the resources.

Social security is the institutional segment that commands the greatest amount of resources and covers the largest number of people. A main feature of Mexican social security is that it is not only a financial instrument, but also operates its own health care facilities and hires its own medical and nursing staff. The dominant institution within this subsystem is the Mexican Institute of Social Security (IMSS), which covers all wage earners outside government and their relatives, plus agricultural labourers during the work season. In addition, federal civil servants and the armed forces have separate social security institutes.

The public assistance health care system provides health services for the rural and urban poor who do not participate in the formal sector of the economy. They work in subsistence agriculture, the underground economy, or are unemployed. The most important institution in this subsystem is the Ministry of Health, which also co-ordinates the ten semi-autonomous National Institutes of Health, in which advanced research and teaching activities are developed. In addition, the non-insured population benefits from the activities of a governmental organization called the National System for the Comprehensive Development of the Family, which is in charge of social assistance for vulnerable groups.

21.2 Science and technology in Mexico

Scientific and technological progress is embedded in a dynamic setting of society. Demographic, epidemiological, and economic changes all affect science and technology, and are affected by it. When the demographic and epidemiologic context is transformed, there is a change in needs which must be addressed. New challenges arise for science and technology that must be confronted. Such challenges have arisen in Mexico. For this reason, an adequate discussion of the scientific and technological policy of Mexico must first analyse its processes of change.

21.2.1 *The demographic transition*

The crude mortality in Mexico fell from 23.5 deaths per 1000 inhabitants in 1940 to 5.0 in 1988, a decrease of almost 80 per cent. There has also been a dramatic fall in the infant mortality rate: from 323 deaths per 1000 births in 1910 to 24 deaths per 1000 in 1985 (263). Furthermore, the fertility rate fell from 6.7 children for each woman of childbearing age in 1970, to 5.7 in 1975–76, to 4.3 in 1981, and 3.8 in 1986 (73). Thanks to this rapid drop in fertility, the population growth rate fell from 3.5 per cent per annum at the beginning of the 1970s—one of the highest in the world—to its present 1.9 per cent.

21.2.2 *The epidemiologic transition*

The classic pattern of the epidemiologic transition involves three fundamental transformations:

(1) a shift from a predominance of common infections as the leading causes of death to a preponderance of non-communicable diseases and injuries;

(2) a change in the age structure of mortality, with a growing importance of adult deaths, especially among the elderly;

(3) a change in the social meaning of disease, which is no longer an acute event that is resolved either by cure or death, but has become instead a chronic condition.

Countries do not necessarily go through the same stages of change in their epidemiology in a linear and unidirectional manner (261). In Mexico, the transitional experience is proceeding in a way different from that of industrialized countries. There are four distinguishing features of this new experience (263,264):

(1) an overlapping of stages (i.e., the simultaneous existence of high levels of 'pre-transitional' and 'post-transitional' pathology);

(2) countertransition (i.e., backward movements whereby some diseases that had been controlled, such as malaria, dengue fever and cholera, re-emerge);

(3) protracted transition (i.e., the lack of a clear resolution of the transition);

(4) epidemiological polarization (i.e., deeper social inequalities in health, as the poor and rural populations continue to suffer primarily from malnutrition and common infections, while urban dwellers face rising levels of chronic diseases and injuries).

This situation has created a protracted and polarized model in which inequalities continue, and may even worsen, resulting in the co-existence of pre- and post-transitional diseases within the ten leading causes of death. For example, by 1980, the leading cause of death in Mexico was diseases of the heart and circulatory system, just as in industrialized countries, but the sixth leading cause was acute respiratory infections and the seventh was intestinal infections (262). In a more detailed analysis, inequality is reflected in the distribution of diseases along different lines: geographic, economic, technological, and occupational (263).

21.2.3 The economic transition

In 1982 Mexico experienced the most serious economic crisis in its history, which gave rise to the implementation of adjustment policies to reactivate the economy (152). As a result, the Mexican economy did not grow for ten years, real wages decreased, reducing purchasing power by 55 per cent, unprecedented inflationary pressures were released, and the burden of the external debt stood in the way of any task undertaken by the government.

Nevertheless, the sacrifice entailed in the adjustment policy is now beginning to bear fruit. Since 1990 the economy has grown at rates higher than 4 per cent, inflation has gone down from three figures in 1988 to 16 per cent in 1991, public finances have been put on a sound footing, the debt burden has diminished, and there are signs of recovery in the real wages of some sectors.

Furthermore, spending on social welfare has been given special support, and health care expenditures have been substantially increased by the government. For example, the 1992 budget for health care increased by 10 per cent in real terms over that of 1991.

As part of its policy of economic opening, Mexico joined the General Agreement on Tariffs and Trade (GATT) in 1986, and in 1991 it began negotiations for a North American Free Trade Agreement with Canada and the USA (272).

A process of tariff deregulation, aimed at entering the so-called harmonized system, was also launched. This made the importation of inputs simpler and less expensive, while at the same time it spurred national industry, including the health care industry, into open competition in terms of quality and cost.

21.3 Consequences of the transitional process for health care demands

The transitions described have profound implications for the patterns of health care demand. A good example is medical attention at childbirth. Although the fertility rate has gone down markedly, the momentum produced by past high rates means that 2 900 000 births are projected for the year 2000, or 400 000 more than in 1988. At present, only 55 per cent of births are attended by qualified personnel, and there is a 45 per cent deficit of beds for confinement. If Mexico wants to achieve universal coverage, it will have to double its number of obstetrical beds by the year 2000. The economic implications of meeting these demands are considerable, and technological advances are needed to implement the most cost-effective measures (262).

Another consequence of the drop in fertility rates is the change in age structure, which is reflected in the rapid ageing of the population. The group aged 15–64 will expand from 53 per cent of the total in 1980 to 65 per cent in 2010, representing about 80 million people. This will increase the demand for care of chronic-degenerative diseases and injuries. In the same period, the population under 15 years of age will drop from 44 per cent to 29 per cent. Nevertheless, in absolute terms the younger age group will still expand from 30.6 million to 35.7 million. Finally, the proportion of people over 65 years will double, rising from 3 per cent to 6 per cent, and their absolute number will triple to more than 7 million, which will substantially increase demands for health care among the elderly (262).

The net result will be a rise in the absolute number of deaths, which will go from 462 000 in 1980 to 665 000 in 2010. There will be marked increases in the number of deaths caused by chronic diseases, accidents, and violence. These changes imply a greater demand for health care that must be met in the various stages of illness—whether in prevention, treatment, or rehabilitation.

The higher costs related to these increases in demand must be added to the additional expense of higher intensity and quality of care. This is true not only for medical attention and rehabilitation, but also in activities promoting health that require large investments of time and money to be effective.

To further complicate the picture, it should be stressed that infectious diseases still figure importantly among the leading causes of death. Therefore, it may be expected that there will be competition among types of pathology for scarce health care resources.

The foregoing projections all converge on one main conclusion: the health scene will grow increasingly complex during the next years. In this context, science and technology will be called on to provide appropriate responses.

21.4 Health care responses

Notwithstanding the economic crisis, the National Health System underwent a substantial transformation during the 1980s. A key element was the legal recognition of health protection as a constitutional right of all Mexicans. This recognition was based on a General Health Law, which explicitly guarantees the quality of services and makes a commitment to support a level of technology adequate to solve the different health care problems.

In order to raise the quality of services and cope with the crisis, the health care sector defined objectives, strategies, and lines of action. It also set priorities for medical inputs and supported the transfer and incorporation of emerging technologies.

21.5 Policies towards research and development

During the 1980s, a clear-cut scientific and technological policy was implemented in Mexico. The policy was expressed in the National Programme for Technological and Scientific Development 1984–1988, which proposed to increase self-determination in technology and to make research part of the flow of resources aimed at improving living conditions in Mexico.

In addition, a Health Research Regulation was enacted. Through this instrument, rules were laid down for the integration of committees on research, ethics, and biosafety in every organization conducting research. In addition, a united model for presenting research protocols was established. A major step was the organization of the National Registration System for Research and Technological Development in Health (115).

Important progress was achieved in collecting information on scientific activities, epidemiology, and health care services. A major effort was launched for the first time to conduct national surveys to document more precisely Mexico's epidemiological and demographic transitions (176,614,615).

As part of these efforts, the information gathered by the 1984 National Survey on Health Research made it possible to create an inventory of scientific and technological institutions and activities, as well as to quantify co-ordination and centralization problems. Thus, the survey revealed that 82 per cent of the country's research was conducted in Mexico City, and 72 per cent in health sector institutions.

This diagnostic exercise led to the creation of the Interinstitutional Commission on Health Research in 1985. The Commission is designed to co-ordinate the efforts of the health and educational sectors, thereby rationalizing the process of research and technological development.

21.6 Financing of research and development

As a result of the economic crisis, public funding of science and technology were progressively reduced from 0.54 per cent of the GDP in 1984 to 0.20 per cent in 1987 (141). There have been recent signs of recovery: by 1991 the budget for science and technology doubled to 0.38 per cent of GDP, which, however, is still insufficient and imprecise since the amount of private expenditures is unknown.

What is known is that between 25 and 35 per cent of public expenditure in science and technology goes to the health care sector. As a consequence, more than 40 per cent of Mexican scientific publications relate to the health field (225).

A fundamental shift in Mexico's science and technology policy has been the development of instruments to selectively channel funds towards projects of excellence and to subsidize high-level researchers. Thus, the larger budget of the National Council on Science and Technology (CONACYT) has been used to strengthen support for projects of excellence. A major effort has been the creation, in 1983, of the National System of Researchers, through which the government grants fellowships to researchers on condition that they remain active in their field and not contribute to the brain drain.

Another form of channelling funds has been through tax incentives to encourage technological innovations in export activities, research, employment, investment, and regional development.

Nevertheless, the private sector faces problems in financing continued technological development in the health field. In a survey of enterprises producing, distributing, and servicing medical equipment, the great majority of businesses reported that their chief problems were the delay and bureaucratic red tape involved in purchasing, the low volume of orders, the high cost of primary material, the lack of trained personnel, the difficulties in obtaining credit, and the high interest charged on bank loans. Moreover, 58.7 per cent of those surveyed stated that they needed financial assistance (151).

Because this situation affects the financial situation of businesses, there is a need to regulate, streamline, and expedite payments for goods sold to the public sector. It is also necessary to expand the market for medical technology by taking every advantage of new export possibilities.

The demand for increasing the percentage of public expenditure allocated to science and technology is not enough. In addition, there is the need to diversify the sources of financing, and this requires the active participation of the private sector. Indeed, research institutions face a dual challenge: on the one hand, to use public funds more efficiently; on the other, to intensify efforts to attract external financing for the development of specific projects, which could derive from national or international non-profit institutions, as well as from private enterprise. For this purpose, it is necessary to implement measures that support the integration of research and development centres with private firms. Mexico has established institutions of international standing that are underutilized by industry; the survival of both depends on their interaction.

Furthermore, in order to stimulate competition, the government, guided by the principle of efficiency, should develop a policy of financing strategic projects to obtain high-quality, low-cost results, regardless of whether these projects are carried out in public or private institutions. This will do away with practices that protect inefficiency in the public sector and will give impetus to scientific–technological development both in government institutions and in the private sector.

Finally, technological research and development should be encouraged in private sector companies. This is not only possible, but will also become imperative after the Free Trade Agreement is signed.

21.7 Technological inputs to health care

Because of the economic crisis, health care authorities had to place the highest priority on the evaluation of decisions concerning the purchase, transfer, and incorporation of inputs for medical use in order to ensure an efficient utilization of resources. The major tool was through the design and application of 'Essential Input Lists', which were established to regulate demand for strategic inputs such as medical devices, supplies, implants, prostheses, and drugs. In addition, a policy of consolidated purchase was adopted so that public sector institutions could obtain better prices by buying in large volume.

Through these actions, the costs of medical care were reduced and, at the same time, Mexican enterprises that were competitive in quality and price benefited, because preference was given to domestic suppliers in awarding contracts. In this way, the government used its purchasing power to stimulate industrial development.

Another area of systematization was the effort to clearly structure the health care system into levels, each with standard facilities according to their technological complexity. Manuals were prepared for each standard facility regulating the material inputs and personnel to be made available and specifying the technology required, according to size, complexity, location, and level of medical care.

As can be seen, there have been significant advances in regulating and controlling key elements of the scientific and technological processes. Nevertheless, there is still much to be done, especially with respect to the process of assessing technology in its different stages.

21.8 Policies towards pharmaceuticals

As a result of the economic crisis, there was an acute shortage of pharmaceuticals at the end of 1982, mainly because 80 per cent of their manufacture depended on importing primary and intermediate products, for which there was no foreign exchange. To remedy this situation, the government implemented the Comprehensive Program for the Development of the Pharmaceutical Industry. Its purpose was to accelerate consolidation of domestic manufacturers in order to continue supplying drugs to the public and to protect national sovereignty (420).

In addition, the government drew up an Essential Drug List, which helped to rationalize prescription. Competitive bidding was organized and consolidated so that the purchase of pharmaceutical products would be conducted openly and without any irregularities. Thanks to these actions, in 1988 it was possible to save 50 per cent of the volume of originally stipulated drugs, which permitted the Ministry of Health to broaden medication coverage. Also, by defining the demand for drugs, it was possible to encourage the domestic industry to promote research and technological development in the pharmaceutical sciences. In this way, Mexican production of the primary and intermediate materials used in drug manufacturing rose from 20 per cent in 1982 to 55 per cent in 1988, under guidelines designed to ensure quality and competitive prices in the world market (636).

None the less, there are still serious problems in applying the Essential Drug List. In 1988 an analysis was made of prescription practices in a survey of 2782 clinical consultations at 164 health care centres in Mexico City and in nine states. It was found that 71 per cent involved medication and that two-thirds of the drugs prescribed did not appear in the Essential Drug List, with a marked use of multiple drugs (196).

Regarding the mechanism of consolidated purchase, initial data indicated that drugs were overpriced in Mexico by 300 per cent as compared to the prices registered in the World Health Organization. Applying the consolidated purchase policy brought prices down to an average of 125 per cent (466).

Another important aspect of pharmaceutical policy was the creation of a centre to concentrate information on reactions. Instruments were further strengthened to raise the quality, safety, and efficacy of drugs. More emphasis was placed on sanitary inspection, analytical sampling, quality control, and process validation in the pharmaceutical industry. This made it possible to prepare a programme for qualification of producers, which by the end of 1988 covered 85 per cent of the industry.

In conclusion, it should be remembered that Mexico's pharmaceutical policy has a solid tradition dating back to 1960 when the Mexican Institute of Social Security created and adopted the concept of essential drugs. This concept preceded the list of essential drugs drawn up by the WHO, and it contains drugs for treatment of 97 per cent of national pathology, serving as a guide for rational prescription. It is still necessary, however, to support more strongly research in clinical pharmacology, herbal medicines, and biotechnology.

21.9 Policies towards medical devices and other inputs

Health care inputs have suffered from weak linkages between industry and research and development centres. The 1984 National Health Research Survey found that 224 research projects were engaged in developing a technological product; of these, 22 were trying to produce a medical prototype or device. In 1987, a follow-up survey was conducted that found that only 18 projects were still active and that none had been transferred to the industrial sector.

In turn, industry has little contact with research and development centres. A survey of businesses found that 39.9 per cent were interested in promoting closer relations and, of these, only 40 per cent were doing something about it (151).

In addition to its lack of interaction with R&D centres, industry has failed to establish specific areas for introducing research findings. This means that such findings are underutilized, opportunity costs are high, there is still a brain drain due to lack of motivation, problems remain unsolved, and mechanisms become outdated due to the absence of effective communication channels.

In order to resolve these problems, a Centre for Technological Innovation was created at the National Autonomous University of Mexico in 1987. In addition, under new policies for financing research, the National Council on Science and Technology made one of its priorities the establishment of a strategy for incorporating scientific–technological advances.

It should be noted that little has been done traditionally to develop technological innovations both in Mexico and Latin America as a whole. About 95 per cent of the technologies incorporated into Latin America's health care services are imported (529). Medical equipment prototypes are primarily designed by agencies affiliated with large foreign companies, and there are few national institutions and domestic firms that have systematically attempted to develop prototypes. A study found that only 23 per cent of the companies selling medical devices in Mexico produced such items, whereas 70 per cent were distributors of products, mainly imported, and the remaining 7 per cent provided installation and maintenance services and sold accessories and spare parts (151).

To give an idea of the magnitude of Mexico's external dependence, in 1984 it was found that 75 per cent of the medical–surgical items listed in the Essential Inputs List of the Health Care Sector were imported. Therefore, they could be included in a strategy of import substitution on competitive terms (639).

There has been scant investment in technological research and development in private industry, with only 59 per cent of businesses planning expansion. Worse yet, the universe of companies surveyed invested very little in research and technological development, with 66 per cent of them making no investment in such activities in 1988.

21.10 Policies towards the assessment of health care technology

An analysis of the processes of manufacturing or of simply importing health care technologies in Mexico highlights two facts: first, the weakness of the material and institutional infrastructure to ensure competitive production; second, the absence of a system for evaluation and follow-up of existing technologies and for assessment of new technologies.

As a consequence, Mexico suffers from the absence of an information system to assist in making present decisions that would also take into account future needs, especially in light of the process of demographic and epidemiologic transition that Mexico is experiencing.

It is also necessary to make a more thorough evaluation of the process of assimilating medical technologies, which is regarded as a simple acquisition without considering such important aspects as morbidity and mortality conditions, cultural and social heterogeneity, and economic consequences.

Typically, the purchase of medical devices and especially of equipment has ignored the need for an infrastructure that guarantees not only the installation and start-up of the equipment, but also its maintenance and continued operation. In other words, the incorporation of technologies is not seen as part of a long and complex process that includes everything from the conditions of the physical installation of equipment to the professional and technical training of those who operate it.

This situation has caused various difficulties in operating equipment and in keeping it working properly. It has been found, for example, that in primary health care units where relatively unsophisticated technology is used, five or six different brands of equipment have been incorporated. This makes maintenance more complicated and means that about 30 per cent of the equipment used in these units is not in working order due to lack of maintenance and shortage of spare parts. The equipment breaks down sooner than expected because those who operate it lack technical training, which also means that more mistakes are made and that the equipment is not operating at full capacity (177).

To face the problems of maintenance and assessment, the Centre for Technological Development and Applications was established by the Ministry of Health in 1983. Guidelines were laid down for operative units that would guarantee the processes of installation, use, and maintenance in order to utilize medical equipment more rationally.

21.11 Conclusions

A first conclusion is that changes in the demographic and epidemiologic profile in Mexico will alter demand at all levels of health care. Therefore, the technology needed will have to change. It is thus imperative to make health care more efficient so that it serves as a means of redistributing income and ensures that everyone has access to services. This will require a number of steps:

(1) a redefinition of priorities;

(2) more emphasis on health promotion and disease and injury prevention;

(3) new approaches to managing chronic diseases, relying on the primary care level;

(4) comprehensive training of providers to meet the new demands;

(5) modification and updating of procedures to build medical facilities and purchase equipment;

(6) more effective processes of supervision and evaluation;

(7) an increase and diversification of the sources of financing, in which the private sector should participate more actively.

A second conclusion is that during the 1980s Mexico was able to establish both a legal framework and effective guidelines for scientific and technological development. The regulation of demand by means of basic lists, consolidated purchase, and standardization of the type of inputs included at each health care level are of special interest. Also worth mentioning are the information policy on and for research and the creation of centres for research and technological development with links to industry. Nevertheless, much remains to be done, such as updating the basic lists, permanently monitoring the standard-setting process, and consolidating the newly created centres.

A third conclusion is that financing sources should be expanded and diversified in order to accelerate technological development and cope with growing demands. This situation calls, first, for an increase in government expenditure on science and technology, with selective channelling of resources towards priority research and excellence groups. The private sector should actively participate both in financing and in developing projects, thereby establishing a plural system.

A fourth conclusion is that there are two strategic areas of intervention regarding health care inputs. The first refers to the need for closer links between industry and research centres. The second deals with the development of interface mechanisms that manage the introduction of research findings and innovation into health care organizations and into industry.

Finally, there is a pressing need to designate a specific authority within the health sector to supervise and evaluate every aspect of the use of technology. Above all, there should be a comprehensive view on acquisitions, taking into account not only price and sales conditions, but also further support services. There should be more emphasis on programmes for preventive and corrective maintenance, and functional inventories should be made to keep track of the state of equipment and devices.

Although much of what is needed to support technological development in health has already been put in place, more attention should be paid to the scientific assessment of technologies in order to make health care services more effective, efficient, and equitable.

The Mexican experience in health care technology can offer alternative solutions to similar problems in other countries. Clearly, we must invent new cooperation strategies that respond to the challenges of an era of global integration.

22. Medical technology in China

H. David Banta and Chen Jie

22.1 The Chinese health care system

China is the most populous country in the world, with more than 1 billion people. During the decades following World War II, Chinese health policy focused on the control of communicable diseases, development of primary health care, and better sanitation and nutrition. Life expectancy increased from an estimated 35 years in 1949 to 69 years in 1986 (746). As a result, China is facing disease patterns typical of more developed countries, with rising rates of chronic diseases.

The Ministry of Public Health (MOPH) is responsible for overall policy direction and implementation. Each province has a provincial bureau of public health that relates to the MOPH. China's system is public, with very limited private practice. Essentially all institutions are publicly owned, and personnel are salaried. They are not directly budgeted, but collect fees for services, including hospitalization days.

Between 1981 and 1986, state expenditures on health increased rapidly. By 1987, total health spending was equivalent to about 20 per cent of the national budget and roughly 4 per cent of gross domestic product (746). Payment sources are very varied and complex, and include government subsidies, insurance payments, and self-pay. As indicated below, public payments to hospitals have been systematically lowered during the last years, which means that private payment has been increasing. In fact, the great majority of rural people now have no health insurance. The majority of urban residents have compulsory, state-subsidized health insurance (746).

22.2 Technology transfer to China

Part of the process of modernization for any developing country is to develop a health care system that incorporates modern health care technology. During the last few decades, China has invested considerably in the health care technology of the West. This has led to certain problems. In particular, Chinese policy-making is not based on information on the benefits, risks, and costs of specific technologies.

Traditional Chinese medicine has developed over the course of thousands of years. Western medicine was imported by missionaries beginning in the 1700s. During this century, Western influences have become more and more important in the Chinese health care system. After national liberation in 1949, international contacts changed mainly to the USSR and Eastern European countries, and contact with the West was very limited (123). A series of agreements with these socialist countries led to importation of some technology. However, this aid ended with the break between China and the USSR in 1961.

Subsequently, trade with Japan increased. The Nixon visit to Chairman Mao, as well as growing contact with other Western countries, opened the possibility of increased trade and imports, including medical imports. From the early 1970s to 1977, China imported a total of US$4 billion worth of equipment and technology in all sectors (123). This may be illustrated by the US experience. According to US Commerce Department figures, US exports of medical equipment to China rose from US$413 thousand in 1978 to US$45.9 million in 1986 (339). In addition, China sought foreign investment, long-term loans, Chinese–foreign joint ventures, and the creation of special economic zones. Since the early 1970s, China has sent an estimated 5000 health care professionals and students to study in the West, both for short and for long periods (339). In particular, the awareness and knowledge of modern medical technology has increased dramatically during this period. Chinese physicians and planners have sought to learn about Western technology and to acquire it (324). Imports of drugs and medical devices increased dramatically. Joint ventures with such drug companies as Squibb, and Smith, Kline and French have been developed. In 1992 there were no joint ventures in the area of medical equipment, although several were being discussed. More recently, China has focused on developing local resources.

22.3 Development of the drug industry

The Western drug industry developed rapidly in China in the period following World War II. Since 1979, the State Pharmaceutical Administration (SPAC) has supervised pharmaceuticals and medical instruments; its National Medical Instrument Corporation is in charge of policy, regulations, and guidelines concerning research, production, distribution, import, and export of medical instruments; its China National Pharmaceutical Corporation is responsible for the production of drugs; its National Drug Corporation is responsible for marketing drugs; and its China National Herbal Medicine Corporation is responsible for overseeing traditional Chinese medicine (27). The great majority of the 1452 manufacturers are under the State Pharmaceutical Administration and its provincial and local components; a few come under the agriculture ministry or other government bodies.

By 1980, although the production of drugs was growing, imports had also grown rapidly and the reputation of Chinese drugs was poor. With the assistance of the World Bank and other Western institutions, including the US Food and Drug Administration (FDA), China set out to modernize its industry.

Modernization involved a series of actions. One was to close marginal factories and merge others. The number of manufacturers fell from about 1900 to

1452, largely because of inability to meet quality standards. At the same time, large investments were made in training and new equipment. The result, according to SPAC spokespeople, is few problems with quality at present. Production is distributed mainly through hospitals (90 per cent), and the remainder through drug stores.

Quality was assured through the passage of a 1984 law developing a regulatory process for safety and efficacy of drugs. The manufacture and regulation of the quality of drugs is based on international standards as stated in the Chinese pharmacopoeia that was based particularly on the British model. The regulatory process is overseen by the Ministry of Public Health (MOPH), through its Drug Biological Production Quality Control Institution and counterpart institutions at all levels of government. The provincial institutes inspect hospitals, factories, and drug stores and carry out tests of drugs. Clinical trials for drugs are carried out at the provincial level, but approval can only be at the national level. The World Bank assisted with loans to purchase precise equipment for testing drugs from the West, and animal laboratories and other facilities have been developed. The MOPH has also developed two national training centres to upgrade staff in drug control institutes.

Production of all drugs rose in value from 10.5 billion RMB in 1984 to 19.2 billion RMB in 1987 (1 RMB = US$3.7). At the same time, imports of drugs have been increasingly limited under the 1984 law. By 1988, only drugs considered essential were imported. China is now self-sufficient in drugs, importing only a few difficult-to-manufacture drugs such as those for cancer chemotherapy. Less than 100 drugs are imported. The total imports of drugs were US$150 million in Western drugs and US$30 million Chinese traditional drugs in 1987. This means that China produces about 99 per cent of the drugs that it uses. In fact, China has become an exporter of drugs. Exports were US$400 million in Western drugs and US$200 million in Chinese traditional drugs in 1987.

The situation with vaccines parallels that of drugs. China is officially self-sufficient in vaccines. These vaccines, however, have quality problems, including low titres of viruses. China has gained outside assistance in improving its manufacturing facilities for vaccines.

Traditional Chinese drugs are another category, not much changed by developments in the Western drug area. Regulators seek methods of assuring quality of traditional drugs, but since in most cases the active ingredients of these products are not known, there is a limited basis for such regulation. Regulation often must fall back on such methods as microscopic examination to assure that herbal preparations are relatively pure.

22.4 Development of the medical device industry

Attempts have also been made to develop a medical device industry (27). These attempts, though, came later and have not been as effective. In part, the problem is the fact that drugs must be developed in a separate industry, whereas devices can be made in general factories, as in the electronics or computer industry.

Thus, in China devices tend not to be well-suited to their specific application. China has obviously not mastered all Western technology. For example, active attempts were made to develop a Chinese computed tomography (CT) scanner, but the national product was very poor (338).

As mentioned above, the National Medical Instrument Corporation plays a key role in production of medical instruments and machines. The National Commission on Machinery has similar responsibilities for non-medical equipment, but which may be needed in the health care system; for example, computers, vehicles, and laundry equipment. The Ministry of Electronic Industry is also involved in certain electronic devices that may be required in the health care system. The number of factories under the National Medical Instrument Corporation producing medical equipment and materials has risen from 240 in 1978 to 373 in 1987. The industry does well in meeting needs for normal equipment, but has problems with producing high-quality sophisticated equipment. A number of examples of poor-quality devices can be identified: X-ray machines above 500 ma, gastroscopes, dental chairs, automatic biochemical analysers, centrifuges, specialized microscopes, ambulances, gamma cameras, and linear accelerators.

A related problem is that of shortages. X-ray film particularly is in short supply, which leads to a pervasive use of fluoroscopy. Spare parts for equipment and reagents for diagnostic equipment are also in short supply. In general, maintenance of equipment seems well-handled by Chinese hospitals. However, the wide variety of equipment in China raises particular problems of servicing, spare parts, and calibration. One large hospital could have equipment from a number of countries, requiring fluency in different languages and raising difficulties of stockpiling spare parts.

The issue of quality, which is acknowledged by officials of SPAC, has not been effectively addressed in China. There is no attempt to regulate the quality of equipment in China. The marketplace is left largely to itself. Training of workers is not adequate, nor are components and materials. Profits for the industry are also poor. The result is a poor product and a strong preference for Western imports.

There has been, however, a small programme for the regulation of radiological devices since 1978. The programme is based on protecting providers and patients from excessive radiation, while replacing X-ray equipment with more adequate machines as rapidly as possible.

In the years 1981–1986, the SPAC estimates that China imported US$880 million in medical equipment, 70 per cent of the Chinese product value. Sources in the Ministry of Public Health estimate 1987 imports as 230 million RMB. According to the United Nations, in 1988 China imported US$34.5 million in medical equipment from the USA, more than US$10 million from Western Europe, and US$72.7 million from Japan (201). In general, Japanese equipment seems to be preferred, both because of lower transportation costs and because of better service. Exports of medical equipment were US$300 million in the same years (1981–1986)—600 items, mostly needles for Chinese traditional medicine, small X-ray machines, electronic medical equipment, and health materials.

The official Chinese policy is to discourage imports of technology and to encourage the development of local industry. In practice, however, imports from outside are not effectively regulated. Decisions concerning imports occur at a multiplicity of levels. For the 13 medical schools that are part of the national Ministry of Public Health, imports come from the budget of the Ministry and are controlled by the Ministry of Finance. In most cases, however, the only effective control is access to foreign currency.

Despite the policy of discouraging imports, the Chinese policy in practice responds to the pressure to obtain Western medical equipment. The fee system for hospitals, to be described below, gives large incentives for the provision of some services based on Western equipment. A hospital administrator can acquire modern equipment and use it to gain additional resources for investment in the hospital sector (339).

22.5 Purchase of medical equipment by hospitals

Domestically made equipment can be purchased with great freedom at all levels, subject to budgetary constraints. Grants are also available from government for equipment purchase. If a hospital obtains approval from its own level of government, it can usually get special support for large equipment, but most equipment is purchased from recurrent costs. The provinces tend to have informal guidelines for medical equipment, but do not have explicit plans. The MOPH has standards for medical equipment intended mainly to encourage the purchase of modern medical equipment.

The principle that imports should only be allowed when a reasonable domestic product is unavailable is administered (or co-ordinated) by the State Economic Commission. Imported equipment is given a priority if the need for equipment cannot be met domestically either because national equipment is of poor quality or because of a serious shortage. Access to foreign currency is controlled by the planning commission of the appropriate level of government. A large number of types of medical equipment are subject to controls by the State Economic Commission, including endoscopes, X-ray machines, ultrasound, electron microscopes, laboratory equipment, and so forth. Some of these are controlled at the provincial level and some by the central government. A prospective purchaser must apply for an import license. Without approval, the import is not possible. In practice, larger and more specialized hospitals can often justify the import because of stated specifications that are not available in Chinese-made equipment. Smaller hospitals must usually buy the national product. Larger hospitals often take out loans for equipment that can be rapidly paid off.

22.6 Payment for health care technology

Physicians and other health care providers have no financial incentives to over-use technology, but the payment to hospitals does include inappropriate incentives. The payment system is state-regulated. Regulation is co-ordinated by the State Price Bureau, which decentralizes actual control to the provincial level.

The principle followed under guidelines of the State Finance Bureau is that the price for new services should be set at the level of cost, minus salaries (which are covered separately). The provincial price bureau sets a fee for each service; prices are typically set for about 1500 separate items, including the day-bed rate. Before the 1960s, medical care costs were basically set according to actual costs. However, in the 1960s, the government stated a general policy that health care should be seen as a social service, and prices were lowered three times during the 1960s. In provincial hospitals, only two thirds of their costs were covered by fees. The result of this action was higher and higher government subsidies, to keep hospitals solvent. In 1985, prices began to be increased. Eventually, they should be restored to the 1952 level. The result is that fees are considerably below cost for most established services such as surgical procedures.

However, the policy for some years has been that the payment for drugs is set above costs at the hospital level. The policy of the price bureau is that hospitals pay a controlled wholesale price for drugs and then can mark them up by 10−18 per cent (13 per cent on average). The mark-up is higher for traditional medicine drugs, about 20 per cent. There is an obvious incentive for over-prescription.

For new procedures it is difficult to establish costs, so prices are often set by negotiation. Hospitals therefore have an incentive to acquire new equipment that can bring in a higher fee. If they can obtain the equipment from outside sources, such as provincial equipment budgets, their incentive is even higher. A number of new technologies have fees set above costs. The CT scanner is the most prominent example. The fee is typically more than 200 RMB per scan, with a cost of perhaps half that amount. Shanghai Medical University evaluated 20 CT body scanners and calculated that the cost of operating the scanners was 384 000 RMB, while they generated an income of 1 547 000 RMB, for a profit of about 1 150 000 RMB. Four MRI machines generated a profit of more than 3 million RMB. Fees for laboratory services (by automated equipment), ultrasound examination, coronary care units, and renal dialysis (and others) are set above costs. The State Price Bureau allows this situation to encourage new technology and to give hospitals income to break even. However, one result is an overuse of those technologies, and, more importantly, it has led to a situation of techno-logical development in large, central hospitals outside the context of any plan or set of priorities. For example, specialized cancer hospitals mainly see far-advanced cancer because there has been limited attention to the problem of early diagnosis or screening at the local level.

22.7 Distribution and use of technology in the Chinese health care system

Drugs are relatively available at all levels of the Chinese health care system. In fact, the utilization of pharmaceuticals is quite high. Pharmaceuticals account for 58 per cent of total health expenditure; Western drugs (made in China) consume 49 per cent of total health expenditure. An average of 2.3 drugs is prescribed at each patient visit. It is generally acknowledged in China that overuse of drugs is a key problem. This particularly applies to antibiotics and tranquilizers. In general, drugs can be bought freely in drug stores without a prescription. In theory, a prescription is required for narcotics and psychotropic drugs; however, at lower levels, these drugs may be dispensed directly by personnel such as rural doctors. Drugs bought in drug stores are paid for by the person directly; drugs acquired by prescription are given out by hospital pharmacies and may be covered by insurance.

High-technology equipment tends to be concentrated in large, urban hospitals. In 1987, the Ministry of Public Health carried out a survey concerning selected pieces of equipment in 13 medical universities and 33 affiliated hospitals. The survey showed an impressive number of medical devices, especially diagnostic equipment, in these institutions. This confirms personal impressions that Chinese physicians have a tendency to be fascinated by diagnosis and pay relatively little attention to the contribution of this technology to therapy or patient outcome (339).

Surveys in provinces have shown a relatively good supply of equipment in medium-level municipal hospitals. Otherwise, medium-level and smaller hospitals are relatively poor in equipment. Local clinics are generally poorly equipped. They have primitive laboratories and X-ray machines are technically inadequate and often out of service. Therapeutic options are limited, although the drug supply is extensive.

There are many questionable investments, especially in diagnostic equipment. Vectorcardiographs and polygraphs for collecting data on multiple cardiac functions are common. Another technology beginning to diffuse into China is electronic fetal monitoring, which is not known to be of value (47,677). Outmoded diagnostic equipment is in widespread use, especially in cardiology.

The CT scanner and MRI scanner may be used as examples of the maldistribution of sophisticated technology (339,338). The Ministry of Public Health estimates that there were 170 CT scanners in China in 1986. CT scanners were unevenly distributed across the country, with the highest number by population in Beijing, with 27, for a population rate of about 2.9 per million population. Shaanxi province, with a population of 29 million, had three CT scanners. By 1992, Beijing had 50 scanners. Apparently, institutions in Beijing have easier access to government resources and can more easily get approval than hospitals in other areas. In 1992, the city of Hongzhou, with 1.5 million people, had 12 CT scanners. In 1991, Shanghai Medical University found that there were 15 CT scanners in Shanghai. The cities of Baoji, Jiujiang, and Jiuhua had no CT scanners in 1991. Shanghai had four MRI machines, while the other three cities had none. There was rapid diffusion of CT scanners in 1991–1992, apparently because of increased prices. Physician bonuses were developed by hospitals, giving physicians a strong financial incentive to use modern technology.

Cardiac monitoring and resuscitation equipment is common. This capability is often underutilized, indicating a lack of planning for appropriate siting and referral. Chronic renal dialysis is another example of an expensive technology in the early phase of diffusion.

22.8 Traditional Chinese medicine

Although the official policy in China is that traditional medicine and Western medicine should be integrated, this policy is not well-developed at the local level. In fact, two establishments have developed: a traditional medicine establishment with its own practitioners and hospitals (also seeking Western equipment and drugs) and a Western medicine establishment in which hospitals include a department of traditional medicine and the pharmacy stocks both Western and traditional drugs.

From the standpoint of technology, Chinese traditional medicine has produced practices of undoubted efficacy, such as acupuncture. Almost all Chinese believe that traditional medicine has many efficacious practices and drugs. Traditional medicine physicians state that their practice cannot be evaluated by Western means, such as controlled clinical trials. The merit of this statement is difficult to see. In the long run, traditional medicine needs to be evaluated for its effects on health in the same way that Western medicine should be evaluated.

22.9 Quality assurance in China

Many actions can be seen as promoting increased quality in health care. For example, improving medical education or building new hospitals are indirectly responsible for promoting better quality of care. Such actions are not considered in this section, which deals only with national policies addressed to assuring quality. Attempts to assure quality of health services in China are quite undeveloped.

There has been some attention to the issue of quality of laboratory testing. Some countries regulate clinical laboratories and evaluate the precision of their test results. In China, a programme modelled on Western efforts using blind testing of samples has been initiated by the Ministry of Public Health. This programme applies only to a few of the largest hospitals.

Although there is a small programme to promote radiation safety in the MOPH, radiological technicians and physicians working with X-rays do not commonly wear film badges or other monitoring devices. Shielding of machines is inadequate. Appropriate gloves and aprons are not available. Patients also are not appropriately shielded.

Peer review in an organized sense does not seem to exist in China. Evaluation of services in terms of outcomes is rarely done outside the area of drug regulation.

22.10 Evaluation and assessment of technology

In China, assessment of health care technology is a new idea. The standard effectiveness tends to be one of personal experience rather than controlled clinical trials. The term 'cost-effective' is unfamiliar to policy-makers and health care providers. Decisions made with regard to the purchase of medical equipment generally do not include an element of scientifically derived information on effectiveness and safety. The situation is somewhat better in the area of pharmaceuticals, as described above, but only at the regulatory level. Use of drugs seems often to be irrational.

The result is that Chinese hospitals are full of technologies that are unproven or obsolete. Industry promotion, especially from Japan, is leading to the rapid diffusion of newer technologies of unknown value. In addition, traditional Chinese medicine is widespread with limited attempts to assess its efficacy.

This situation may be changing. For several years, the national Ministry of Public Health (MOPH) has supported studies of medical technology, focusing on financial issues. The Medical University of Shanghai has been studying health technology diffusion and cost-effectiveness. Policy-makers in Beijing have shown a strong interest in the principles and implications of such tools as cost-effectiveness analysis.

The World Bank has given strong encouragement to this effort. In its current health loan project, carried out in three provinces, technology assessment has been part since the beginning. Each province was expected by the MOPH to establish a technology assessment activity. The MOPH itself has established a small office for this purpose. In 1991, the MOPH sponsored a national seminar on technology assessment, aimed primarily at staff of the three provinces and the MOPH itself. In 1992, another national seminar was held. At that seminar, the MOPH announced that national centres for health care technology assessment would be developed at Shanghai Medical University and Beijing Medical University.

22.11 Conclusions

Modernization of health care in China has been rapid. However, much of the investment in technology has been without real attention to its benefits and costs.

The decision was made to develop and import modern technology. In implementing this policy, China has aggressively sought Western technology. The result is a system of large specialized hospitals, often with quite modern medical equipment, but with an inadequate supporting infrastructure of community hospitals and clinics. The greatest policy problem is the nature of the payment system, which gives large and inappropriate incentives for purchase and utilization of certain 'high' technologies.

China has taken certain steps to develop a mechanism for guiding decisions based on best available knowledge on risks, benefits, costs, and social implications of specific health care technologies. There is now a need to address problems in the policy structure, particularly the issue of inappropriate incentives.

23. Selected experiences of other countries

The development of health care technology is an international activity. Biomedical researchers in different specialized fields work hard to know exactly the state of research in their own areas, especially through reading journals and attending international conferences. Industry is international as well, with a large multinational industry dealing with health products. A health research finding anywhere in the world may lead to a technology.

Likewise, health care technology itself is international. Only a small minority of countries export more drugs and medical devices than they import. Technology flows readily anywhere in the world through commercial and professional channels. Physicians may adopt a practice from another country, perhaps one they have heard about at an international conference.

Health care technology assessment, too, is becoming an international activity. No country in the world can assess all health care technology used or likely to be used in its health care system. The need for international sharing of research methods and results and of experiences with specific technologies seems obvious.

No strong international activity has developed in health care technology assessment as yet. Most observers seem to feel that the best course is to encourage national efforts and then ensure sharing of information and co-ordination of efforts. The development of the International Society for Technology Assessment in Health Care in 1985, with the simultaneous development of its official journal, *The International Journal of Technology Assessment in Health Care*, is consistent with this perspective. Activities by international organizations will, in any case, be a welcome aid to national efforts.

The development of the field of health care technology assessment is still in its infancy. However, as this chapter will demonstrate, enough national activities have developed to make international co-ordination well worth the effort.

23.1 An international perspective on health-related research

In 1979, the world's total public and private R&D budget was estimated to be roughly US$150 billion (482). About one-third of that amount was invested by the USA and another third by Western Europe and Japan combined. Six nations (the USA, the Soviet Union, Japan, West Germany, France and the UK) employed nearly 70 per cent of the world's R&D manpower and spent nearly

85 per cent of R&D funds. The investment in this area by the USA rose from $8.8 billion in 1981 to $22.6 billion in 1990 (479). In 1986, the world investment in health R&D was estimated to be about $30 billion (137).

Overall, 7–18 per cent of the R&D expenditure is related to health (14,43,482) (see Table 14). Several European countries declared during the 1970s that health R&D was one of their top priorities in coming years (514).

The highest investments in health research on a per capita basis are in Switzerland, Sweden, and Germany. In both Germany and Switzerland, more than half of the expenditure is made by private industry, primarily the drug industry. In Sweden, in contrast, about 90 per cent of the investment is in public funds. In the USA, almost 40 per cent of the health research expenditure is by industry, while the National Institutes of Health alone makes up about 30 per cent of the total (480).

Generally, basic research is not planned or targeted centrally. Even so, in recent years a number of countries have developed programmes to specify allocation of their research resources, especially in the applied areas of epidemiology, development of certain technologies, and technology assessment.

Finally, an important part of research policy is how the government resources for biomedical research are distributed between universities and university hospitals, medical research councils and government departments (158). In general, in Europe the major part of the funds is channelled directly to universities and university hospitals. The general European system has the advantage of providing stable on-going research support, but does not encourage flexible use of the research resources. Analysing available data, Danielsson (158) concluded that too much of the research resources are given directly to universities and teaching hospitals.

Table 14. Total national expenditure on health-related research, percentage of GDP, selected countries, 1979.

	Expenditure excluding private enterprise (%)	Private enterprise (%)	Total (%)
Denmark	0.14	0.06	0.20
Finland	0.09	0.04	0.13
Germany	0.20	0.25	0.40
Ireland	0.03	0.02	0.05
Netherlands	0.22	0.03	0.25
Norway	0.14	—	0.14
Sweden	0.20	0.02	0.22
Switzerland	0.12	0.17	0.29

Source: ref. (158), Tables I and II.

Biomedical research has implications for all countries, wherever it is done. Rapid developments in biotechnology are an outstanding present example. Historically, the international impact of such technologies as the computed tomography (CT) scanner, developed in the UK, and of renal dialysis, developed in The Netherlands, illustrate this point (43). In many cases, the critical decision for policy-makers is how to react to a new technology developed elsewhere and not whether or when to develop it as a national product. This is particularly true for a small country such as Sweden or The Netherlands.

23.2 The multinational industry

World commerce is now dominated by giant multinational firms. This is well-recognized in the case of the pharmaceutical industry, but the medical devices or equipment industry has not received the same degree of attention.

The industrialized countries account for about 23 per cent of the world's population, but their combined share of the world GDP is more than 80 per cent. Their level of wealth and development is also shown by the fact that they produce the lion's share of pharmaceuticals and medical devices for the entire world.

The global market for health care technology products in 1990 was around US$65 billion. The market was heavily concentrated in the USA (43 per cent), Western Europe (31 per cent), and Japan (16 per cent) (583).

23.2.1 *The pharmaceutical industry*

Seventy per cent of the world's production of pharmaceuticals, valued at US$95.6 billion in 1985 (750), is produced in the industrialized capitalist countries that are concentrated in Western Europe and North America. The three largest drug manufacturing countries—the USA, Japan, and Germany—together represent half of the output of pharmaceutical products (693). In total, in 1980 the industrialized countries exported US$13.2 billion and imported US$9.5 billion in drugs. Table 15 shows the distribution of drug imports and exports by region in 1984.

The top 50 drug companies supply nearly two-thirds of all the pharmaceutical products shipped for human use, while the top 25 companies supply about one-half (283). In 1980, the top 13 companies in the world were US, German, or Swiss (see Table 16). By 1988, Japanese companies were becoming more prominent, and one had moved into the top 15 (Table 17). All of the 50 largest firms are transnational corporations that sell in foreign markets and usually engage in manufacturing and research and development activities abroad as well. The European firms are the most internationalized in terms of drug sales. Almost all of the main European firms have more than 50 per cent of their sales outside their home country. The combined share of sales by the top eight Western European markets was just over 20 per cent in 1985 (Table 18).

Table 15. Distribution of drug imports and exports by region, 1984.

	Imports (%)	Exports (%)
Africa	10.2	0.2
Latin America	6.5	1.7
Asia	18.9	3.6
Total developing countries	35.6	5.5
European countries	42.4	77.5
North America	10.9	14.0
Japan	7.5	0.9
Other developed countries	3.6	2.1
Total developed countries	64.4	94.5

Source: ref. (750), p. 26.

Table 16. The world's 15 largest pharmaceutical companies, 1980.

Company	Country of origin	Pharmaceutical sales (US$ millions)	Research and development (US$ millions)
Hoechst	FRG	2.413	660
Merck and Co.	USA	2.287	234
American Home Prod.	USA	2.193	603
Bayer	FRG	2.182	630
Warner-Lambert	USA	1.926	72
Bristol-Myers	USA	1.905	379
Ciba-Geigy	SWI	1.805	217
Pfizer	USA	1.644	160
Roche-Sapac	SWI	1.461	389
Eli Lilly	USA	1.426	201
SmithKline	USA	1.376	468
Sandoz	SWI	1.339	170
Boehringer-Ingelheim	FRG	1.267	139
Rhone-Poulenc	FRA	1.255	302
Glaxo	UK	1.214	106

Source: ref. (347), p. 4.

At the same time, the countries that produce drugs also tend to consume them. Seventy-nine per cent of the world production was consumed by the industrialized countries in 1985 (750). The two largest national drug markets, the USA and Japan, accounted for 28 per cent and 15 per cent, respectively, of worldwide pharmaceutical sales in 1985 (Table 18). Consumption varies greatly from country to country. Table 19 shows numbers of pharmacists by population,

Table 17. The world's 15 largest pharmaceutical companies, 1988.

Company	Country of origin	Pharmaceutical sales (US$ millions)
Merck and Co.	USA	4984
Hoechst	FRG	3958
Bayer	FRG	3713
Glaxo	UK	3706
Ciba-Geigy	SWI	3532
American Home Prod.	USA	3218
Sandoz	SWI	3147
SmithKline	USA	2975
Takeda	JAP	2841
Eli Lilly	USA	2680
Abbott	USA	2599
Pfizer	USA	2539
Warner-Lambert	USA	2509
Bristol-Myers	USA	2509
Kodak	USA	2500

Source: ref. (750).

pharmaceuticals as a percentage of total health expenditures, and pharmaceutical expenditures per capita for a number of countries. Table 20 gives similar figures from another source.

23.2.2 *The medical device and equipment industry*

The medical device and equipment industry is not nearly as large as the pharmaceutical industry. The Institute of Development Studies estimated that the total world market for medical equipment and supplies, not including pharmaceuticals, was about US$30 billion in 1985 (71). The market is dominated by demand from the USA and Europe, which together account for almost 80 per cent of total sales, with the USA accounting for 53.3 per cent and Europe for 25 per cent.

Table 20 gives figures for health expenditures by category, comparing pharmaceuticals and medical aids and equipment. It can be seen that the expenditure on equipment is substantial, but not as large as that on drugs. In the USA, the expenditure on equipment is almost 50 per cent of that for pharmaceuticals, and the percentage in The Netherlands is even higher. In France, on the other hand, the expenditure on equipment is only about 24 per cent of that for pharmaceuticals.

The dominance of the industrialized countries in equipment may be illustrated by the fact that the USA exported more than US$1 billion in all types of scientific apparatus to Latin America in 1988, while only Colombia was able to

Table 18. The 20 largest world drug markets, 1985 (excludes centrally planned economies).

Country	Sales (US$ billions)	Percentage of world market
USA	$26.4	28.1
Japan	14.9	14.9
FRG	6.0	6.4
China	4.7	5.0
France	4.5	4.7
Italy	3.7	3.9
UK	2.3	2.5
India	1.8	1.9
Canada	1.7	1.8
Brazil	1.4	1.5
Spain	1.4	1.5
Mexico	1.2	1.3
Argentina	1.2	1.3
Republic of Korea	1.0	1.1
Egypt	0.71	0.75
Belgium	0.70	0.70
Switzerland	0.60	0.65
Australia	0.58	0.60
Iran	0.51	0.55
Netherlands	0.51	0.50
Total for top 20 markets	75.0	80
Total worldwide	94.1	100.0

Source: ref. (750), Table 2, p. 9.

sell such equipment to the USA. Colombia sold US$1.5 million in such equipment to the US that year (201).

Table 21 shows figures for most of the large developers and users of medical devices. The total exports of these countries was less than US$4 billion in 1985, compared to about US$13 billion in pharmaceutical exports from a roughly comparable group of countries in 1980. Table 22 gives figures for the world market for diagnostic imaging equipment. The figure of US$4.1 billion is dwarfed by the pharmaceutical sales of US$84 billion (see above).

The medical device industry has grown dramatically since World War II. In the USA, sales of medical devices grew from less than US$1 billion in 1958 to more than US$17 billion in 1983, an annual increase of more than 12 per cent (495, p. 17). There were at least 3000 companies selling medical devices in the USA in 1983, and this figure too had dramatically increased. Employment in the industry grew from 129 000 to 200 000 during this period. Figures given here

Table 19. Availability, use, and expenditures for pharmaceutical services in industrialized countries, 1988.

	Pharmacists per 1000 population	Pharmaceuticals as percentage of total health expenditures	Pharmaceutical expenditures per capita (US$)
Australia	0.66	8.3	92
Austria	0.25	11.6	121
Belgium	1.18	17.4	161
Canada	0.80	11.6	175
Denmark	0.29	9.3	78
Finland	0.86	9.5	95
France	0.91	16.7	196
Germany	0.56	20.7	258
Greece	0.69	26.3	90
Iceland	0.74	12.9	174
Ireland	0.31	11.2	68
Italy	—	18.2	179
Japan	0.69	18.4	179
Luxembourg	0.77	15.5	178
Netherlands	0.15	9.6	103
New Zealand	0.67	14.3	115
Norway	0.45	5.3	65
Portugal	1.08	18.2	60
Spain	0.87	18.8	106
Sweden	0.51	6.7	89
Switzerland	—	12.3	159
UK	—	11.3	88
USA	0.66	8.3	182
Average	0.65	13.6	129

Source: ref. (598).

are taken from Department of Commerce surveys of US industry. They are not complete because of certain exclusions, including multiproduct companies.

United Nations statistics (200) show that exports and imports of electro-medical equipment in 24 countries have generally increased rapidly during the period 1978–1985. In Sweden, for example, exports in 1978 were about US$74 million; in 1985 they had risen to US$110 million. Imports in 1978 were almost US$30 million; in 1985 they had risen to more than US$47 million.

Exports to less developed countries also grow. In 1981, the Department of Commerce reported that the USA exported US$400 million to Latin America and the Caribbean. By 1986, the figure had grown to $1.5 billion (309).

Table 20. Health expenditures for selected categories in industrialized countries, total in billion US dollars, per capita in US dollars, 1988.

	Total	Per capita	Drugs	Per capita	Medical aids and equipment	Per capita
Austria	7.59	1000	0.71	93	0.22	29
Belgium	9.05	917	1.46	148	0.46	47
Canada	38.76	1495	4.74	183	1.52	59
Denmark	5.60	1090	0.42	83	0.18	36
France	64.46	1154	11.04	201	2.66	48
Germany	73.94	1200	12.18	198	5.38	87
Ireland	2.33	658	0.27	77	0.13	37
Italy	57.10	996	10.30	180	2.57	45
Japan	121.28	989	21.27	173	5.60	46
Luxembourg	0.53	1419	0.08	227	0.03	83
Netherlands	15.68	1063	1.45	98	0.77	52
Spain	25.61	657	4.70	121	1.11	28
Sweden	11.24	1329	0.76	90	0.44	52
Switzerland	9.17	1385	0.96	145	0.32	49
UK	48.84	858	6.64	116	1.07	19
USA	494.20	1006	41.90	170	20.10	82
Mean		1138		144		69

Source: ref. (584).

23.2.3 *Regulation of industrial products*

The first regulation to control drugs was enacted in England a little more than a century ago. Switzerland developed legislation in 1900 and the USA in 1906 (409). Norway and Sweden were the first countries (in the 1920s) to develop regulation relevant to efficacy and safety of drugs. In 1938, the US Food, Drug and Cosmetic Act gave physicians the central role as agents for consumers (599). After the Thalidomide tragedy in Europe in the late 1950s and early 1960s, virtually all European nations developed regulations regarding safety and efficacy, and the USA strengthened its regulatory legislation.

Pharmaceutical products are regulated on a pre-marketing basis. First, the manufacturer applies for an investigational drug license (IND in the United States), which allows clinical investigation of the drug. After completion of the investigations, which include controlled clinical trials in humans, the industry applies for permission to market the new drug (NDA in the USA). If the data presented are deemed to be sufficient, the drug is licensed for marketing.

Probably all countries now have a system analagous to this for pharmaceutical products although these systems are weak in many ways. Many countries do

Table 21. Exports and imports of electromedical equipment, selected countries, 1985, thousands of US dollars.

Country	Exports	Imports	Balance
Australia	5 425	81 365	– 75 940
Belgium and Luxembourg	43 294	57 583	– 14 289
Canada	23 120	159 900	– 136 780
Denmark	94 868	25 079	+ 69 789
Finland	27 428	25 363	+ 2 065
France	138 144	166 045	– 27 901
FRG	734 574	300 893	+ 433 681
Israel	115 016	37 506	+ 77 510
Italy	69 443	105 014	– 35 571
Japan	659 423	153 003	+ 506 420
Netherlands	347 820	140 190	+ 207 630
Norway	10 300	27 985	– 17 685
Sweden	109 919	47 243	+ 62 676
Switzerland	52 171	50 486	+ 1 685
UK	161 751	136 157	+ 25 594
USA	1 149 739	1 081 326	+ 68 413

Source: United Nations Statistics. Comtrade Database. Taken from ref. (200).

little clinical testing, but rely on information from tests in other countries. It may be quite difficult for developing countries to acquire such information.

Medical devices are also regulated increasingly often. Such regulation has been carried out in the USA since 1976, where pre-marketing approval of devices important to life and death is done in a manner similar to that for pharmaceuticals (495). Only a few countries, including the UK and France, scrutinize devices carefully. In the European Community, however, a common approach to device regulation is being developed (see Section 23.4.3).

23.3 National efforts in health care technology assessment

In recent years, a number of countries initiated national efforts in health care technology assessment (43,353). In most cases, these efforts have been coupled with changes in the regulatory or financing structure of the health services. Diffusion of technology has become a subject of many studies. Tables 23–25 show the international distribution of certain forms of transplant, and Table 26 gives figures for the distribution of radiotherapy machines per capita. Again, the fact that the USA generally has the highest rates of advanced technology is a striking finding.

Table 22. The world market for diagnostic imaging equipment, 1984, millions of US dollars.

Company	X-ray	CT	Nuclear medicine	Ultra-sound	NMR	Total
General Electric	380	210	35	20	25	670
Siemens	340	210	50	25	20	645
Philips*	300	50	—	65	20	435
GEC/Picker	160	80	25	20	45	330
Toshiba	180	60	10	55	12	317
Technicare (J&J)	35	110	30	45	70	290
CGR +	200	40	—	10	6	256
Hitachi	80	40	—	20	8	148
Elscint	10	80	25	10	20	145
Diasonics	15	—	—	75	30	120
All others	450	30	65	200	15	760
Total	2150	910	240	545	271	4116

Source: Biomedical Business International, Volume VIII, p. 153. Taken from ref. (200), p. 81.

* A spokesman for Philips has stated that the figures in this Table are wrong for Philips, and that Philips does in fact make and sell nuclear medicine equipment. (Philips does not release sales figures.) For this reason, this Table should be considered as indicative, and not necessarily accurate.

+ CGR was purchased by General Electric in 1987.

23.3.1 France

France has considerable expertise in health care technology assessment. The sick funds have become more and more concerned about the costs of health care and financed some studies of efficacy. The concern is particularly felt in CNAM, the National Sickness Insurance Fund under the central government. CNAM has also sought evaluations, especially from INSERM (The National Institute of Health and Medical Research). INSERM too has made health care technology assessment a priority issue. INSERM has a number of units that fund and carry out assessments of efficacy and cost-effectiveness. In addition, The Programme for Economic and Social Evaluation (La Mission de Valorisation Economique et Social) of INSERM funds studies of the consequences of technology for the health and social services.

In 1982 the French Parliament passed a law establishing an Office Parlementaire d'Evaluation des Choix Scientifiques et Technologiques (Parliamentary Office of Evaluation of Scientific Choices and Technologies). This small office began work in 1984, summarizing information on science and technology of interest to the Parliament.

Table 23. Numbers and rate (per million population) of kidney transplants by country and year.

Country	Number transplants		Transplants per million pop.	
	1988	1990	1988	1990
USA	9150	9491	39.7	40.0
France	1808	1949	32.5	34.9
Belgium	375	372	38.3	38.5
West Germany	1770	1979	29.1	33.0
Netherlands	418	401	28.5	29.1
England	1790	1969	31.5	32.5
Italy	658	533	11.5	9.2
Spain	1018	1240	26.2	32.2

Source: ref. (80).

Table 24. Numbers and rate (per million population) of heart transplants by country and year.

Country	Number transplants		Transplants per million pop.	
	1988	1990	1988	1990
USA	1647	2007	7.2	8.2
France	600	636	10.8	11.4
Belgium	96	107	9.8	10.7
West Germany	250	457	4.1	7.5
Netherlands	45	39	3.1	2.6
England	278	329	4.9	5.4
Italy	196	184	3.4	3.2
Spain	72	164	1.8	4.3

Source: ref. (80).

Other permanent structures in France have become increasingly involved in issues concerning health care technology. In 1983, the Comite Consultatif National d'Ethique pour les Sciences de la Vie et de la Sante (National Consultative Committee on Ethics for Health and Life Sciences) issued a much-discussed report on reproductive technologies.

Table 25. Numbers and rate (per million population) of liver transplants by country and year.

Country	Number transplants		Transplants per million pop.	
	1988	1990	1988	1990
USA	1680	2541	7.3	10.4
France	409	663	7.3	11.8
Belgium	121	140	12.3	14.0
West Germany	166	316	2.7	5.2
Netherlands	22	40	1.5	2.7
England	261	359	4.6	5.9
Italy	81	119	1.4	2.1
Spain	136	313	3.5	8.1

Source: ref. (80).

Table 26. Numbers of radiotherapy centres and machines by country, 1990.

Country	RT centres	Cobalt	Lin. accel.	Total	Per million pop.
USA	1293	507	1874	2381	9.5
EEC	706	624	648	1272	3.9
Belgium	36	37	26	63	6.4
France	198	195	140	335	5.9
West Germany	150	100	187	287	4.7
Denmark	10	1	23	24	4.7
Netherlands	21	5	48	53	3.6
England	70	67	124	191	3.4
Greece	16	20	10	30	3.0
Spain	90	90	23	113	2.8
Italy	100	93	59	152	2.6
Ireland	5	4	3	7	2.1
Portugal	7	12	5	17	1.7
Luxembourg	0	0	0	0	0
Sweden	18	13	39	52	6.2
Finland	12	5	20	25	5.6
Switzerland	14	13	15	38	4.2
Austria	13	12	13	25	3.7
Norway	10	2	15	17	2.5
Poland	35	40	16	56	2.5
Turkey	20	19	9	28	0.5

Source: refs (80), (518).

Despite this activity, the government felt that routine technology and quality of care were not adequately assessed. After the election in 1988, active discussions began in policy circles concerning strengthening the French approach to health care technology assessment. The government decided to establish the Agence pour le developpement de l'evaluation medicale (Agency for the Development of Medical Evaluation) as a national body in France beginning 20 April 1990. ANDEM is a private, non-profit organization. The 1991 budget for ANDEM was 20 million francs, of which 50 per cent came from the Ministry of Health. The 1992 budget was about 24 million francs.

The main purpose of ANDEM is to develop the field in France. There is limited knowledge of health care technology assessment in France, particularly among clinical physicians. Until recently, decisions were based primarily on pressures—politics, industry, and on expert opinion. Thus, ANDEM is putting an emphasis on educational and standard-setting activities.

ANDEM's Study Department has done technology assessments either for social security to assist reimbursement decisions or for the Ministry of Health. In the Ministry of Health, the Minister or any Director can ask for a study. The Study Department follows an explicit method of synthesis of scientific literature and expert opinion. The Department has the capacity to do about 5 studies a year, and in 1991 studied such technologies as osteodensitometry, prevention of non-A non-B hepatitis, treatment of menopause, and gall bladder lithotripsy. The Study Department also developed a document giving standards for consensus conferences and distributed 5000 copies. This was necessary because of the proliferation of such conferences in France. ANDEM will co-sponsor such conferences if they conform to the standards. ANDEM co-sponsored about 4 meetings of this type in 1992. ANDEM also has a Communication Department and an Education Department that concentrates on seminars and programmes for policy-makers.

Another important body carrying out health care technology assessment in France is the Assistance Publique de Paris. The central office operates a technology assessment activity. The office does syntheses of information on subjects of importance to the Assistance Publique, combined with expert specialist opinion. A recent example was an assessment of hyperthermia treatment of prostatic hypertrophy. The office has also sponsored some data analyses, such as a retrospective study of the results of renal stone lithotripsy in its own services.

In the meantime, France has become very active with consensus conferences. Four or five different institutions (including the Assistance Publique, the Assurance Maladie, and different medical associations) have organized conferences, and they are being held almost every month. ANDEM co-sponsors 4–6 of these conferences each year.

The health system of France allows a high degree of freedom to physicians, yet has a complex regulatory structure concerning technology. The most visible part of this regulatory structure is the carte sanitaire, a system of health facilities and services charts that is used for health planning. Much medical equipment is regulated under the carte sanitaire, including a specific list of 'heavy' equipment. Sometimes an assessment is done before standards are set for the carte sanitaire. In addition, procedures for equipment purchase by public hospitals have been modified to require prior assessment of clinical efficacy. Hospitals function under a global budget, which requires choices among competing technologies.

23.3.2 Denmark

In 1980, the Danish Parliament commissioned a Danish physician to examine the technology problems facing the health services and to suggest solutions. The report to the Parliament recommended the establishment of an office of technology assessment as part of the Danish Parliament, modelled after the US Congressional Office of Technology Assessment (97). In 1985, the Parliament decided to proceed with the plan and the office, organized as a 15-member Council on Technology, was established with a budget of 4 million Danish crowns a year. The Council does broad assessments of technological development with the basic aim of supporting and stimulating public debate on technology.

The Committee on Planning of the Danish National Board of Health instituted a subcommittee on technology assessment in 1984. The Committee has carried out several activities, including initiation of assessments in medical imaging, ultrasound in pregnancy, and appropriate technology for primary health care. The major activity, however, has been the development of a card giving the principles of technology assessment—this has been widely distributed within the health services in Denmark. After the 1988 Danish election this subcommittee became less active.

The Danish Medical Research Council (MRC) also established a Committee on Health Technology Assessment and Health Services Research and has made technology assessment a priority. The Committee began to support consensus conferences in 1983 by examining the early detection of breast cancer. Since then, the Committee has supported 1 or 2 consensus conferences each year. In 1988 a Danish Society for Medical Priority Setting was formed involving prominent physicians, policy-makers, and others. One area of consideration for this new Society is health care technology assessment. However, this illustrates a problem in Denmark. Technology assessment has been seen by some as a part of the field of quality assurance, preventing the development of a clear-cut area of technology assessment.

Decision-making in the Danish health care system is quite decentralized, encouraging an educational approach to health care technology assessment.

23.3.3 Finland

Health care technology assessment has been widely discussed in Finland as a method of improving health care. Perhaps the most important event was the statement in the Cabinet long-range health plan of March 1985 that 'the effectiveness and economy of health care should be evaluated and improved'. In June 1985 the Medical Research Council of Finland appointed the Medical Technology Assessment Advisory Committee to review the status of medical technology assessment and to make proposals for strengthening this field in Finland. The Committee examined the structure of institutions in Finland, including the Medical Research Council, the medical faculties, the Finnish Medical Association and other professional societies, the Ministry of Social Affairs and Health, the National Board of Health, and the Hospital League. In its 1986 report, the Committee proposed that the Medical Research Council establish an 'initiative group' for medical technology assessment consisting of 5–7 experts to promote the field of technology assessment, with an education and research budget from the Medical Research Council. Further, the Committee proposed that co-ordination committees be established to ensure that medical technology assessment activities are well-planned and the results effectively used (2). A number of technology assessments have been planned and carried out in Finland, especially by the National Public Health Institute. Consensus development conferences have also been supported (411). A Finnish Society for Technology Assessment in Health Care was formed in 1987. In 1992, it had more than 300 members.

The Ministry of Social Affairs and Health oversees the Finnish health services, preparing long-term plans, budgetary proposals to the parliament, and so forth (21). The municipalities actually deliver the health services. The national government subsidizes the municipalities in this function. Equipment must generally be in the hospital plan approved by the municipality, under municipal and national requirements. Expensive equipment (more than US$200 000) must usually be in the national five-year health plan. Procedures are not directly controlled.

23.3.4 Norway

Interest is growing in health care technology assessment in Norway, although it does not have a national programme. The Norwegian Hospital Institute in Trondheim has initiated some studies, and the Council for Medical Research has considerable interest in promoting technology assessment. Officials of the Ministry of Health and the National Institute for Public Health have also expressed an interest in seeing the field develop in Norway.

Norway initiated a study on future health care technology in early 1985, sponsored by the Council for Medical Research (289). The project identified future technologies with the help of groups of medical specialists. The project also examined special research areas, such as biotechnology and immunology. Part of the project was to carry out economic analyses in selected technological areas, such as treatment of end-stage renal disease and of diabetes. The final report synthesized this material and pointed out many important implications of future health care technology for Norway's health care system.

23.3.5 *Canada*

The central Canadian government has considered establishing a health care technology assessment activity for some years. In 1989, the decision was made to establish a Canadian Co-ordinating Office for Health Care Technology Assessment (CCOHTA) with a budget of $500 000 shared by central, provincial, and territorial governments. The Office publishes a newsletter on health care technology assessment and has published a number of documents on specific technologies. It also has monitored some technologies, such as the diffusion of laparoscopic cholecystectomy.

A number of Canadian provinces have become increasingly active in health care technology assessment. The most organized is Quebec. In early 1988, Quebec created a Council on Health Care Technology Assessment, made up of 12 individuals with expertise in different disciplines, including biomedical engineering, administration, bioethics, sociology, and clinical research. During 1989, the Council was organized. In 1990 and 1991, it published studies on a number of subjects.

In 1991, Saskatchewan formed a Technology Advisory Committee (TAC), which has evaluated several technologies. The province of British Columbia established an Office of Health Technology Assessment (BCOHTA) 1 December, 1990.

23.3.6 *Australia*

Health care technology assessment is an area with considerable visibility in Australia. The major organization is the National Health Technology Advisory Panel (NHTAP), formed in 1982 primarily to advise the national government on technology issues. The NHTAP was made up of representatives of national and provincial governments, manufacturers, physicians, and hospitals, and also included experts on economics and technology assessment. In 1984, the NHTAP developed a permanent secretariat, located at the Australian Institute of Health and Welfare in Canberra. In 1991, The Australian National Health Technology Advisory Panel (NHTAP), following a proposal from the Australian Health Ministers Advisory Council (AHMAC), was merged with the Superspecialty Services Subcommittee of the AHMAC to form a new body to be called the Australian Health Technology Advisory Committee to advise both on health technologies and specialty services. The new Committee reports to the National Health and Medical Research Council and may also report to the AHMAC. The Committee will continue to be serviced by the Australian Institute of Health and Welfare.

The NHTAP has published reports on a number of technologies. For example, a prominent example has been a study of magnetic resonance imaging (MRI), in which only five MRI scanners have been allowed in Australia under a requirement to participate in a prospective trial of cost-effectiveness. So far, the study has developed useful cost information, and has demonstrated the utility of

MRI in certain areas, especially with brain and spinal disorders; however, the Australian study has not confirmed advantages claimed for other areas of the body. NHTAP also studied lithotripsy and suggested three machines for Australia. Finally, a completed study dealt with desk-top (dry chemistry) analysers in general practice, which showed that tests were not done with a high degree of precision and tended to be additional to those ordered from central laboratories.

The Australian health care system is rather open, although budget constraints, especially on public hospitals, restrain rapid technological change. Equipment is rather tightly controlled, but medical practice is not.

23.3.7 Japan

As can be seen in many of the tables, Japan generally has high rates of advanced technology such as CT scanners and MRI scanners. New health care technology is generally accepted with enthusiasm by Japan's health care system (335). Costs of health care have been rising rapidly in Japan, and these rises have been attributed to medical technology. In 1988, the International Symposium of Medical Technology Assessment was held in Tokyo. Officials of the Ministry of Health and Welfare, researchers and journalists have paid increasing attention to issues concerning technology assessment since this Symposium. A Japanese Society for Medical Technology Assessment was established in 1985. In 1990, the Health Policy Bureau of the Ministry of Health and Welfare began to support technology assessments, beginning with assessments of medical imaging and medical informatics (334). Still, health care technology assessment is at an early phase in Japan.

23.4 International efforts in health care technology assessment

23.4.1 Overall support for health care technology assessment

No overall figures are available on national and international support for health care technology assessment. It is clear that the United States supports a substantial percentage of assessments, probably more than half.

The US Institute of Medicine (350) estimated the amount of US sources for health care technology assessment in that country as US$1.3 billion in 1984. By far the largest amount was US$1.1 billion for clinical trials, mostly of drugs. Of that amount, US$750 million was estimated as the industry expenditure. Only US$35 million was estimated as the expenditure of the medical device industry for the assessment of devices. Other than industry, government is by far the largest supporter of assessments.

The National Institutes of Health (479) releases figures on its own support for clinical trials. The total US support for health research and development in 1990 was US$22.6 billion, of which US$7.1 billion represented the NIH budget. That

Table 27. Obligations of the National Institutes of Health for clinical trials, by component of NIH, 1990 (thousands of US dollars).

National Institute on Aging	7 686
National Institute of Allergy and Infectious Diseases	145 749
National Institute of Arthritis, and Musculoskeletal and Skin Diseases	5 288
National Cancer Institute	245 954
National Institute of Child Health and Human Development	38 701
National Institute of Dental Research	7 102
National Institute of Diabetes and Digestive and Kidney Diseases	32 400
National Eye Institute	24 082
National Heart, Lung, and Blood Institute	74 396
National Institute of Neurological Disorders and Stroke	23 987
Total	609 738

Source: ref. (479).

same year, NIH invested US$609.7 million in clinical trials, about 8.6 per cent of its overall budget, compared to 6.3 per cent in 1986. The amount rose from US$197 million in 1981 to US$316 million in 1986, indicating modest growth. The investment in clinical trials by different components of NIH in 1990 is shown in Table 27.

23.4.2 *The World Health Organization*

The central office of WHO in Geneva has no formal programme in technology assessment. A global programme in appropriate technology began development during the 1980s, but it was abolished in 1988. However, a small programme for technology transfer was established in 1991. In addition, many of WHO's programmes are involved in assessments of technologies pertinent to their areas of interest, especially when these affect the less developed countries (more details are given below).

An important related activity in WHO is the essential drugs programme, developed from 1975. In 1977, WHO prepared a model list of essential drugs, including about 200 generic drugs and vaccines (521,749). Naturally, such a list requires assessment of both the drug and its application to specific important health problems. The WHO initiative followed development of national programmes in a number of countries, including Mexico, as mentioned earlier (374). In 1981, a WHO Action Programme on Essential Drugs (APED) was established to promote the availability of low-cost, high-quality essential drugs for the poor majorities in developing countries. APED attempted to improve procurement, storage, and distribution of drugs (374,752). During the last decade, WHO, in co-operation with other United Nations agencies such as

UNICEF, national governments, and consumer organizations, has succeeded in legitimizing the essential drugs concept. This concept, however, is generally used by a national government only in its public health care sector, but not in its private sector.

Theoretically, it should also be possible to list essential medical equipment. WHO has initiated the development of a basic radiology system (BRS) that is highly applicable to the situation in less developed countries. The BRS X-ray machine was designed by an advisory group of WHO to comply with economic, technological, and manpower considerations in developing countries (545). Otherwise, WHO has not gone very far to analyse what is needed.

The European office of the World Health Organization adopted as one of its targets for 1990 the realization of a central focus in health care technology assessment in all member states. In addition, another target states that by 1990 all member states should have built effective mechanisms for ensuring quality of patient care within their health care systems. All countries in Europe endorsed that goal (755). In the 1992 targets, technology assessment was made part of a target on improving quality of care.

The Pan American Health Organization (PAHO—AMRO of the World Health Organization) has stimulated development of health care technology assessment throughout Latin America, and Mexico, Brazil, Uruguay, and Argentina (at least) have been particularly active in this field. PAHO has also developed a manual describing methods of health technology assessment for developing countries (522).

As a small organization, the major role of WHO is to foster the dissemination of information through publications, conferences, and development of networks of interested individuals.

23.4.3 *The European Community (EC)*

In 1984, the EC Committee on Medical and Public Health Research approved a proposal by a special working group on health services research (COMAC—HSR) to develop a programme on the broader aspects of health technology assessment. Three activities were approved: (1) examination of economic appraisal, including specific case studies of open heart surgery, genetic screening, and lasers (46); (2) investigations of variations of use of technology, especially lithotripsy (372); and (3) examinations of policies towards health care technology. The third area has included studies of diffusion of transplants (79), prenatal screening (554), and renal stone treatment (387) in Europe.

The EC is gradually expanding its activities in health care technology assessment. However, the nature of the organization dictates that these activities should take into account the needs of industry. Still, Directorate-General XII of the EC for Science, Research, and Development is developing plans to become actively involved in applying technology assessment (specifically economic analysis) to selected health care technologies. These plans may be accelerated by the inclusion of public health as an EC activity in the treaty of Maastricht.

The EC is also interested in encouraging networks to exchange information, as shown by its support to the University of Birmingham (Professor Michael Drummond) to collect information on health care technology assessment and by its interest in developing a clearing house for technical evaluations of equipment.

Another EC activity is the COMETT–ASSESS programme (University–Industry Partnership in the Training for Medical Technology Assessment), which started in 1990 and is made up of a network of organizations and individuals in Europe. The main tool of COMETT–ASSESS is educational. In addition to actually supporting courses and seminars, COMETT–ASSESS has developed a set of training materials in medical technology assessment.

The EC has supported a working group on biomedical engineering (COMAC–BME), focusing on the safety of medical equipment, for several years. The Advanced Informatics in Medicine (AIM) programme and the Forecasting and Assessment of Science and Technology (FAST) programme have also funded assessments, oriented to informatics.

In 1992, the BIOMED 1 programme was announced as the EC structure for health-related research. Health care technology assessment was stated as a priority of the programme.

In 1991, in the Maastricht meeting of heads of European states that developed the treaty for economic integration of Europe in 1993, the decision was made to expand and co-ordinate activities in the health sector (572). Health Ministers in Europe have recognized the importance of technology assessment. These moves mean that health care technology assessment will grow in Europe, but its future course is not clear, nor is the rapidity of change.

One certainty, however, is that the development of economic integration will result in European approaches to the regulation of pharmaceuticals and medical devices. The essential objective of the EC is to establish a common market within which there is free movement of goods, services, and capital. In particular, the free movement of goods must not be obstructed by tariff or non-tariff barriers. In so far as differences in national legislation create obstacles to trade, these must be eliminated by a process of harmonization of legislation. The harmonization or 'approximation' is achieved through a long series of consultations and negotiations and the final results are likely to be untidy. Pharmaceuticals and medical devices are treated essentially as any other consumer good and thus fall within the scope of harmonization, although it is recognized that there must be a system of regulatory control.

A major question of how the drug registration process can be harmonized has been the subject of many discussions and papers, and still is—especially considering that some of the 12 countries have very rigorous regulatory systems (e.g., the UK and The Netherlands), while others have weak systems. Two opposite poles have defined the debate: either a central registration authority (something like the American FDA) or a system of 'mutual recognition'. The first alternative is not acceptable because of the loss of national sovereignty and the expensive bureaucracy that would be needed, perhaps duplicating national efforts. Mutual recognition is not acceptable because it would mean accepting the lowest standards for drug safety and efficacy to be found in Europe for any particular drug. The EC has sought a middle path, and the final system is likely to be one in which a European Medicines Agency (EMA) deals with the so-called high-tech new drugs and would arbitrate on differences between the member states. If a company applied for registration in one country that was not challenged by another state, the registration would be accepted throughout Europe. Naturally, any manufacturer could seek local registration for drugs only intended for the local market. It is envisaged that most drugs would take this route, that is, seeking registration in one country as a path to registration throughout Europe. This means a gradual increase in the volume of work and the power of the EMA, since disagreements and challenges are likely to be frequent. The exact composition of the EMA, where it is to be situated, what language(s) it will use, and so forth, is still being discussed.

As with drugs, the aim of the European Community economic integration is to make one marketplace without regulatory or other barriers to sales with the Community. The EC is actively engaged in developing a 'global approach' to device quality. Part of this work means developing regulations for quality where there have often been no regulations at all. Thus, the overall situation may very well improve. At the same time, the EC standards will be quite general overall, so standards in some countries may fall. The countries with the strongest programmes at present are the UK, Germany, and France. The EC approach depends strongly on industry to meet good manufacturing practices. Only in the case of industry failures are governments expected to engage in direct activities regulating devices.

23.4.4 *The World Bank*

The World Bank began direct lending for health in 1980. By 1983, the Bank had become one of the largest funders of health projects in developing countries, lending more than $100 million annually (744). The usual Bank procedure is to respond to a request for a loan by doing a systematic study of the health sector as a whole. Lending operations have focused on the development of basic health care programmes, including expansion of primary health care, provision of drugs, and support for training and technical assistance.

A problem with the Bank's loans is that the motivation at the country level for seeking a loan is primarily to obtain foreign currency. This foreign currency can then be used for imports, particularly for medical equipment. Earlier, the Bank paid little systematic attention to the issue of what equipment was purchased. This situation has gradually changed. In China, for example, the Bank has encouraged development of a technology assessment capability since 1988. Still, this seems to be the exception. Most divisions of the Bank still pay relatively little attention to the effectiveness or cost-effectiveness of investments in health care equipment.

23.4.5 *The International Monetary Fund (IMF)*

The International Monetary Fund is often in the news, especially concerning relations between developed and less developed countries. Because these stories are often based on misconceptions about the IMF (356), and because the IMF has a great deal to do with economic development and thus with health care technology in developing countries (483), it will be briefly discussed.

The IMF is a co-operative institution in which more than 150 countries have voluntarily joined because they see the advantage of developing and maintaining a stable system of buying and selling their currencies (185). The IMF lends money to members having trouble meeting their financial obligations to other members, but only on condition that they undertake economic reforms. Thus, the IMF does not suggest what percentage of a national budget can be spent on health care. The IMF might, however, set a standard that would prevent import controls over medical equipment, as happened in the case of Mexico (259). In general, the IMF, in co-operation with the General Agreement on Tariffs and Trade (GATT), promotes an international trading system free from controls and restrictions (483). The IMF believes that its system is beneficial to all member states (355). Whether this is true or not, there is little doubt that developing countries can have severe problems, at least in the short run, meeting the IMF standards. The IMF argues that all countries must participate on an equal basis in world trade.

It is also important to note that it is not necessary for a country to use import controls to encourage local industry. Health care resources can be used to encourage or discourage international trade. The Mexican case, described above, shows how resources for health care can be directed to the purpose of encouraging local industry.

23.4.6 *The European Medical Research Council (EMRC)*

The EMRC was formed in 1971 to promote an exchange of information between medical research councils and corresponding bodies in Western Europe concerning research policies and activities. The EMRC is empowered by its statutes to stimulate international collaboration in medical research. EMRC is aware that medical research is inherently international, and sets stringent criteria for any international initiative. The main criterion is a definite need for the initiative.

In 1980 the EMRC began to discuss the need for initiatives in the area of assessment of health care technologies. This field was seen as important, both in research and to the member countries. As a result, a conference was held in September 1981 on 'Assessment of Biomedical Technology in the Health Care Field: International Perspectives in Methodology'. The experience with this conference was such that the EMRC decided to set up a Planning Committee on Technology Assessment. The Committee is made up of representatives of the member organizations, the US National Institutes of Health, and the European Office of WHO (EURO). A survey was done of research projects dealing with diagnostic technologies, but there seemed to be limited interest in the results, so this activity was not continued. A second conference on methods of technology was held in Copenhagen in May 1985. A third conference, on transfer of information from technology assessment, was held in October 1986, and the papers were published in the *International Journal of Technology Assessment in Health Care* in 1988.

23.4.7 The Organization for Economic Co-operation and Development (OECD)

OECD has shown some interest in health care technology assessment. In 1980 it sponsored an international consultation on the subject and subsequently distributed a position paper on the subject to all member states (513). At present, OECD is not active in this field.

23.4.8 *The Nordic Council*

The Nordic Council, made up of representatives of Denmark, Finland, Norway, and Sweden has become interested in technology assessment. In August 1985 the Council funded a course in health care technology assessment. About 50 people participated in the course.

In addition, there is now a Nordic Committee for Technology Assessment in Health Care. The Committee consists of representatives from four Nordic institutes: SPRI from Sweden; the Danish Hospital Institute; the Norwegian Institute for Hospital Research; and the Finnish Hospital League. The Committee began its work by reviewing and assessing the organizational, clinical, and economic impact of nuclear magnetic resonance (NMR) from a four-country perspective. In 1991, it completed a report on screening and treatment for prostatic cancer. In addition, this body presents courses on technology assessment.

23.4.9 *The International Society for Technology Assessment in Health Care*

In 1985 a new professional Society was formed to foster communication among the rapidly growing group of those interested in health care technology assessment. The organizational meeting of the Society was held in Copenhagen in May 1985. Meetings were held yearly from 1986 (in Washington D.C.), alternating between North America and Europe. The 1992 meeting was in Vancouver, Canada, and the 1993 meeting in Sorrento, Italy. In 1992, the Society had about 800 members in more than 30 countries.

Simultaneously, a new professional journal, the *International Journal of Technology Assessment in Health Care*, was inaugurated: this is the official journal of the Society.

23.5 Conclusions

While a great amount of national and international activity in the field of health care technology assessment has been started, the present amount of activity will surely not be enough to meet the needs for information. At the same time, the proliferation of programmes has produced significant problems of communication and co-ordination. A considerable amount of duplication is already taking place. For example, large studies of the cost-effectiveness of heart transplants have been funded in the USA, Sweden, the UK, and The Netherlands, all coming to similar conclusions. With large gaps in information still existing, such duplication is wasteful. All countries need to develop mechanisms to share information concerning health care technology internationally.

24. Conclusions

All countries are faced with rapid technological change in the health care field. In addition, all countries have limited resources for health care.

Health care technology has become an increasingly visible issue in almost all countries in the world. The very successes of health care have made it a policy issue. The control of infectious disease, and the resulting ageing of the population, have brought ever-increasing burdens on the health care and social security systems. At the same time, the health care system staggers under an ever-increasing outpouring of new technology—and no end is in sight. Technological change is becoming more rapid, driving costs of health care higher and forcing more and more uncomfortable choices.

Until fairly recently, technology was not an explicit issue. Health planning attempted to increase the efficiency of the health care delivery system, but did not become involved in the effectiveness of health care interventions. Those days are gone. Policy-makers are now deeply interested in the benefits that one can expect from new technology. And those benefits must be put in relation to the potential costs.

The field of technology assessment has developed rapidly as a part of changes in approaches to new technology, and implicitly, to older technology as well. For if resources are limited, the new technology must replace something. The new technology must be compared to the old, and if it is more effective, and more cost-effective, steps should be taken to assure that it comes rapidly into use. If it is not more effective, it will be discouraged. If it is less effective, it will not find a place at all.

During its rapid development, perhaps the field of health care technology assessment has paid inadequate attention to problems of the health care system. What are the goals of technology assessment activities? Who must assessors relate to? Who are the clients? What are the hoped-for outcomes? What are the main problems? How can the growing number of individuals and organizations be harnessed to societal goals?

24.1 Policies towards health care technology

Public policies have developed in such a way that they influence the various stages in the life cycle of a technology. Public policies can be made explicit at the stage of basic research, because almost all of the funding comes from government. Public policies affect aspects of applied research and development, although this stage is left largely to industry and clinical physicians (government investments in applied research and development are small). Drugs must be shown to be efficacious and safe before they can be marketed in almost all countries. Certain expensive technologies are regulated and centralized. Health care systems and insurance programmes have explicit packages defining what is covered and what is not covered and how much reimbursement there will be. Policies are beginning to appear concerning cost-effectiveness evidence.

Public policies such as these provide a mechanism for any society to influence technological change in health care. However, diffusion is difficult to control, for a variety of reasons. Physicians want the latest technology for their patients, and patients often share the wish, or even demand the technology. Patients learn about new technologies in the media and ask their specialists for such services. The industry brings pressures against control, arguing both that people's health will be harmed by slow diffusion, and that their products provide jobs and exports. And the ministries dealing with health policy tend to be weak compared with other parts of the government.

It must also be recognized that explicit policies cannot deal with all of the thousands of technologies in health care. The policy framework is a general one. Its mechanisms must provide incentives to push behaviour in certain directions and to protect the public's safety.

A particular problem is that assessment of the consequences of decisions has not generally been a part of policy-making until fairly recently. A second problem is that clinicians have not always relied on the best scientific information as a guide to clinical practice.

This book does not suggest solutions to all of the problems of the health care system. It is clear that an appropriate framework for policy and clinical decisions is necessary in every country. The problem remains that good scientific information is often not available to assist policy (and clinical) decisions.

Well-validated information on benefits, risks, costs, and social effects of health care technology is generally not available. If adoption and use of health care technology are to be based on such information, the information must be developed systematically and to be made available at the appropriate time to the individuals and groups who need it. A process or system for assessing health care technology to meet such goals is described in this book.

24.1.1 *Health care technology assessment*

Although information is still insufficient to guide decision-making, the main achievement of health care technology assessment during the 15 or so years of its life is to greatly increase the amount of valid and useful information on the benefits, risks, and costs of health care technology.

Aside from this achievement, the disciplines associated with technology assessment, including physicians, economists, psychologists, and sociologists, have substantial experience in developing methods of assessment, including randomized trials, cost-effectiveness analysis, and health status assessment. Some, such as health status assessment, are still being developed. There are refinements in other methods that are needed, such as including cost-effectiveness analysis in clinical trials. The critical method of information synthesis continues to need a great deal of development. Nevertheless, methods are generally available and have been found useful in many settings.

24.2 Technology transfer

A relatively small number of countries are producers of the world's health care technology. The rest must depend on 'technology transfer'. Technology transfer refers to the process of transferring technology from the place it develops to where it is applied. Technology transfer takes place between governments, academic and private institutions, and producers. In the case of health care technology, the point of application is the health care system. The health care technology may be a practice or procedure, in which the knowledge and skills are the critical element. The technology may be a machine or a drug, in which case the point of origin is usually in industry. The important point is that technology always includes a 'software' element. A machine is of limited value if personnel are not trained in its use.

Effective technology transfer is 'a process of transferring from one production entity to another the know-how required to successfully utilize a particular technology' (Teece, quoted in (64)).

Conceptually speaking, technology transfer to less-developed countries is no different from technology transfer within an industrialized country or transfer between industrialized countries. In reality, however, there are a number of important practical differences. Perhaps the most important point is that less-developed countries are technology dependent. Their capability for developing technology through biomedical and health-related research is limited. Their local industry is weak (360). Furthermore, and in part because of these facts, they lack the expertise and information sources to identify needed technologies. The technological base and infrastructure is often lacking, so the importing country must develop the capability to absorb and productively utilize foreign technology (288). Finally, they obviously have serious problems because they are poor. Their resources are limited. Because of these differences, technology assessment should be less of a technology-oriented activity in less-developed countries and more oriented to solving problems (20,701).

Despite these difficulties, technology transfer from industrialized countries to less-developed countries is critically important. Technology—applied knowledge—is the path to a healthier population, whether the technology is a vaccine, a diagnostic tool, or a surgical procedure. This is a time of rapid technological change, and health care technology is becoming more effective and more cost-effective. Less-developed countries may be left even further behind if concerted efforts are not made to assure technological change in their health services.

Because the health care resources of less-developed countries are seriously limited, they must make hard choices. Any country that is importing technology needs to ask a series of questions. They need to know what technology is available and what technology is in development. They need to ask how such technology can be acquired and what it will cost. They need to know what the effect of the technology will be on health and on the health care system itself. They need to ask what training, supportive systems, and so forth are necessary for efficient implementation and use of the technology. And they need to be able to judge if the technology will be socially and culturally acceptable.

The answers to these questions—and other related questions—are available through the field of technology assessment. Indeed, the field of technology assessment developed to answer policy questions such as these.

24.3 Western industrialized countries

The previous chapters have described the situation in a number of countries. Basically, industrialized countries produce the technology that is used by the rest of the world. In addition, they are heavy users of such technology themselves.

Faced with cost rises, most of these countries have developed various policies to control costs. These policies have addressed costs directly. It has been recognized for some years that costs could be controlled by prospective budgets (43). For example, the UK has had fewer problems of increasing costs because of the structure of its system (661,662). Other countries have followed the lead of the UK. The Netherlands and France, for example, have developed global, controlled hospital budgets. The result was that costs did not rise in most of these countries during the late 1980s. In fact, in The Netherlands, the relative level of resources for health declined from 1989 to 1990 (515).

However, partial policies such as controlling hospitals probably do not work in the long run. As noted in this book, costs in The Netherlands are now rising. The same is true in France. Ultimately, a budgeting system covering all services is probably necessary.

In the USA, costs continue to rise rapidly, mainly because of the open nature of the US health care system. Proposals for a national health scheme were made in 1992 and are being debated in 1993 after the Presidential election, but their outcome is uncertain. Many people in the US believe that a closed budget system will be necessary to control costs effectively.

Controlling costs does not solve the problem with technology. In fact, a controlled budget discourages innovation, and in an unselected manner. A tight, controlled budget can have the result of stopping technological change and leaving health care practice just as it is. How then can progress be assured? Health care technology assessment fits in this context. Chapter 17 on the UK best illustrates this point.

24.4 Central and Eastern European countries

Central and Eastern European countries and the former Soviet Union show deteriorating health status, particularly in middle-aged adults (249). One reason is that they are far behind the West in terms of health care technology. In Poland, for example, chronic underfunding has created shortages of basic tools at all levels of health care. In addition, the national industry is weak, meaning that imports are necessary. Yet the resources for purchases are extremely limited (745). Other countries such as Romania are in an even worse condition (747).

Countries such as Poland have sophisticated health care providers and other supporting staff such as engineers, so they can absorb technological investment. None the less, careful choice is necessary. Concepts such as effectiveness are not necessarily well understood in the same terms as presented in this book. There is no tradition of assessing health care technology for effectiveness or for financial costs.

How health care system reform will proceed in these countries is not clear, but it is clear that the centralized planning and regulatory structures typical of the Soviet period are generally not acceptable. National health insurance is being considered as an answer. The main problem is that Eastern Europe may retrace developments in the West, with rapidly increasing costs of health care and severe strains on their economies.

The lessons learned by some of the developed countries described in this book, including the UK, apply well in this area of the world. The first priority is to establish a payment system capable of controlling expenditures. Another priority is to establish effective mechanisms such as technology assessment bodies that can guide investments within limited budgets.

24.5 Middle-income (developing) countries

Countries such as Mexico and China illustrate some of the issues and problems for countries that are developing. These countries, and others such as Brazil (26), are increasing health care expenditures and developing policy structures to guide such expenditures (32).

Mexico and China have largely controlled infectious diseases, which means that they are now faced with an ageing population and a growing rate of chronic disease. Both countries now are beginning to become deeply involved in technology transfer to make modern Western technology available to their populations.

Most countries at this level have not been able to develop an effective national health products industry (133). It is a great achievement of China that it has followed a set of policies towards its pharmaceutical industry that has made the country almost entirely self-sufficient in drugs. However, it has not been successful with medical equipment or with other areas of medical technology. Mexico also has had problems in attempting to encourage national industry. For example, in 1980, Mexico had only 69 medical device companies, producing about US$6.7 million in value, about 15 per cent of domestic consumption (567). Both countries illustrate the use of health care resources to stimulate local industry. This policy is applicable in many countries in the world.

As an average, all developing countries produced less than 10 per cent of the world's drugs and accounted for less than one quarter of the annual world expenditure on drugs in 1984 (752). Two-thirds of that production came from India, Cuba, Egypt, Argentina, Brazil, and Mexico (excluding China).

Countries at this level import substantial amounts of technology. This means that they must choose among competing priorities. What can guide choice? Technology assessment should be quite useful for this purpose. Population health needs must be a central part of this assessment. In other words, technology choice needs to be guided by information on health status, such as that obtained by epidemiological studies as well as costs.

It is also worth noting that these exports are significant for industrialized countries. The USA exported US$93.6 million in medical equipment to Mexico in 1988, and US$31.1 million to Venezuela (163). The Health Industry Manufacturers' Association projected a 1988 health care technology product market of US$208 million in Argentina, $546 million in Brazil, $507 million in Mexico, and $60 million in Venezuela, exclusive of pharmaceuticals (583).

Part of choosing the appropriate technologies has to do with necessities to support the technology (e.g., maintenance and spare parts), correct location for the technology in the system, and appropriate use. Mexico has gone farther than most countries in developing such standards. Such decisions must be supported by a reasonable assessment of the technology, as well as of the needs of the community.

Recently, interest has been growing in the transfer of clinical technology, including both advanced skills and biomedical equipment (32). Studies have demonstrated the widespread diffusion of imported technology without careful planning (133,571). In Latin America, technology transfer has '. . . consisted in the uncritical acceptance and indiscriminate, wholesale acquisition of technologies rather than of knowledge, without any regard for the actual usability, suitability, efficiency, or effectiveness' (520). Technology is often concentrated in the private sector, where access by the whole population is limited. For example, in 1985 in Argentina, 93 per cent of the computed tomography scanners, 84 per cent of the gamma cameras, 70 per cent of the linear accelerators, and 76 per cent of the cobalt units were located in the private sector, which serves a minority of the population (68). Another problem is maintenance and spare parts. A study in a South American country of 1289 pieces of equipment bought with European aid during the period 1974–1979 found that 95 per cent was not functioning. Reasons included inadequate numbers of maintenance personnel, poorly trained maintenance personnel, lack of spare parts, and lack of clinical expertise (133).

It is often not recognized that countries at the middle level of development have access to reasonable levels of modern technology and may have resulting cost problems. In fact, countries at the middle level of development in the 1980s and 1990 often experience cost escalation as they attempt to modernize. For example, the experience of Korea has paralleled that of China and Mexico in this regard (162). In fact, in 1990, Korea had more lithotripters on a population basis than Canada or Germany. Mexico has a rather high level of technology, even in health centres (571). Technology assessment could be very helpful in such countries. In Colombia, a study showed under-utilization of personnel and facilities in surgery, and a general low level of complexity of in-patient surgical services (700). Developing an out-patient surgery programme was seen as leading to considerable efficiency. A recent analysis (616) examined the cost-effectiveness of treatment for end-stage renal disease in Brazil. A cost-effectiveness analysis of neonatal intensive care has been carried out in Rio de Janeiro, showing serious problems in applying high technology in that country (626).

24.6 Poor countries

Many countries in the world have extremely limited resources to invest in health care. For example, the poorest countries may invest as little as US$3 per capita per year (744,748). The per capita expenditure on pharmaceuticals is below US$1 per capita in many countries (374). In fact, slow economic growth and budget deficits have forced reductions in public spending. Public and private spending on health care together in developing countries is on average less than 5 per cent of that spent in developed countries per capita (744). Obviously, the small expenditure limits their choice severely. It has long been recognized that poor countries do not allocate money well in the direction of cost-effective activities (744). One problem in this regard is industry promotion of inappropriate products (409). Effective technology assessment policy can be useful in countering these marketing efforts.

Primary health care and prevention of high incidence diseases with cost-effective intervention have been promoted in poor countries (220,709). The impact of public health measures such as immunization is greater in poor countries and should be the priority (325). Health planning in poor countries could be much more based on programme effectiveness and cost-effectiveness than it in fact is. Previously, such programmes were centrally planned and offered to the community without much consultation. However, it has been increasingly recognized that community concerns need to receive attention for programmes to be successful (75). Such issues as management, the health infrastructure, lack of community mobilization, and insufficient political commitment may lead to failure of a programme that otherwise would be very cost-effective.

In other words, technology assessment needs to be modified depending on the situation. In poorer countries, explicit attention to the conditions under which technologies will be used is essential (75).

Little is known in general about how poor countries allocate their health care resources. It is known that 30 per cent and even more of national health budgets go to purchase pharmaceuticals (374). It is ironic and probably inappropriate that industrialized countries allow the export of some drugs not approved for use in their own country (409).

Technology assessment has also been used in poorer countries. Because of the nature of the health problems in less-developed countries, few technology assessments done to date have dealt with modern technology. Shepard (619) was able to identify 25 exemplary studies applying cost-benefit or cost-effectiveness analysis of health programmes in developing countries. The studies dealt with such programmes as malaria eradication, family planning, schistosomiases control, sanitation, immunization, cholera control, and nutrition. The World Health Organization has encouraged such analyses in its immunization and diarrhoea control programmes (145,146,620).

There has been relatively little experience with using assessment as part of programmes of traditional medicine. In poor countries, this approach might be quite valuable. In north-east Brazil, Araujo and his co-workers (18) transferred modern obstetric technology to traditional birth attendants, mainly through developing a process of education and referral channels for complicated deliveries.

24.7 Final comment

In this book, we have tried to describe and analyse the development and diffusion of health care technology. Our approach has been aimed at intervention. We do not believe that technology is autonomous. It can be guided. Processes of development can be controlled. We take the perspective that technology is a tool that offers capabilities. It is then up to people to use technology well.

We have also tried to take a truly international perspective toward health care technology. In such a global orientation, some problems will be left out or only mentioned superficially. Our aim has not been to discuss all issues. Specifically, we have identified technology transfer and methods of improving choice, particularly for poorer countries, as a key issue. The potentials of health care technology assessment have barely begun to be realized in this area.

References

1. Aaronson N, Bullinger M, Ahmedzai S. A modular approach to quality-of-life assessment in cancer clinical trials. *Recent Reviews of Cancer Research* 1988; **111**: 231–248.
2. Academy of Finland. *Medical technology assessment in Finland—present status and prospects for the future.* Helsinki, 1986.
3. d'Adler M A. The transfer of medical information, a journalist's view. *International Journal of Technology Assessment in Health Care* 1988; **4**: 59–63.
4. Advisory Group on Health Technology. *Assessing the effects of health technologies, principles, practice, proposals.* Assessment for the Director of Research and Development. London: Department of Health, 1992.
5. Albritton R B. Cost benefits of measles eradication: effects of federal intervention. *Policy Analysis* 1978; **4**: 1–22.
6. Allen T J. The role of person-to-person communications in the transfer of technological knowledge. In: Robert E B, Levy R I, Finkelstein S N, Moskowitz J, Sondik E J, eds. *Biomedical innovation.* Cambridge, Massachusetts: MIT Press, 1981: pp. 352–378.
7. Altman S, Blendon R eds. *Medical technology: the culprit behind health care costs?* Hyattsville, Maryland: National Center for Health Services Research and Bureau of Health Planning, 1979. (DHEW Publication No. (PHS) 79–3216).
8. Ambrose J, Gooding M, Uttley D. E.M.I. scan in the management of head injuries. *Lancet* 1976; **1**: 847–850.
9. Ambroz A, Chalmers T C, Smith H, *et al.* Deficiencies of randomized control trials. *Clinical Research* 1978; **26**: 280–285.
10. American College of Physicians. *Hospital clinical privileges, guidelines for procedures in gastroenterology and nephrology.* Philadelphia, 1988.
11. Anderson C, Cassidy B, Rivenburgh P. Implementing continuous quality improvement (CQI) in hospitals: lessons learned from the International Quality Study. *Quality Assurance in Health Care* 1991; **3**: 141–146.
12. Andersson F *et al. Potential for economic and health benefits in France through biomedical and behavioral advances.* Washington, DC: Battelle Medical Technology Assessment and Policy Research Center, (Report No. BHARC-013/92/23), 1992.
13. Andriessen J, ter Haar Romeny B, Barneveld Binkhuysen F, van der Horst-Bruinsma I. Savings and costs of a picture archiving and communication system in the University Hospital Utrecht. *Proceedings of the Medical Imaging Conference SPIE III.* 1989; **1093**: 578–584.
14. Annerstedt J. *On the present global distribution of R&D resources.* Vienna: Vienna Institute for Development, 1979.
15. Anon. Effectiveness of UK pharma reps. *Scrip*, No. 15966, 6 March 1991, p. 4.

16. Apfel R J, Fisher S M. *To do no harm: DES and the dilemmas of modern medicine.* London: Yale University Press, 1984.

17. Apolone G, Alfieri V, Braga A, *et al.* A survey of the necessity of the hospitalization day in an Italian teaching hospital. *Quality Assurance in Health Care* 1991; **3**: 1–9.

18. Araujo G, Araujo L, Janowitz B, Wallace S, Potts M. Improving obstetric care in Northeast Brazil. *Bulletin of the Pan American Health Organization* 1983; **17**: 233–244.

19. Arnstein S. Technology assessment: opportunities and obstacles. *IEEE Transactions on Systems, Man, and Cybernetics* 1977; **SMC-7**: 571–585.

20. Attinger E O, Panerai R B. Transferability of health technology assessment with particular emphasis on developing countries. *International Journal of Technology Assessment in Health Care* 1988; **4**: 545–554.

21. Backman G. Health policy in Finland: organization, planning, and high technology development. *International Journal of Technology Assessment in Health Care* 1988; **4**: 375–384.

22. Bailar J C, Mosteller F eds. *Medical uses of statistics.* Waltham, Massachusetts: NEJM Books, 1986.

23. Banta H D. The diffusion of the computed tomography (CT) scanner in the United States. *International Journal of Health Services* 1980; **10**: 251–269.

24. Banta H D. Diffusion of minimally invasive therapy in Europe. *Minimally Invasive Therapy* 1992; **1**: 189–195.

25. Banta H D. Embracing or rejecting innovations: clinical diffusion of health care technology. In: Reiser S J, Anbar M, eds. *The machine at the bedside.* London: Cambridge University Press, 1984: pp. 65–92.

26. Banta H D. Medical technology and developing countries: the case of Brazil. *International Journal of Health Services* 1986; **16**: 363–373.

27. Banta H D. Medical technology in China. *Health Policy* 1990; **14**: 127–137.

28. Banta H D, ed. *Minimally invasive therapy in five European countries.* Amsterdam: Elsevier, 1993.

29. Banta, H D, ed. *Resources for health: technology assessment for policy making.* New York: Praeger, 1982.

30. Banta H D. Developing outcome standards for quality assurance activities. *Quality Assurance in Health Care* 1992; **4**: 25–32.

31. Banta H D. Social dimensions of biotechnology: the case of vaccines. In: Yoxen E, Di Martino V eds. *Biotechnology in future society: scenarios and options for Europe.* Luxembourg: Office for Official Publications of the European Communities, 1989: pp. 47–53.

32. Banta H D. The uses of modern technologies: problems and perspectives for industrialized and developing countries. *Bulletin of the Pan American Health Organization* 1984; **18**: 139–150.

33. Banta H D, van Beekum W T eds. *Anticipating and assessing health care technology,* Volume 7. *Computer assisted medical imaging: the case of picture archiving and communications systems (PACS).* Dordrecht: Kluwer Academic Publishers, 1988.

34. Banta H D, van Beekum W T eds. *Anticipating and assessing health care technology.* Volume 8. *Potentials for home care technology.* Dordrecht: Kluwer Academic Publishers, 1988.

35. Banta H D, Behney C J. Policy formulation and technology assessment. *Milbank Memorial Fund Quarterly/Health and Society* 1981; **59**: 445–479.

36. Banta D, Brown S, Behney C. Implications of the 1976 Medical Devices Legislation. *Man and Medicine* 1978; **3**: 131–143.
37. Banta H D, Behney C J, Willems J S. *Toward rational technology in medicine*. New York: Springer Publishing Company, 1981.
38. Banta H D, Buch Andreasen P. The political dimension in health care technology assessment programs. *International Journal of Technology Assessment in Health Care* 1990; **6**: 115–124.
39. Banta H D, Gelijns A. *Anticipating and assessing health care technology*, Volume 1. *General considerations and policy conclusions*. Dordrecht: Martinus Nijhoff Publishers, 1987.
40. Banta H D, Gelijns A, eds. *Anticipating and assessing health care technology*, Volume 6. *Applications of the new biotechnology, the case of vaccines*. Dordrecht: Kluwer Academic Publishers, 1988.
41. Banta, H D, Gelijns, A, eds. *Anticipating and assessing health care technology*, Volume 5. *Developments in human genetic testing*. Dordrecht: Kluwer Academic Publishers, 1988.
42. Banta H D, Gelijns A, Griffioen J, Graaff P J. *Anticipating and assessing health care technology*, Volume 2. *Future technological changes*. Dordrecht: Kluwer Academic Publishers, 1988.
43. Banta H D, Kemp K eds. *The management of health care technology in nine countries*. New York: Springer Publishing Company, 1982.
44. Banta H, Luce B. Assessing the cost-effectiveness of prevention. *Journal of Community Health* 1983; **9**: 145–152.
45. Banta H D, Saxe L. Reimbursement for psychotherapy: linking efficacy research and public policy-making. *American Psychologist* 1983; **38**: 918–922.
46. Banta H D, Schou I eds. *Lasers in health care, effectiveness, cost-effectiveness and policy implications*. Copenhagen: Academic Publishing, 1991.
47. Banta H D, Thacker S B. Assessing the costs and benefits of electronic fetal monitoring. *Obstetrical and Gynecological Survey* 1979; **34**: 627–642.
48. Banta H D, Thacker S B. The case for reassessment of health care technology, once is not enough. *Journal of the American Medical Association* 1990; **264**: 235–240.
49. Barber B. The ethics of experimentation with human subjects. *Scientific American* 1976; **234**: 25–34.
50. Barnes B A. Discarded operations: surgical innovation by trial and error. In: Bunker J P, Barnes B A, Mosteller F eds. *Costs, risks, and benefits of surgery*. New York: Oxford University Press, 1977: pp. 109–123.
51. Barofsky I, Sugarbaker P. Cancer. In: Spilker B ed. *Quality of life assessments in clinical trials*, Raven Press, New York, 1990.
52. Battelle. *Analysis of CBA/CEA literature*. London: Battelle MEDTAP Research Center, 1992.
53. Battelle. *Analysis of selected biomedical research programs*. Vol 2. Columbus Ohio: Battelle Columbus Laboratories, 1976.
54. Battelle. *Interactions of science and technology in the innovative process. Some case studies*. Prepared for the US National Science Foundation. Columbus, Ohio: Battelle Columbus Laboratories, 1973.
55. BAZIS. *Concluding report, Dutch PACS Project*. Leiden, The Netherlands: BAZIS, 1990.
56. Beeson K P B. Changes in medical therapy during the past half century. *Medicine* 1980; **59**: 79–99.
57. Behney C. Personal communication, 1992.

58. Bell R, Loop J. The utility and futility of radiographic skull examination for trauma. *New England Journal of Medicine* 1971; **284**: 236–239.

59. Bennett C. The remedy for drugs. *Marketing Week*, 8 June 1984, p. 42.

60. Bergner M. Quality of life, health status, and clinical research. *Medical Care* 1989; **27**(suppl): S148–S156.

61. Bergner M, Rothman M L. Health status measures: an overview and guide for selection. *Annual Review of Public Health* 1987; **8**: 191–210.

62. Bergner M, Bobbitt R, Carter W, *et al*. The Sickness Impact Profile: development and final revision of a health status measure. *Medical Care* 1981; **19**: 787–805.

63. Berkelbach van D, Sprenkel J, Mauser H, *et al*. MRI in neurosurgical diagnosis and management of craniocervical junction and cervical spine pathology. *Clinical Neurology and Neurosurgery* 1986; **84**: 245–251.

64. de Bettignies H C. The management of technology transfer: can it be learned? *Impact of Science on Society* 1978; **28**: 321–327.

65. Bezold C ed. *Pharmaceuticals in the year 2000, the changing context for drug R&D*. Alexandria, Virginia: Institute for Alternative Futures, 1983.

66. Bijl K, Koens M, Bakker A, de Valk J. Medical PACS and HIS: integration needed. In: Schneider R, Dwyer S eds. *Proceedings Medical Imaging Conference*. The International Society for Optical Engineering (SPIE) 1987; **767**: 89.

67. Biles B, Schramm C J, Atkinson J G. Hospital cost inflation under state rate setting. *New England Journal of Medicine* 1980; **303**: 664–668.

68. Binseng R, Boncai V, Canitrot C, *et al*. *Informe preliminar sobre relevamiento básico en tecnología de equipamiento en Argentina*. Buenos Aires: Pan American Health Organization, 1986.

69. Black N. Medical litigation and the quality of care. *Lancet* 1990; **335**: 35–37.

70. Bloom B S. Controlled studies in measuring the efficacy of medical care: a historical perspective. *International Journal of Technology Assessment in Health Care* 1986; **2**: 299–310.

71. Bloom G, Temple-Bird C. *Medical equipment in Sub-Saharan Africa: a framework for policy formulation*. IDS research Report, Brighton, UK, The University of Sussex. Geneva, Switzerland: World Health Organization, 1990. WHO/SHS/ NHP/90.6.

72. Blume S S. The significance of technological change in medicine: an introduction. *Research Policy* 1985; **14**: 173–177.

73. Bobadilla J, Frenk F, Lozano R, Stern C. The epidemiological transition and health priorities. In: Jamison D, Mosley W eds. *Evolving health sector priorities in developing countries*. Washington, DC: World Bank, 1990.

74. Bombardier C, Ware J, Russell I, *et al*. Auranofin therapy and quality of life in patients with rheumatoid arthritis: results of a multicenter trial. *American Journal of Medicine* 1986; **81**: 565–578.

75. Bonair A, Rosenfield P, Tengvald K. Medical technologies in developing countries: issues of technology development, transfer, diffusion and use. *Social Science and Medicine* 1989; **28**: 769–781.

76. Bonchek L. Are randomized trials appropriate for evaluating new operations? *New England Journal of Medicine* 1979; **301**: 44–45.

77. Bonsel G J. *Methods of medical technology assessment with an application to liver transplantation*. Doctoral thesis. Erasmus University Rotterdam, 1991.

78. Bos M A. Advising and deciding on medical technology (in Dutch). In: *Grenzen van medische technologie*. Justitiële verkenningen 6/91. The Hague, WODC, 1991.

79. Bos M A. *The diffusion of heart and liver transplantation across Europe.* London: King's Fund Centre, 1991.

80. Bos M. Personal communication, 1992.

81. Boyle M, Torrance G, Sinclair J, Horwood S. Economic evaluation of neonatal intensive care of very-low-birth weight infants. *New England Journal of Medicine* 1983; **308**: 1330−1337.

82. Bradley W G. Comparing costs and efficacy of MRI. *American Journal of Radiology* 1986; **146**: 1307−1310.

83. Braun P. Need for timely information justified NCHCT. *Medical Instrumentation* 1981; **15**: 302−304.

84. Bricker E. Industrial marketing and medical ethics. *New England Journal of Medicine* 1989; **320**: 1690−1692.

85. Britton M, Jonsson E, Marke L A, Murray V. Diagnosing suspected stroke: a cost-effectiveness analysis. *International Journal of Technology Assessment in Health Care* 1985; **1**: 147−158.

86. Brook R H. Quality: can we measure it? *New England Journal of Medicine* 1977; **296**: 170−172.

87. Brook R, Park R, Chassin M, *et al.* Predicting the appropriate use of carotid endarterectomy, upper gastrointestinal endoscopy, and coronary angiography. *New England Journal of Medicine* 1990; **323**: 1173−1177.

88. Brook R, Ware J, Rogers W, *et al.* Does free care improve adults' health? results from a randomized controlled trial. *New England Journal of Medicine* 1983; **309**: 1426−1434.

89. Brooks R G. *Health status and quality of life measurement: issues and developments.* Lund, Sweden: Swedish Institute for Health Economics, 1991.

90. Brown R, Luce, B. *Technology assessment in decision making by health care providers and payers.* Washington, DC: Battelle Medical Technology Assessment and Policy Research Center, 1992.

91. Brown R, Luce B. *The value of pharmaceuticals: a study of selected conditions to measure the contribution of pharmaceuticals to health status.* Washington, DC: Battelle Medical Technology Assessment and Policy Research Center, (Report No. BHARC-013/90/10), 1990.

92. Brown R, *et al. The value of pharmacuticals: an assessment of future costs for selected conditions.* Washington, DC: Battelle Medical Technology Assessment and Policy Research Center, (Report No. BHARC-013/90/25), 1990.

93. Brown R E, Elixhauser A, Corea J, Luce B R, Sheingold S. *National expenditures for health promotion and disease prevention activities in the United States.* Washington DC: Battelle Medical Technology Assessment and Policy (MEDTAP) Research Center, (Report No. BHARC-013/91-019), 1991.

94. Brown R E, Taylor W R, Luce B R, Elixhauser A, Sheingold S. *Prevention spending in the United States,* 1988. (submitted for publication 1992).

95. Bryce R. Support in pregnancy. *International Journal of Technology Assessment in Health Care* 1991; **7**: 478−484.

96. Buch Andreasen P. Consensus conferences in different countries. *International Journal of Technology Assessment in Health Care* 1988; **4**: 305−308.

97. Buch Andreasen P. *Medicinsk teknologivurdering.* Rapport til Folketingets Udvalg Andaende Videnskabelig Forskning. Copenhagen, 1980.

98. Bulpitt C, Fletcher A. Quality of life evaluation of antihypertensive drugs. *Pharmacoeconomics* 1992; **1**: 95−102.

99. Bunker J P, Barnes B A, Mosteller F. *Costs, risks, and benefits of surgery*. New York: Oxford University Press, 1977.
100. Burhenne H. The history of interventional radiology of the biliary tract. *Radiological Clinics of North America* 1990; **28**: 1139–1144.
101. Burkhardt R, Kienle G. Controlled clinical trials and medical ethics. *Lancet* 1978; **2**: 1356–1359.
102. Bush J, Chen M, Patrick D. Health status index in cost- effectiveness: analysis of PKU program. In: Berg R L ed. *Health status indexes*. Chicago: Hospital Research and Educational Trust, 1973.
103. Buxton M J. *Problems in economic appraisal of new health technology: the case of heart transplants*. Presented at an European Community Workshop on the Methodology of Economic Appraisal of Health Technology, Birmingham, England, 23–26 September 1985.
104. Buxton M, Acheson R, Caine N, Gibson S, O'Brien B. *Costs and benefits of the heart transplant programmes at Harefield and Papworth Hospitals*. London: Her Majesty's Stationery Office, 1985.
105. Byar D, Simon R M, Friedewald W T, *et al.* Randomized clinical trials. *New England Journal of Medicine* 1976; **295**: 74–80.
106. Calltorp T. Consensus development conferences in Sweden: effects on health policy and administration. *International Journal of Technology Assessment in Health Care* 1988; **4**: 75–88.
107. Cameron J, Gadacz T. Laparoscopic cholecystectomy. *Annals of Surgery* 1991: **213**: 1–2.
108. Canadian Coordinating Office for Health Technology Assessment (CCOHTA). *CCOHTA Update*. Ottawa, Canada, January 1991.
109. Canadian Erythropoietin Study Group. Association between recombinant human erythropoietin and quality of life and exercise capacity of patients receiving haemodialysis. *British Medical Journal* 1990; **300**: 573–578.
110. Casparie A F, van Everdingen J J E. Consensus development conferences in The Netherlands. *International Journal of Technology Assessment in Health Care* 1985; **1**: 905–912.
111. Cassell E J. Ideas in conflict: the rise and fall (and rise and fall) of new views of disease. *Daedalus* 1986; **115**: 19–41.
112. Centers for Disease Control. Measles prevention: recommendations of the Immunization Practices Advisory Committee (ACIP). *Morbidity and Mortality Weekly Report* (MMWR) 1989; **38**(s-9): 1–18.
113. Centers for Disease Control. Measles vaccination levels among selected groups of preschool-aged children—United States. *MMWR* 1991; **40**: 36–39.
114. Centers for Disease Control. Update: measles outbreak—Chicago 1989. *MMWR* 1990; **39**: 317–319, 325–326.
115. Centro Nacional de Informacion y Documentacion en Salud. *Catalogo de proyectos registrados en institucions publicas del sistema nacional de salud*. Mexico City: Secretariat of Health, 1991.
116. Chalmers I. Under-reporting research is scientific misconduct. *Journal of the American Medical Association* 1990; **263**: 1405–1408.
117. Chalmers I, Enkin M, Keirse M eds. *Effective care in pregnancy and childbirth*. Oxford: Oxford University Press, 1989.
118. Chalmers I, Hetherington J, Elbourne D, *et al.* Materials and methods used in synthesising evidence to evaluate the effects of care during pregnancy and

childbirth. In: Chalmers I, Enkin M, Keirse M eds. *Effective care in pregnancy and childbirth*. Oxford: Oxford University Press, 1989: pp. 39–65.

119. Chalmers T C. The impact of controlled trials on the practice of medicine. *Mount Sinai Journal of Medicine* 1974; **41**: 753–759.

120. de Charro F, Banta, D. Transplant policy in The Netherlands. *International Journal of Technology Assessment in Health Care* 1986; **2**: 507–531.

121. Chassin M, Kosecoff J, Solomon D, Brook R. How coronary angiography is used, clinical determinants of appropriateness. *Journal of the American Medical Association* 1987; **258**: 2543–2547.

122. Chetley A. *A healthy business? World health and the pharmaceutical industry.* London: Zed Books Ltd, 1990.

123. *China, Facts and Figures, China's economic and technical cooperation with foreign countries.* Foreign Language Press, Beijing (no date).

124. Chren M, Landefeld C S, Murray T. Doctors, drug companies and gifts. *Journal of the American Medical Association* 1989; **262**: 3448–3451.

125. Christensen E, Juhl E, Tygstrup N. Treatment of duodenal ulcer: randomized clinical trials of a decade (1964–1974). *Gastroenterology* 1977; **73**: 1170–1178.

126. Chu F, Cotter D. PPS policies should reflect payment adjustments for new technologies. *Business and Health* 1986; **4**: 60.

127. Churchill D, Wallace J, Ludwin D, Beecroft M, Taylor D W. A comparison of evaluative indices of quality of life and cognitive function in hemodialysis patients. *Controlled Clinical trials* 1991; **12**: 159S–167S.

128. Cleary P, Greenfield S, McNeil B. Assessing quality of life after surgery. *Controlled Clinical Trials* 1991; **12**: 189S–203S.

129. Cluff L. Chronic disease, function and quality care. *Journal of Chronic Disease* 1981; **34**: 299–304.

130. Coates J. Technology assessment. In Teich A ed. *Technology and man's future.* New York: St. Martin's Press, 1977: 251–270.

131. Coates J. Technology assessment: the benefits . . . the costs . . . the consequences. *Futurist* 1971; **5**: 225–231.

132. Cochrane A. *Effectiveness and efficiency*. Abingdon, England: Burgess & Son, 1972.

133. Coe G, Banta H D. Health care technology transfer in Latin America and the Caribbean. *International Journal of Technology Assessment in Health Care* 1992; **89**: 255–267.

134. Cohen E P. Direct-to-the-public advertisement of prescription drugs. *New England Journal of Medicine* 1988; **318**: 373–376.

135. Cohen D, Henderson J. *Health, prevention and economics.* Oxford: Oxford Medical Publications, 1988.

136. Coleman J S, Katz E, Menzel H. *Medical innovations: a diffusion study.* Indianapolis: Bobbs-Merrill, 1966: pp. 11–12, 59–60.

137. Commission on Health Research for Development. *Health research: essential link to equity in development.* Oxford: Oxford University Press, 1991.

138. Committee on the Life Sciences and Social Policy, Assembly of Behavioral and Social Sciences, National Resarch Council. *Assessing biomedical technologies: an inquiry into the nature of the process.* Washington, DC: National Academy of Sciences, 1975.

139. Committee on Technology and Health Care. Institute of Medicine. *Medical technology and the health care system.* Washington, DC: National Academy of Sciences, 1979.

140. Commonwealth of Australia. *Guidelines for the pharmaceutical industry on preparation of submissions to the Pharmaceutical Benefits Advisory Committee: including submissions involving economic analysis.* Canberra: Department of Health, Housing and Community Services, 1990.

141. Consejo Nacional de Ciencia y Tecnologia. CONACYT en cifras 1987. *Ciencia y Tecnologia* 1990; **16**: 55–67.

142. Cooper L S, Chalmers T C, McCally M, Berrier J, Sacks H S. The poor quality of early evaluations of magnetic resonance imaging. *Journal of the American Medical Association* 1988; **259**: 3277–3280.

143. Copenhagen Collaborating Center. *Bibliography on regional variation in health care.* Copenhagen, Number 2: 1987.

144. Copenhagen Collaborating Center. CCC *Bibliography on regional variation in health care* 1985. Copenhagen.

145. Creese A. The economic evaluation of immunization programmes. In: Lee K, Mills A eds. *The economics of health in developing countries.* Oxford: Oxford University Press, 1983: 146–166.

146. Creese A, Henderson R H. Cost-benefit analysis and immunization programmes in developing countries. *Bulletin of the World Health Organization* 1980; **58**: 491–497.

147. Croog S H, Levine S, Testa M A, *et al.* The effects of antihypertensive therapy on the quality of life. *New England Journal of Medicine* 1986; **314**: 1657–1664.

148. Crowe B. Overview of some methodological problems in assessment of PACS. Presented at the International Workshop on Technology Assessment of PACS, Enkhuizen, The Netherlands, May 26–27, 1991.

149. Crues J, Mink J, Levy T, Lotysch M, Stoller D. Meniscal tears of the knee: accuracy of magnetic resonance imaging. *Radiology* 1987; **164**: 445–448.

150. Cruz C, Arredondo A, Faba G, *et al. Informe tecnico de la investigacion sobre oferta de aparatos medicos en Mexico.* Mexico: National Institute of Public Health/ Panamerican Health Organization, 1991.

151. Cruz C, Arredondo A, Hernandez B, *et al. La oferta de aparatos medicos en Mexico.* Salud Publica Mexica (in press).

152. Cruz C, Lozano R, Querol J. *The impact of economic crisis and adjustment on health care in Mexico.* Italy: International Child Development Centre, UNICEF, 1991 Innocenti Occasional Papers 13.

153. Culyer A. Assessing cost-effectiveness. In: Banta D ed. *Resources for health.* New York: Praeger, 1982: pp. 107–120.

154. Culyer A, Horisberger B. Medical and economic evaluation: a postscript. In: Culyer A, Horisberger B eds. *Economic and medical evaluation of health care technologies.* Berlin: Springer-Verlag, 1983: pp. 347–358.

155. Cuschieri A, Dubois F, Mouiel J, *et al.* The European experience with laparoscopic cholecystectomy. *American Journal of Surgery* 1991; **161**: 285–287.

156. Cwikiel W, Ivances K, Lunderquist A. Metallic stents. *Radiological Clinics of North America* 1990; **28**: 1202–1210.

157. Daddario E Q. Statement of the chairman. In: *Technology assessment.* Washington, DC: US Congress, House of Representatives, Committee on Science and Astronautics, Subcommittee on Science, Research, and Development. 90th Congress, 1st Session, 1967.

158. Danielsson H. *Functioning and funding of medical research, European Medical Research Councils.* Manuscript Prepared by the President of the European Medical Research Councils, 1985.

159. Davidoff F, Goodspeed R, Clive J. Changing test-ordering behavior, a randomized controlled trial comparing probabilistic reasoning with cost-containment education. *Medical Care* 1988; **27**: 48–58.

160. Davis J. The future of major ambulatory surgery. *Surgical Clinics of North America* 1987; **67**: 893–901.

161. DCCT Research Group. Reliability and validity of a diabetes quality-of-life measure for the diabetes control and complications trial (DCCT). *Diabetes Care* 1988; **11**: 725–732.

162. De Geyndt W. *Managing health expenditures under national health insurance, the case of Korea*. Washington, DC: The World Bank, 1991.

163. Department of Commerce. *Reports on exports and imports*, 1988.

164. Department of Community Services & Health, Commonwealth of Australia. *Pharmaceutical benefits scheme (PBS) cost-effectiveness guidelines*, August 28, 1990.

165. Department of Health. *Research for health, a research and development strategy for the NHS*. London: Department of Health, 1991.

166. De Simone D, Kundel H, Arenson R, Seshadn S, *et al*. Effect of a digital imaging network on physician behavior in an intensive care unit. *Radiology* 1988; **169**: 41–44.

167. Deyo R, Diehr P, Patrick D. Reproducibility and responsiveness of health status measures: statistics and strategies for evaluation. *Controlled Clinical Trials* 1991; **12**: 142S–158S.

168. Deyo R, Diehl A, Rosental M. How many days of bed rest for acute low back pain? A randomized clinical trial. *New England Journal of Medicine* 1986; **315**: 1064–1070.

169. Deyo R, Patrick D. Barriers to the use of health status measures in clinical investigation, patient care, and policy research. *Medical Care* 1989; **27**(suppl): S254–S268.

170. Diagnostic and Therapeutic Technology Assessment (DATTA). Laparoscopic cholecystectomy. *Journal of the American Medical Association* 1991; **265**: 1585–1587.

171. Diamond J, Kramer S, Hanks G. Trends in radiation therapy demographics— 1974–1983. *International Journal of Radiation Oncology, Biology and Physics* 1986; **12**: 1673–1674.

172. Dickersin K, *et al*. Perusing the literature. Comparison of MEDLINE searching with a perinatal trials database. *Controlled Clinical Trials* 1985; **6**: 306–317.

173. DiMasi J A, *et al*. Cost of innovation in the pharmaceutical industry. *Journal of Health Economics* 1991; **10**: 107–115.

174. Dimond E, Kittle C, Crockett J. Comparison of internal memmary artery ligation and sham operation for angina pectoris. *American Journal of Cardiology* 1960; **5**: 483–486.

175. Dinkel R. Cost-cost comparisons of Nitroderm TTS in Switzerland and Australia. In van Eimeren W, Horisberger B eds. *Socioeconomic evaluation of drug therapy*. Berlin: Springer-Verlag, 1988: 110–118.

176. Direccion General de Epidemiologia. *Encusta nacional de salud*. Mexico: Secretariat of Health, 1988.

177. Direccion General de Investigacion y Desarrollo Tecnologico. *Inventario funcional de equipos medicos en unidades de primer nivel de atencion*. Mexico: Secretariat of Health, 1987.

178. Donabedian A. Evaluating the quality in medical care. *Milbank Memorial Fund Quarterly* 1966; **44** (Part 2): 166–206.

179. Donabedian A. *Explorations in quality assessment and monitoring*, Volume 1, *The definition of quality and approaches to its assessment*. Ann Arbor, Michigan: Health Administration Press, 1980.

180. Donaldson M, Sox H eds. *Setting priorities for health technology assessment, a model process*. Washington, DC: National Academy Press, 1992.

181. Doty P. *Memo to the Interstate and Foreign Commerce Committee*. Washington, DC: Office of Technology Assessment, 1980.

182. Doubilet P, Abrams H L. The cost of underutilization. *New England Journal of Medicine* 1984; **310**: 95–101.

183. Dowling H. *Medicines for man*. New York: Alfred A. Knopf, 1970.

184. Drew P. *Picture archiving and communication systems*. Chicago: American Hospital Association, 1985.

185. Driscol D. *What is the International Monetary Fund?* Washington, DC: International Monetary Fund, 1991.

186. Drummond M. *Principles of economic appraisal in health care*. London: Oxford University Press, 1980.

187. Drummond M, Hutton J. *Economic appraisal of health technology in the United Kingdom*. Prepared for the European Community Workshop on the Methodology of Economic Appraisal of Health Technology, Birmingham, England, September 1985.

188. Drummond M, Stoddart B. Economic analysis and clinical trials. *Controlled Clinical Trials* 1984; **5**: 115–124.

189. Drummond M, Brandt A, Luce B, Rovira J. Standardizing methodologies for economic evaluation in health care: practice, problems and potential. *International Journal of Technology Assessment in Health Care* 1993; **9**: 26–36.

190. Drummond M F, Stoddart G L, Torrance G W. *Methods for the economic evaluation of health care programmes*. Oxford: Oxford Medical Publications, 1987.

191. Dubois F, Icard P, Berthelot G, Levard H. Coelioscopic cholecystectomy, preliminary report of 36 cases. *Annals of Surgery* 1990; **211**: 60–62.

192. Dubois R W, Brook R H. Preventable deaths: who, how often, and why? *Annals of Internal Medicine* 1988; **109**: 582–589.

193. Dubois R W, Brook R H, Rogers W H. Adjusted hospital death rates: a potential screen for quality of medical care. *American Journal of Public Health* 1987; **77**: 1162–1166.

194. Duke R, Bloch R, Turpie A, Trebilcock R, Bayer N. Intravenous heparin for the prevention of stroke progression in acute partial stable stroke: a randomized controlled trial. *Annals of Internal Medicine* 1986; **105**: 825–828.

195. Dunning A, Chairman. Committee on Choices in Health Care. *Choices in Health Care* (Kiezen and Delen). Rijswijk: Ministry of Health, 1991.

196. Duran-Gonzalez L, Becerra-Aponte J, Franco F, *et al*. Uso del cuadro basico de medicamentos en el primer nivel de atencion. *Salud Publica Mexica* 1990; **32**: 543–551.

197. Dutrée M A. *The introduction and diffusion of expensive medical technology in The Netherlands* (in Dutch). Doctoral thesis. Erasmus University, Rotterdam, 1991.

198. Dutton D. *Worse than the disease, pitfalls of medical progress*. Cambridge: Cambridge University Press, 1988.

199. The EC/IC Bypass Study Group. Failure of extracranial-intracranial arterial bypass to reduce the risk of ischemic stroke. *New England Journal of Medicine* 1986; **313**: 1191–1200.

200. Economic Commission for Europe. Working Party on Engineering Industries and Automation. *Digital imaging in health care*. New York: United Nations, 1987.

201. Economic Commission for Europe. *Bulletin of statistics on world trade in engineering products*. Table 9. New York: United Nations, 1990: pp. 524–529.

202. ECRI. *Computer-processed EEG monitoring during surgery*. Issues in health care technology. New technology briefs/5.E.4 (rev.), 1986.

203. Eddy D ed. *Common screening tests*. Philadelphia, Pa: American College of Physicians, 1991.

204. Eddy D. Designing a practice policy, standards, guidelines and options. *Journal of the American Medical Association* 1991; **266**: 3077–3084.

205. Eddy D. Oregon's plan, should it be approved? *Journal of the American Medical Association* 1991; **266**: 2439–2445.

206. Eddy D. Practice policies, what are they? *Journal of the American Medical Association* 1990; **263**: 877–880.

207. Eddy D. *Screening for cancer: theory, analysis, and design*. Englewood Cliffs, NJ: Prentice-Hall, 1980.

208. Eddy D. Selecting technologies for assessment. *International Journal of Technology Assessment in Health Care* 1989; **5**: 485–501.

209. Eddy D. Variations in physicians practice. *Health Affairs* 1984; **3**: 74–89.

210. Edelson J, Weinstein M, Tosteson A, *et al*. Long-term cost-effectiveness of various initial monotherapies for mild to moderate hypertension. *Journal of the American Medical Association* 1990; **263**: 408–413.

211. Eisenberg J. *Doctor's decisions and the cost of medical care*. Ann Arbor, Michigan: Health Administration Press, 1986.

212. Eisenberg J. Substituting diagnostic services, new tests only partly replace older ones. *Journal of the American Medical Association* 1989; **262**: 1196–1200.

213. Ekelman K B ed. *New medical devices, invention, development, and use*. Washington, DC: National Academy Press, 1988: 35–47.

214. Elixhauser A, Luce B, Taylor W, Reblando J. *Health care cost-benefit and cost-effectiveness analysis from 1979 to 1990: a bibliography*. Submitted for publication, 1992.

215. Ellul J. *The technological society*. Translated from the 1954 French version by John Wilkinson. New York: Random House, 1964: p. 18.

216. Ellwood P. Outcomes management, a technology of patient experience. *New England Journal of Medicine* 1988; **318**: 1549–1546.

217. Erickson P, Kendall E, Anderson J, Kaplan R. Using composite health status measures to assess the nation's health. *Medical Care* 1989; **27** (suppl): S66–S76.

218. Erp van W F M, Bruyninckx C. De eerste ervaringen met laparoscopische cholecystectomie. *Nederlands Tijdschrift voor Geneeskunde* 1991; **135**: 272–276.

219. The EuroQoL Group. EuroQoL—a new facility for the measurement of health-related quality of life. *Health Policy* 1990; **16**: 199–208.

220. Evans J, Hall K, Warford J. Health care in the developing world: problems of scarcity and choice. *New England Journal of Medicine* 1981; **305**: 1117–1127.

221. Evans R W. Health care technology and the inevitability of resource allocation and rationing decisions. *Journal of the American Medical Association* 1983; **249**: 2041–2053, 2208–2219.

222. Evans R, Rader B, Manninen D, *et al*. The quality of life of hemodialysis recipients treated with recombinant human erythropoietin. *Journal of the American Medical Association* 1990; **263**: 825–830.

223. Evens R. Economic costs of nuclear magnetic resonance imaging. *Journal of Computer Assisted Tomography* 1984; **3**: 200–203.
224. van Everdingen J J E. Consensus ontwikkeling in de geneeskunde (*Consensus development in medicine*). Thesis, University of Amsterdam. Antwerp: Bohn, Scheltema en Holkema, 1988.
225. Faba G. *Protocolo de investigacion sobre la produccion cientifica y tecnologica en salud*. Mexico: Secretariat of Health, 1989.
226. Fairbank J, Couper J, Davies J, O'Brien J. Oswestry low-back pain disability questionnaire. *Physiotherapy* 1980; **66**: 271–272.
227. Fakes R. Doctors and the drug industry. *British Medical Journal* 1986; **293**: 905–906.
228. Fanshel S, Bush J. A health status index and its application to health-services outcomes. *Operations Research* 1970; **18**: 1021–1066, 1970.
229. Feeny D, Torrance G. Incorporating utility-based quality-of-life assessment measures in clinical trials. *Medical Care* 1989; **27**: S190–S204.
230. Feeny D. Neglected issues in the diffusion of health care technologies: the role of skills and learning. *International Journal of Technology Assessment in Health Care* 1985; **1**: 681–692.
231. Feeny D, Guyatt G, Tugwell P. *Health care technology: effectiveness, efficiency & public policy*. Montreal: The Institute for Research on Public Policy, 1986.
232. Feinstein A P. A survey of the statistical procedures in general medical journals. *Clinical Pharmacology and Therapeutics* 1975; **15**: 97–107.
233. Feldstein M, Taylor A. *The rapid rise of hospital costs*. Washington, DC: The President's Council on Wage and Price Stability, 1977.
234. Ferguson F, Davey A, Topley W. The value of mixed vaccines in the prevention of the common cold. *Journal of Hygiene* 1927; **26**: 98–109.
235. Fibiger J. Om Serumbehandlung af Difteri. *Hospitalstidende* 1898; **4**: 309,337.
236. Field M, Lohr K eds. *Guidelines for clinical practice*. Washington, DC: National Academy Press, 1992.
237. Fineberg H V. Clinical chemistries: the high cost of low-cost diagnostic tests. In: Altman S, Blendon R eds. *Medical technology: the culprit behind health care costs?* Hyattsville, Maryland: National Center for Health Services Research and Bureau of Health Planning, 1979. (DHEW Publication No. (PHS) 79-3216): pp. 144–165.
238. Fineberg H V. Effects of clinical evaluation on the diffusion of medical technology. In: *Institute of Medicine. Assessing medical technologies*. Washington, DC: National Academy Press, 1985: pp. 176–210.
239. Fineberg H V. Gastric freezing: a study of diffusion of a medical innovation. In: Committee on Technology and Health Care. *Medical technology and the health care system*. Washington, DC: National Academy of Sciences, 1979: pp. 173–200.
240. Fineberg H V, Bauman R, Sosman M. Computerized cranial tomography: effect on diagnostic and therapeutic plans. *Journal of the American Medical Association* 1977; **238**: 224–227.
241. Fineberg H V, Hiatt H. Evaluation of medical practices: the case for technology assessment. *New England Journal of Medicine* 1979; **301**: 1086–1091.
242. Fink A, Brook R, Kosecoff J, *et al*. *Sufficiency of clinical literature on the appropriate use of six medical and surgical procedures*. Santa Monica, California: RAND, 1991.
243. Fisher L, Kennedy J. Randomized surgical clinical trials for treatment of coronary artery disease. *Controlled Clinical Trials* 1982; **3**: 235–258.

244. Fitzgibbons R, Schmid S, Santoscoy R. *Paper on laparoscopic cholecystectomy*, submitted for publication (described in ref. 273).
245. Flagle C, Gremy F, Perry S eds. *Assessment of medical informatics technology*. Montpellier, France: Editions ENSP, 1991.
246. Fletcher R H, Fletcher S W. Clinical research in general medical journals. *New England Journal of Medicine* 1979; **301**: 180–183.
247. Fletcher S W, Fletcher R, Greganti A. Clinical research trends in general medical journals, 1946–1976. In: Roberts E B, Levy R I, Finkelstein S N, Moskowitz J, Sondik E J eds. *Biomedical innovations*. Cambridge Massachusetts: MIT Press, 1981: 284–300.
248. Food and Drug Administration, US Department of Health and Human Services. *General considerations for the clinical evaluation of drugs*. Washington, DC, US Government Printing Office.
249. Forster D, Jozan P. Health in Eastern Europe. *Lancet* 1990; **335**: 458–460.
250. Foss L, Rothenberg K. *The second medical revolution: from biomedicine to info-medicine*. Boston: Shambhala Publications and Random House, 1987.
251. Fowler F, Wennberg J, Timothy R, *et al.* Symptom status and quality of life following prostatectomy. *Journal of the American Medical Association* 1988; **259**: 3018–3022.
252. Fox R C. The medicalization and demedicalization of American society. *Daedalus* 1977; **106**: 9–22.
253. Fox R C. A preface. *International Journal of Technology Assessment in Health Care* 1986; **2**: 189–194.
254. Fox R C, Swazey J P. *The courage to fail*. Chicago: The University of Chicago Press, 1974.
255. Freeland M, Schendler C. National health expenditure growth in the 1980s: an aging population, new technologies, and increasing competition. *Health Care Financing Review* 1983; **3**: 1–58.
256. Freeman R. Cost containment. *Journal of Medical Education* 1977; **51**: 157–158.
257. Freidson E. *Patients' views of medical practice*. New York: Russell Sage Foundation, 1961.
258. Freidson E. *The profession of medicine*. New York: Dodd, Mead & Company, 1972.
259. Frenk J. Personal communication, 1991.
260. Frenk J. The political economy of medical underemployment in Mexico: corporatism, economic crisis and reform. *Health Policy* 1990; **15**: 143–162.
261. Frenk J. The public/private mix and human resources for health. In: Jardiel J, Good E eds. *Saitama Public Health Summit*. Geneva: World Health Organization (in press).
262. Frenk J, Bobadilla J. Los futuros de la Salud. *Nexos* 1991; **157**: 63.
263. Frenk J, Bobadilla J, Sepulveda J, Lopez-Cervantes M. Health transition in middle-income countries: new challenges for health care. *Health Policy and Planning* 1989; **4**: 29–39.
264. Frenk J, Frejka T, Bobadilla J, *et al.* La transicion epidemiologica en America Latina. *Bolletin Senataria Panamericana* 1991; **111**: 485–496.
265. Frieds J. Aging, natural death, and the compression of morbidity. *New England Journal of Medicine* 1980; **303**: 130–135.
266. Fries J, Spitz P, Young D. The dimensions of health outcomes: the health assessment questionnaire, disability, and pain scales. *Journal of Rheumatology* 1982; **9**: 789–793.

267. Froberg D, Kane R. Methodology for measuring health-state preferences—I: measurement strategies. *Journal of Clinical Epidemiology* 1989a; **42**: 345–354.

268. Froberg D, Kane R. Methodology for measuring health-state preferences—II: scaling methods. *Journal of Clinical Epidemiology* 1989b; **42**: 459–471.

269. Froberg D, Kane R. Methodology for measuring health-state preferences—III: population and context effects. *Journal of Clinical Epidemiology* 1989c; **42**: 585–592.

270. Froberg D, Kane R. Methodology for measuring health-state preferences—IV: progress and a research agenda. *Journal of Clinical Epidemiology* 1989d; **42**: 675–685.

271. Fuchs V R ed. *The growing demand for medical care*. New York: Columbia University Press, 1972.

272. Gabinete de Comercio Exterior. *Proceso de adhesion de Mexico al Acuerdo General Sobre Aranceles Aduaneros y Comercio (GATT)*. Mexico: Secretariat of Commerce and Industrial Promotion, 1976.

273. Gadacz T, Talamini M, Lillemoe K, Yeo C. Laparoscopic cholecystectomy. *Surgical Clinics of North America* 1990; **70**: 1249–1262.

274. Gaensler E H L, Jonsson E, Neuhauser D. Controlling medical technology in Sweden. In: Banta H D and Kemp K B eds. *The management of health care technology in nine countries*. New York: Springer Publishing Company, 1982: pp. 167–192.

275. Galbraith J. *The new industrial state*. New York: The New American Library, Inc., 1977: p. 31.

276. Ganz P, Schag C, Lee J, Sim M. The CARES: a generic measure of health-related quality of life for patients with cancer. *Quality of Life Research* 1992; **1**: 19–30.

277. Garnick D, Hendricks A, Brelin N. Can practice guidelines reduce the number and costs of malpractice claims. *Journal of the American Medical Association* 1991; **266**: 2856–2860.

278. Geertsma R H, Parker R C, Whitbourne S K. How physicians view the process of change in their practice behavior. *Journal of Medical Education* 1982; **57**: 752–761.

279. Gelijns A C. *Innovation in clinical practice, the dynamics of medical technology development*. Washington, DC: National Academy Press, 1991.

280. Gelijns A C, Rigter H. Health care technology assessment in The Netherlands. *International Journal of Technology Assessment in Health Care* 1990; **6**: 157–163.

281. Gelijns A, Thier S. Medical technology development: an introduction to the innovation-evaluation nexus. In: *Modern methods of clinical investigation*, Vol. 1, *Medical innovation at the crossroads*. Washington, DC: National Academy Press, 1990: pp. 1–15.

282. Gennip van E, van Poppel B, Bakker A, Ottes F. *Comparison of worldwide opinions on the costs and benefits of PACS*. Presented at the International Workshop on Technology Assessment of PACS, Enkhuizen, The Netherlands, May 26–27, 1991.

283. Gereffi G. *The pharmaceutical industry and dependency in the Third World*. Princeton, New Jersey: Princeton University Press, 1983.

284. Gewecke J, Weisbrod B A. Clinical evaluation vs. economic evaluation: the case of a new drug. *Medical Care* 1982; **20**: 821–830.

285. Gifford R H, Feinstein A R. A critique of methodology in studies of anticoagulant therapy for acute myocardial infarction. *New England Journal of Medicine* 1969; **280**: 351–357.

286. Gilbert J P, McPeek B, Mosteller F. Progress in surgery and anesthesia: benefits and risks of innovative therapy. In: Bunker J P, Barnes B A, Mosteller F eds. *Costs, risks, and benefits of surgery.* New York: Oxford University Press, 1977: pp. 124–169.

287. Gilling E, Cannon P. Pathogenic effects of elixir of sulfanilamide (diethyleneglycol) poisoning. *Journal of the American Medical Association* 1938; **111**: 919.

288. Girvan N. *Notes on technological capability.* Presented to the Caribbean Technology Policy Studies Workshop, Port-of-Spain, Trinidad, May 5–9, 1981.

289. Gjone E. *Presentation at the meeting on future health scenarios,* World Health Organization, Copenhagen, 5 November 1985.

290. Glass G V. Primary, secondary, and meta-analysis of research. *Educational Researcher* 1976; **5**: 3–8.

291. Goodman C. It's time to rethink health care technology assessment. *International Journal of Technology Assessment in Health Care* 1992; **8**: 335–358.

292. Goodman C, Baratz S eds. *Improving consensus development for health technology assessment: an international perspective.* Washington, DC: National Academy Press, 1990.

293. Goodwin J S, Goodwin J M. The tomato effect: rejection of highly efficacious therapies. *Journal of the American Medical Association* 1984; **251**: 2387–2390.

294. Gore S M, Jones I G, Rytter E C. Misuse of statistical methods: critical assessment of articles in BMJ from January to March 1976. *British Medical Journal* 1977; **1**: 85–87.

295. Grabowski H G, Vernon J M. *The regulation of pharmaceuticals, balancing the benefits and risks.* Washington, DC: American Enterprise Institute, 1983.

296. Greenberg E R, Chute C G, Stukel T, Baron J A, Freeman D H, Yates J, Korson R. Social and economic factors in the choice of lung cancer treatment. *New England Journal of Medicine* 1988; **318**: 612–617.

297. Greenberg S. The challenges and opportunities that quality assurance rasies for technology assessment. In Lohr K, Rettig R eds. *Quality of care and technology assessment.* Washington, DC: National Academy Press, 1989: pp. 134–141.

298. Greer A L. Adoption of medical technology: the hospital's three decision-systems. *International Journal of Technology Assessment in Health Care* 1985; **1**: 669–680.

299. Greer A L. Advances in the study of diffusion of innovation in health care organizations. *The Milbank Memorial Fund Quarterly* 1977; **55**: 505–532.

300. Greer A L. *Deus ex machina: physicians in the adoption of hospital medical technology.* Milwaukee: Urban Research Center, the University of Wisconsin-Milwaukee, 1981.

301. Greer A L. Medical conservatism and technological acquisitiveness: the paradox of hospital technology adoptions. In: Roth J, Ruzak S eds. *Research in the sociology of health care. IV: the adoption and social consequences of medical technology.* Greenwich, Connecticut: JAI Press, 1986: pp. 185–235.

302. Greer A L. Medical technology and professional dominance theory. *Social Science and Medicine* 1984; **18**: 809–817.

303. Greer A L. The state of the art versus the state of the science: the diffusion of new medical technologies into practice. *International Journal of Technology Assessment in Health Care* 1988; **4**: 5–26.

304. Griner P F. Treatment of acute pulmonary edema: conventional or intensive care? *Annals of Internal Medicine* 1972; **77**: 501–506.

305. Griner P F. Use of laboratory tests in a teaching hospital: long-term trends: reductions in use of relative cost. *Annals of Internal Medicine* 1979; **75**: 157–163.

306. Groot L M F. *Diffusion of medical technology, a Dutch case study*. Presented at the EEC Workshop on Regulatory Mechanisms Concerning Expensive Health Technology, London, 22—25 April 1986.

307. Groot L M J. Medical technology in the health care system of The Netherlands. In: Banta D, Kemp K eds. *The management of health care technology in nine countries*. New York: Springer Publishing Company, 1982: pp. 150—166.

308. Groot L M J. *Study on regulatory mechanisms of the diffusion of expensive health technology in the member states of the European Community*. Interim Report to the European Commission. August 1986.

309. Guerrero, M. *Importación y exportación de tecnología médica en América Latina y el Caribe*. ICMDRA. Washington, DC: WHO/PAHO/FDA, 1986.

310. Guther B. Transdermal nitrate therapy in coronary heart disease from the patient's point of view—a quality of life study in the Federal Republic of Germany. In: van Eimeren W, Horisberger B eds. *Socioeconomic evaluation of drug therapy*. Berlin: Springer-Verlag, 1988: pp. 181—187.

311. Guyatt G H, Drummond M F. The ethics and feasibility of randomized trials of diagnostic technology: a reply. *International Journal of Technology Assessment in Health Care* 1985; **1**: 901—904.

312. Guyatt G, Jaeschke R. Measurements in clinical trials: choosing the appropriate approach. In: Spilker B ed. *Quality of life assessments in clinical trials*, Raven Press, New York, 1990.

313. Guyatt G, Berman L, Townsend M, Pugsley S, Chambers L. A measure of quality of life for clinical trials in chronic lung disease. *Thorax* 1989; **42**: 773—778.

314. ter Haar Romeny J, van der Wielen A, Achterberg F, *et al*. PACS efficiency: a detailed quantitative study to the distribution process of films in a clinical environment in the Utrecht University Hospital. *Proceedings of the Medical Imaging Conference* SPIE III. 1989; **1093**: 259—271.

315. Haley L R W. *Managing hospital infection control for cost-effectiveness: a strategy for reducing infectious complications*. Chicago: American Hospital Publishing Inc., 1986.

316. Harris J. The internal organization of hospitals: some economic implications. *Bell Journal of Economics* 1977; **8**: 467—482.

317. Hatziandrieu E, Brown R, Revicki D. *Cost-effectiveness of sertraline maintenance treatment for recurrent major depression*. Washington, DC: Battelle Medical Technology Assessment and Policy Research Center, 1992.

318. Hatziandreu E, Shakespeare A, Andersson F, *et al*. *The status and future of socioeconomic studies in Europe: a survey and analysis*. London: Battelle Medical Technology Assessment and Policy Research Centre, 1992.

319. Health Action International. *Promoting health or pushing drugs?* Amsterdam, 1992.

320. Health Care Financing Administration (HCFA). *Federal Register*, Vol. 54, No. 18, January 30, 1989.

321. Health Council of The Netherlands. *Medicine at the crossroads* (in Dutch). The Hague, 1991.

322. Health Council of The Netherlands (Gezondheidsraad). *NMR—vorming en opleiding*. The Hague, 13 July 1985.

323. Health Industry Manufacturers Association. *Personal communication*, 1992.

324. Henderson G, Liu Yuanli, Guan Xiaoming, Liu Zongxziu. The rise of technology in Chinese hospitals. *International Journal of Technology Assessment in Health Care* 1987; **3**: 253—264.

325. Henderson R. *Putting vaccines to work in the Expanded Programme on Immuniza-tion*. Paper presented at Conference on Immunization—New Horizons. Geneva: World Health Organization, 19–20 March, 1987.

326. Hendryx M. A review of the literature on quality assurance programmes. Reported outcomes and intervention types. *Quality Assurance and Utilization Review* 1991; **6**: 123–126.

327. Henry D. Economic analysis as an aid to subsidisation decisions. The development of Australian guidelines for pharmaceuticals. *PharmacoEconomics* 1992; **1**: 54–67.

328. Hilborne L, Leape L, Kahan J, *et al. Percutaneous transluminal coronary angio-plasty*. Santa Monica, California: RAND, 1991.

329. Hillman A. Sounding board: avoiding bias in the conduct and reporting of cost-effectiveness research sponsored by pharmaceutical companies. *New England Journal of Medicine* 1991; **324**: 1362–1365.

330. Hillman A, *et al. Collaborative Task Force to Establish Clinical Economics Research and Reporting Guidelines: operating plan and grant proposal*. Philadel-phia: Center for Health Policy, Leonard Davis Institute of Health Economics, March, 1992.

331. Hilsenrath P, Smith W, Berbaum K, *et al.* Analysis of the cost-effectiveness of PACS. *American Journal of Radiology* 1991; **156**: 177–180.

332. Hinman A. What will it take to fully protect all American children with vaccines? *American Journal of Diseases of Children* 1991; **145**: 559–562.

333. Hirschfeld E. Should practice parameters be the standards of care in malpractice litigation? *Journal of the American Medical Association* 1991; **266**: 2886–2891.

334. Hisashige A. *The introduction and evaluation of MRI in Japan*. Presented at the Meeting of the International Society for Technology Assessment in Health Care, Vancouver, Canada, June 15–17, 1992.

335. Hisashige A, Sakurai T, Kaihara S. Medical technology assessment and medical information in Japan: present and future. In: Flagle C, Gremy F, Perry S eds. *Assessment of medical informatics technology*. Montpellier, France: Editions ENSP, 1991: 509–519.

336. Hoare J ed. *Report of the Caversham Conference*. London: King's Fund Centre, 1992.

337. Hollandsworth J G. Evaluating the impact of medical treatment on the quality of life: a 5-year update. *Social Science and Medicine* 1988; **26**: 425–434.

338. Hsiao, Teh-ku, Tsai, Jen-hwa. An assessment of the management and utilization of CT scanners—a survey of CT in the City of Shanghai. *Weisheng Jingi (Health Economics)* 1986, pp. 53–56.

339. Hu, Teh-wei, Diffusion of Western medical technology in China since the eco-nomic reform. *International Journal of Technology Assessment in Health Care* 1988; **4**: 345–358.

340. Huang H. *Elements of digital radiology*. New York: Prentice-Hall, 1986.

341. Hunt S, McKenna S, McEwen J, Backett E, Williams J, Papp E. A quantitative approach to perceived health status: a validation study. *Journal of Epidemiology and Community Health* 1980; **34**: 281–286.

342. Huse D, Oster G, Weisbrod B, Read J, *et al.* The cost effectiveness of transdermal nitroglycerin in the Michigan Medicaid Program: a preliminary report. In: van Eimeren W, Horisberger B eds. *Socioeconomic evaluation of drug therapy*. Berlin: Springer-Verlag, 1988: pp. 119–131.

343. Hutter Am, Sidel V W, Shine K I, DeSanctis R W. Early hospital discharge after myocardial infarction. *New England Journal of Medicine* 1973; **288**: 1141–1144.

344. Hutton J, Fagnani F, Joergensen T, *et al.* ASSIST: Assessment of information systems and technologies in health care. In: Noothoven van Goor J, Christensen J. *Advances in medical informatics.* Amsterdam: IOS Press, 1992: pp. 30–38.

345. Hutton J, Persson J, Saranummi N, *et al. Project A 1016: ASSIST (Assessment of Information Systems and Technologies in Medicine), Final report: summary and conclusions.* Deliverable No. 6. Brussels: CEC DG XIII/F AIM Programme, January, 1991.

346. Illich I. *Medical nemesis: the expropriation of health.* New York: Pantheon Books (Random House, Inc.), 1976.

347. *IMS Pharmaceutical Marketletter.* London. 11 January 1982.

348. Inlander C, Levin L, Weiner E. *Medicine on trial.* London: Prentice Hall Press, 1988.

349. Inman W. Prescription event monitoring. *Acta Medica Scandinavica* 1987; **683** (suppl): 119–130.

350. Institute of Medicine. *Assessing medical technologies.* Report of the Committee for Evaluating Medical Technologies in Clinical Use. Washington, DC: National Academy Press, 1985.

351. Institute of Medicine. *Consensus development at the NIH: improving the program.* Washington, DC: National Academy Press, 1990.

352. Institute of Medicine. *A consortium for assessing medical technology.* Washington, DC: National Academy Press, 1983.

353. Institute of Medicine. *Medical technology assessment directory.* Washington, DC: National Academy Press, 1988.

354. Instituto Nacional de Geografia, Estadistica e Informatica. *Resultados preliminares del XI censo general de poblacion y vivienda 1990.* Mexico: National Institute of Geography, Statistics, and Informatics, 1990.

355. International Monetary Fund (IMF). *Annual report.* Washington, DC, 1991.

356. International Monetary Fund (IMF). *Ten common misconceptions about the IMF.* Washington, DC, 1988.

357. Jacoby I. The consensus development program of the National Institutes of Health. *International Journal of Technology Assessment in Health Care* 1985; **1**: 420–432.

358. James A, Carroll F, Pickens D, *et al.* Medical imaging management. *Radiology* 1986; **160**: 411–416.

359. Jennett B. *High technology medicine, benefits and burdens.* London: The Nuffield Provincial Hospitals Trust, 1983.

360. Jequier N. *Appropriate technology: problems and promises*, part 1, *the major policy issues.* Paris: Development Centre of the OECD, 1976.

361. Johnsson M. Evaluation of the consensus development program in Sweden: its impact on physicians. *International Journal of Technology Assessment in Health Care* 1988; **4**: 89–94.

362. Jonas S. *Medical mystery.* New York: W.W. Norton & Company, 1978.

363. Jonas S. *Quality control of ambulatory care: a task for health departments.* New York: Springer, 1977.

364. Jonsson B, Bjork S, Hofvendahl S, Levin, J. Quality of life in angina pectoris: a Swedish randomized cross-over comparison between Transderm-Nitro and long-acting oral nitrates. In: van Eimeren W, Horisberger B eds. *Socioeconomic evaluation of drug therapy.* Berlin: Springer-Verlag, 1988: pp. 166–180.

365. Jonsson E. Broadening the concepts of cost and effectiveness. In: Banta H D ed. *Resources for health.* New York: Praeger, 1982: pp. 121–125.

366. Jonsson E. *Studies in health economics.* Stockholm: The Economic Research Institute, Stockholm School of Economics, 1980.

367. Joskow P L. *Controlling hospital costs: the role of government regulation.* Cambridge, Massachusetts, MIT Press, 1981.

368. Kahan J P, Danouse D E, Winkaler J D. Stylistic variations in National Institutes of Health consensus statements, 1979–1983. *International Journal of Technology Assessment in Health Care* 1988; **4**: 289–304.

369. Kaluzny A. Innovation of health services: a comparative study of hospitals and health departments. *Milbank Memorial Fund Quarterly/Health and Society* 1974; **9**: 101–114.

370. Kaluzny A, Barhyte D Y, Reader G G. Health systems. In: Gordon G, Fisher L eds. *The diffusion of medical technology.* Cambridge, Massachusetts: Ballinger Publishing Company, 1975:29–43.

371. Kamlet M. *A framework for cost-utility analysis of government health care programs.* Washington, DC: Department of Health and Human Services, Office of Disease Prevention and Health Promotion, 1992.

372. Kamper Jorgensen F, Challah S, Folmer Andersen T. *Technology assessment and new kidney stone treatment methods.* Oxford: Oxford University Press, 1988.

373. Kane N, Manovkian P. The effect of the Medicare Prospective Payment System on the adoption of new technologies: the case of cochlear implants. *New England Journal of Medicine* 1989; **32**: 1378–1383.

374. Kanji N, Hardon A, Harnmeijer J, *et al. Drugs policy in developing countries.* London: Zed Books Ltd, 1992.

375. Kanouse D E, Jacoby I. When does information change practitioners' behavior. *International Journal of Technology Assessment in Health Care* 1988; **4**: 27–33.

376. Kanouse D, Winkler J. Kosecoff J, *et al. Changing medical practice through technology assessment.* Santa Monica, California: RAND, 1989.

377. Kaplan R, Bush J. Health-related quality of life measurement for evaluation research and policy analysis. *Health Psychology* 1982; **1**: 61–80.

378. Kaplan R, Anderson J, Wu A, *et al.* The Quality of Well-Being Scale: Applications in AIDS, cystic fibrosis, and arthritis. *Medical Care* 1989; **27**: S27–S43.

379. Kass L R. The new biology: what price relieving man's estate? *Science* 1971; **174**: 779–788.

380. Katz J. Why doctors don't disclose uncertainty. *Hastings Center Report* 1984; **1**: 35–44.

381. Katz S, Ford A, Moskowitz R, Jaffee M. Studies of illness in the aged. The index of ADL: a standardized measure of biological and psychosocial function. *Journal of the American Medical Association* 1963; **185**: 914–919.

382. Kaye H L. The biological revolution and its cultural context. *International Journal of Technology Assessment in Health Care* 1986; **2**: 275–283.

383. Kent D L. Clinical efficacy of MR needs rigorous study. *Diagnostic Imaging* 1990; 69–71,161.

384. Kent D L, Larson E B. Magnetic resonance imaging of the brain and spine. Is clinical efficacy established after the first decade. *Annals of Internal Medicine* 1988; **108**: 402–424.

385. Kessner D, Kalk C E, Singer J. Assessing health quality—the case for tracers. *New England Journal of Medicine* 1973; **288**: 189–194.

386. King L. Clinical laboratories become important, 1870–1900. *Journal of the American Medical Association* 1983; **249**: 3025–3029.

387. Kirchberger S. *The diffusion of two technologies for renal stone treatment across Europe*. London: King's Fund Centre, 1991.

388. Kirscher B, Guyatt G. A methodological framework for assessing health indices. *Journal of Chronic Disease* 1985; **38**: 27–36.

389. Klein L, Charache P, Johannes R, Lewis C. Effect of physician tutorials on prescribing patterns and drug cost in ambulatory patients. *Clinical Research* 1980; **28**: 296–301.

390. Knapp D A, Speedie M K, Yaeger D M, Knapp D A. Drug prescribing and its relation to length of hospital stay. *Inquiry* 1980; **17**: 254–259.

391. Kohn A. *False prophets, fraud and error in science and medicine*. Oxford: Basil Blackwell, 1986.

392. Koplan J, White C. An update on the benefits and costs of measles and rubella immunization. In: Gruenberg E M, Lewis C, Goldston S eds. *Immunizing against mental disorders: progress in the conquest of measles and rubella*. Oxford: Oxford University Press, 1985.

393. Kosekoff J, Kanouse D, Rogers W, McCloskey L, Winslow C, Brook R. Effects of the National Institutes of Health consensus development program on physician practice. *Journal of the American Medical Association* 1987; **258**: 2708–2713.

394. Kravitz R, Greenfield S, Rogers W, *et al*. Differences in the mix of patients among medical specialities and systems of care: results from the medical outcomes study. *Journal of the American Medical Association* 1992; **267**: 1617–1623.

395. Krowczynski L. The development of pharmaceutical technology (chronological tabulated facts). *Pharmazie* 1985; **40**: 346–349.

396. Krugman S. The conquest of measles and rubella. *Natural History* 1983; **92**: 16–20.

397. Kuhn L T S. *The structure of scientific revolutions*. Chicago: University of Chicago Press, 1970.

398. Kupperman M, Luce B, McGovern B, *et al*. An analysis of the cost effectiveness of the implantable cardiac defibrillator. *Circulation* 1990; **81**: 91–100.

399. Lambert E C. *Modern medical mistakes*. Bloomington, Indiana: Indiana University Press, 1978.

400. Lammer J, Klein G, Kleinert R, *et al*. Obstructive jaundice: use of expandable metal endoprosthesis for biliary drainage. *Radiology* 1990; **177**: 789–792.

401. Lara M, Goodman C eds. *National priorities for the assessment of clinical conditions and medical technologies: report of a pilot study*. Washington, DC: National Academy Press, 1990.

402. Larson G, Vitale G, Casey J, *et al*. Multipractice analysis of laparoscopic cholecystectomy in 1,986 patients. *American Journal of Surgery* 1992; **163**: 221–226.

403. Lasch K, Maltz A, Mosteller F, Tosteson T. A protocol approach to assessing medical technologies. *International Journal of Technology Assessment in Health Care* 1987; **3**: 103–122.

404. Laupacis A, Feeny D, Detsky A, Tugwell P. How attractive does a new technology have to be to warrant adoption and utilization? Tentative guidelines for using clinical and economic evaluations. *Canadian Medical Association Journal* 1991; **146**: 473–481.

405. Laupacis A, Sackett D L, Roberts R S. An assessment of clinically useful measures of the consequences of treatment. *New England Journal of Medicine* 1988; **318**: 1728–1733.

406. Laupacis A, Wong C, Churchill D, Canadian Erythropoietin Study Group. The use of generic and specific quality-of-life measures in hemodialysis patients treated with erythropoietin. *Controlled Clinical Trials* 1991; **12**: 168S–179S.

407. Lauper P. The socioeconomic study program on Nitroderm TTS. In: van Eimeren W, Horisberger B eds. *Socioeconomic evaluation of drug therapy.* Berlin: Springer-Verlag, 1988: pp. 101–109.

408. Lawless E C. *Modern medical mistakes.* Indiana University Press, Bloomington, Indiana, 1977.

409. Lee P. *Drug promotion and labelling in developing countries: an update.* Presented at the Conference on Availability and Use of Therapeutic Agents and Vaccines in Developing Countries, Bellagio, Italy, April 16–20, 1990.

410. Lehman A, Burns B. Severe mental illness in the community. In: Spilker B ed. *Quality of life assessments in clinical trials.* Raven Press, New York, 1990.

411. Lehtinen V, Panelius M, Tienari P. Finnish consensus development conference on the treatment of schizophrenia. *International Journal of Technology Assessment in Health Care* 1989; **5**: 269–281.

412. Lenz W. Malformations caused by drugs in pregnancy. *American Journal of Diseases of Children* 1966; **112**: 99.

413. Levine R. *Ethics and regulation of clinical research.* Urban & Schwarzenberg, 1981.

414. Levine S, Croog S. What constitutes quality of life? A conceptualization of the dimensions of life quality in healthy populations and patients with cardiovascular disease. In: Wenger N K, Mattson M E, Furberg C D, Elinson L eds. *Assessment of quality of life in clinical trials of cardiovascular therapies.* New York: Le Jacq, 1984.

415. Levy R, Sondik E. The management of biomedical research: an example for heart, lung, and blood diseases. In: R. Levy *et al.* eds. *Biomedical innovation.* Cambridge, Massachusetts: The MIT Press, 1981: pp. 10–22.

416. Lewin and Associates. *A forward plan for Medicare coverage and technology assessment, final report.* Contract No. 282-45-0062. Prepared for the Assistant Secretary for Planning and Evaluation, Department of Health and Human Services, Washington, DC, 1986.

417. Lewis C, Pantell R, Kieckhefer G. Assessment of children's health status: field test of new approaches. *Medical Care* 1989; **27**(suppl): S54–S65.

418. Liang M, Katz J, Ginsberg K. Chronic rheumatic disease. In: Spilker B ed. *Quality of life assessments in clinical trials.* New York: Raven Press, 1990.

419. Liebenau J. Innovation in pharmaceuticals: industrial R&D in the early twentieth century. *Research Policy* 1985; **14**: 179–187.

420. Lieberman M. *Formulacion e implementacion de las politicas farmaceuticas.* El caso de Mexico. Memorias de la Conferencia Latinoamericana sobre Politicas Farmaceuticas y Medicamentos Esenciales. Mexico: National Institute of Public Health/World Health Organization, 1988.

421. Lister J. By the London Post. *New England Journal of Medicine* 1980. **302**: 733.

422. Lohr K ed. Advances in health status assessment: conference proceedings. *Medical Care* 1989; **27**(suppl).

423. Lohr K ed. Advances in health status assessment: fostering the application of health status measures in clinical settings. *Medical Care* 1992; **30**(suppl).

424. Lohr K ed. *Breast cancer: setting priorities for effectiveness research.* Washington, DC: National Academy Press, 1990.

425. Lohr K N ed. *Medicare: a strategy for quality assurance.* Volume 1. Washington, DC: National Academy Press, 1990.

426. Lohr K, Heithoff K eds. *Hip fracture: setting priorities for effectiveness research.* Washington, DC: National Academy Press, 1990.

427. Lohr K, Rettig R eds. *Effectiveness initiative: setting priorities for clinical conditions.* Washington, DC: National Academy Press, 1989.

428. Lohr K, Rettig R. *Quality of care and technology assessment.* Washington, DC: National Academy Press, 1989.

429. Lohr K, Winkler J, Brook R. *Peer review and technology assessment in medicine.* Santa Monica, California: RAND, 1981.

430. Loo van der R, van Gennip E. *Evaluation of personnel savings through PACS: a modelling approach.* Presented at the International Workshop on Technology Assessment of PACS, Enkhuizen, The Netherlands, May 26–27, 1991.

431. Luce B, Brown R. *Technology assessment in decision-making by health care providers* (Submitted for publication, 1992).

432. Luce B, Elixhauser A. *Standards for socioeconomic evaluation of health care products and services.* Berlin: Springer-Verlag, 1990.

433. Luce B, Weschler J, Underwood C. *The use of quality of life measures in the private sector.* Washington, DC: National Academy Press, 1989.

434. Luft H. HMO's and medical costs: the rhetoric and the evidence. *New England Journal of Medicine* 1978; **298**: 1336–1340.

435. Luiten A L. The birth and development of an innovation: the case of magnetic resonance imaging. In: F F H Rutten and S J Reiser eds. *The economics of medical technology.* Berlin: Springer Verlag, 1988: pp. 99–108.

436. Lundberg G D. The role and function of professional journals in the transfer of information. *International Journal of Technology Assessment in Health Care* 1988; **4**: 51–58.

437. McDowell I, Newell C. *Measuring health: a guide to rating scales and questionnaires.* Oxford University Press, New York, 1987.

438. McGrady G A. The controlled clinical trial and decision making in family practice. *Journal of Family Practice* 1982; **14**: 739–744.

439. McNeil B. Values and preferences in the delivery of health care. In: *Committee for Evaluating Medical Technologies in Clinical Use.* Assessing Medical Technologies. Washington, DC: National Academy Press, 1985: pp. 535–541.

440. McNeil B, Abrams H. *Brigham and Women's Hospital handbook of diagnostic imaging.* Boston, Mass.: Little, Brown, 1986.

441. McPherson K, Wennberg J E, Hovind O B, Clifford P. Small-area variations in the use of common surgical procedures: an international comparison of New England, England, and Norway. *New England Journal of Medicine* 1982; **307**: 1310–1314.

442. McWhinney I R. Through clinical method to a more human medicine. In: White K L. *The task of medicine, dialogue at Wickenburg.* Menlo Park, California: The Kaiser Family Foundation, 1988: pp. 218–231.

443. Mahler D, Weinberg D, Wells C, Feinstein A. The measurement of dyspnea. contents, interobserver agreement, and physiologic correlates of two new clinical indexes. *Chest* 1984; **85**: 751–758.

444. Mahoney T. *The merchants of life.* New York: Harper & Brothers, 1959.

445. Manco L, Berlow M. Meniscal tears—comparison of arthrography, CT and MRI. *Critical Reviews in Diagnostic Imaging* 1989; **29**: 151–179.

446. Mansfield E, Rapoport J, Schnee J, Wagner S, Hamburger M. *Research and innovation in the modern corporation*. New York: WW Norton & Co, 1971.
447. Marcus S H, Grover P L, Revicki D A. The method of information synthesis and its use in the assessment of health care technology. *International Journal of Technology Assessment in Health Care* 1987; **3**: 491–493.
448. Martens L. Personal communication, 1990.
449. Martens L, Rutten F, Erkelens D, Ascoop C. Cost effectiveness of cholesterol-lowering therapy in the Netherlands, Simvastatin versus cholestyramine. *American Journal of Medicine* 1989; **87**: 54S–58S.
450. Marton K I. Modification of physician use of diagnostic imaging. Presented at the Meeting of the International Society for Technology Assessment in Health Care, Rotterdam, The Netherlands, 1987.
451. Mattingly P, Lohr K eds. *Acute myocardial infarction: setting priorities for effectiveness research*. Washington, DC: National Academy Press, 1990.
452. Mechanic D. The growth of medical technology and bureaucracy: implications for medical care. *Milbank Memorial Fund Quarterly/Health and Society* 1977; **55**: 61–74.
453. Mechanic D. *Politics, medicine, and social science*. New York: John Wiley & Sons, 1974.
454. Medical Research Council. The prevention of whooping cough by vaccination. *British Medical Journal* 1951; **1**: 1462–1471.
455. Medical Research Council. Streptomycin treatment of pulmonary tuberculosis. *British Medical Journal* 1948; **2**: 769–82.
456. Medical Research Council. Clinical trials of antihistaminic drugs in the prevention and treatment of the common cold. *British Medical Journal* 1950; **2**: 425–429.
457. Medicare program. Criteria and procedures for making medical services coverage decisions that relate to health care technology. *Federal Register*, Jan 30, 1989; **54**(18): 4302–4318.
458. Meenan R, Anderson J, Kazis L, *et al*. Outcome assessment in clinical trials. *Arthritis and Rheumatism* 1984; **27**: 1344–1352.
459. Mehrez A, Gafni A. Quality adjusted life years (QALYs), utility theory and healthy years equivalent. *Medical Decision Making* 1989; **9**: 142–149.
460. Meinert C. Toward more definitive clinical trials. *Controlled Clinical Trials* 1980; **1**: 249–261.
461. Melnick G A, Wheeler J, Feldstein P G. Effects of rate regulation on selected components of hospital expenses. *Inquiry* 1981; **18**: 240–246.
462. Mesthene E. The role of technology in society. In: Teach A ed. *Technology and man's future*. New York: St. Martin's Press, 1977: p. 158.
463. Ministry of Health, Welfare and Cultural Affairs. *Care in The Netherlands 1992*. Rijswijk, 1992.
464. Modic M, Masaryk R, Boumphrey F, Goormastic M, Bell G. Lumbar herniated disk disease and canal stenosis: prospective evaluation by surface coil MR, CT, and myelography. *American Journal of Neuroradiology* 1986; **7**: 709–717.
465. Modic M, Masaryk R, Mulopulos G, Bundschuh C, Han J, Bolhman H. Cervical radiculopathy: prospective evaluation with surface coil MR imaging, CT with metrizamide, and metrizamide myelography. *Radiology* 1986; **161**: 753–759.
466. Molina R. *Sobreprecio de los medicamentos en Mexico—el caso del cuadro basico*. Memorias de la Conferencia Latinoamericana sobre Politicas Farmaceuticas y Medicamentos Esenciales. Mexico: National Institute of Public Health/World Health Organization, 1988.

467. Moses L. Framework for considering the role of data bases in technology assessment. *International Journal of Technology Assessment in Health Care* 1990; **6**: 183–193.

468. Moskowitz G, Chalmers T C, Sacks H, *et al*. Deficiencies of controlled trials of alcohol withdrawal. *Alcoholism Clinical and Experimental Research* 1981; **5**: 162–166.

469. Mozes B, Schiff E, Modan B. Factors affecting inappropriate hospital stay. *Quality Assurance in Health Care* 1991; **3**: 211–217.

470. Mulley A. Assessing patient's utilities: can the ends justify the means? *Medical Care* 1989; **27**: S269–S281.

471. Mulrow C. The medical review article: state of the science. *Annals of Internal Medicine* 1987; **104**: 485–488.

472. Mushkin S J, Paringer L C, Chen M M. *Returns to biomedical research, 1900–1975: an initial assessment of impacts on health expenditures*. Washington, DC: Georgetown University Public Services Laboratory, 1977 (mimeograph).

473. Mushkin S. *Biomedical research: costs and benefits*. Cambridge, Massachusetts: Ballinger Publishing Company, 1979.

474. Myers L P, Schroeder S A. Physician use of services for the hospitalized patient: a review, with implications for cost containment. *Milbank Memorial Fund Quarterly/Health and Society* 1981; **59**: 481–507.

475. Nash D, Goldfield N eds. *Providing quality care*. Philadelphia: American College of Physicians, 1989.

476. Nathanson L, Shimi S, Cuehieri A. Laparoscopic cholecystectomy: the Dundee experience. *British Journal of Surgery* 1991; **78**: 150–154.

477. National Health Service. *NHS research and development strategy*. London: National Health Service, 1991.

478. National Heart and Lung Institute. *The totally implantable artificial heart*. Report of the Artificial Heart Assessment Panel. Bethesda, Maryland: National Institutes of Health, 1973.

479. National Institutes of Health. *Annual report, 1991*. Bethesda, Maryland.

480. National Institutes of Health. *NIH data book*. Bethesda, Maryland, 1992.

481. National Institutes of Health, Office of Medical Applications of Research, personal communication, 1992.

482. Norman C. The world's research & development budget. *Environment* 1979; **21**: 6–7.

483. Nowzad B. *Promoting development, the IMF's contribution*. Washington, DC: International Monetary Fund, 1991.

484. Noz M, Erdman W, Maguire G, *et al*. Modus operandi for a picture archiving and communication system. *Radiology* 1984; **152**: 221–223.

485. Nunnally J. *Psychometric theory*. McGraw-Hill, New York, 1978.

486. Oberender P. Cost-benefit analysis of angina prophylaxis in the Federal Republic of Germany. In: van Eimeren W, Horisberger B eds. *Socioeconomic evaluation of drug therapy*. Berlin: Springer-Verlag, 1988: pp. 132–140.

487. Office of Technology Assessment. *Assessing the efficacy and safety of medical technologies*. Washington, DC: US Government Printing Office, 1978.

488. Office of Technology Assessment. *Commercial biotechnology: an international analysis*. Washington, DC: US Government Printing Office, 1984.

489. Office of Technology Assessment. *Cost effectiveness of influenza vaccination*. Washington, DC: US Government Printing Office, 1981.

490. Office of Technology Assessment. *Costs and effectiveness of cholesterol screening in the elderly*. Washington, DC: US Government Printing Office, 1989.

491. Office of Technology Assessment. *Costs and effectiveness of colorectal cancer screening in the elderly*. Washington, DC: US Government Printing Office, 1990.

492. Office of Technology Assessment. *Development of medical technology: opportunities for assessment*. Washington, DC: US Government Printing Office, 1976.

493. Office of Technology Assessment. *Effects of Federal policies on extracorporeal shock wave lithotripsy*. Washington, DC: US Government Printing Office, 1986.

494. Office of Technology Assessment. *Evaluation of the Oregon Medicaid proposal*. Washington, DC: US Government Printing Office, 1992.

495. Office of Technology Assessment. *Federal policies and the medical devices industry*. Washington, DC: US Government Printing Office, 1984.

496. Office of Technology Assessment. *The impact of randomized clinical trials on health policy and medical practice*. Washington, DC: US Government Printing Office, 1983.

497. Office of Technology Assessment. *The implications of cost-effectiveness analysis of medical technology*. Washington, DC: US Government Printing Office, 1980.

498. Office of Technology Assessment. *The implications of cost-effectiveness analysis of medical technology*. Background paper # 1. Methodological issues and literature review. Washington, DC: US Government Printing Office, 1980.

499. Office of Technology Assessment. *Medical technology and costs of the Medicare program*. Washington, DC: US Government Printing Office, 1984, pp. 41–53.

500. Office of Technology Assessment. *Medicare's prospective payment system*. Washington, DC: US Government Printing Office, 1985.

501. Office of Technology Assessment. *Nuclear magnetic resonance imaging technology, a clinical industrial, and policy analysis*. Health Technology Case Study 27. Washington, DC: US Government Printing Office, 1984.

502. Office of Technology Assessment. *Policy implications of the computed tomography (CT) scanner*. Washington, DC: US Government Printing Office, 1978.

503. Office of Technology Assessment. *Policy implications of the computed tomography (CT) scanner: an update*. Washington, DC: US Government Printing Office, 1981.

504. Office of Technology Assessment. *Preventive health services for Medicare beneficiaries: policy and research issues*. Washington, DC: US Government Printing Office, 1990.

505. Office of Technology Assessment. *The quality of medical care, information for consumers*. Washington, DC: US Government Printing Office, 1988.

506. Office of Technology Assessment. *A review of selected Federal vaccine and immunization policies*. Washington, DC: US Government Printing Office, 1979.

507. Office of Technology Assessment. *Screening for open-angle glaucoma in the elderly*. Washington, DC: OTA, 1988.

508. Office of Technology Assessment. *Strategies for medical technology assessment*. Washington, DC: US Government Printing Office, 1982.

509. Office of Technology Assessment. *Update of federal activities regarding the use of pneumococcal vaccine*. Washington, DC: US Government Printing Office, 1984.

510. Olsson G, Lubsen J, Van Es G, Rehnqvst N. Quality of life after myocardial infarction: effect of long term metoprol on mortality and morbidity. *British Medical Journal* 1986; **292**: 1491–1493.

511. Ontario. *Guidelines for preparation of economic analysis to be included in submission to drug programs branch for listing in the Ontario drug benefit formulatory/comparative drug index.* Ministry of Health, Drugs Programs Branch, Ontario, Canada, October 15, 1991 (draft).

512. Ontario. *Status report on Ontario's draft guidelines for economic analysis of drugs.* Ministry of Health, Drug Programs Branch, Ontario, Memorandum Subject, May 7, 1992.

513. Organisation for Economic Co-operation and Development (OECD). *Assessing medical technology to aid policy-making.* (Note by the Secretariat) Paris, 1981.

514. Organisation for Economic Co-operation and Development (OECD). *Changing priorities for government R&D.* Paris, 1975.

515. Organisation for Economic Co-operation and Development (OECD). *New OECD health data on diskette.* Press release. Paris, 25 September 1991.

516. Otten A. Reuse of devices by hospitals and doctors stirs debate over cost savings and safety. *Wall Street Journal*, 14 September 1984, p. 24.

517. Overbeek van G. *In-vitro-fertilisatie* (in Dutch). Amsterdam: Free University Publisher, 1992.

518. Owen J, Loia L, Hanks G. Recent patterns of growth in radiation therapy facilities in the United States. *International Journal of Radiation Oncology, Biology, and Physics* 1991; **21**(suppl. 1): 223.

519. Pacey A. *The culture of technology.* Cambridge, Massachusetts: MIT Press, 1983.

520. Pan American Health Organization. *Health for all by the year 2000: strategies.* PAHO Official Document 179. Washington, DC, 1980.

521. Pan American Health Organization. *Policies for the production and marketing of essential drugs.* Prepared for the Technical Discussions of the XXIX Meeting of the Directing Council of PAHO. Washington, DC, 1984. (Scientific Publication No. 462)

522. Panerai R, Pena Mohr J. *Health technology assessment, methodologies for developing countries.* Washington, DC: Pan American Health Organization, 1989.

523. Patrick D, Deyo R. Generic and disease-specific measures in assessing health status and quality of life. *Medical Care* 1989; **27**: S217–S232.

524. Patrick D, Erickson P. *Health Status and Health Policy: Allocating Resources to Health Care.* New York: Oxford University Press (in press).

525. Pauker S G. Decision analysis as a synthetic tool for achieving consensus in technology assessment. *International Journal of Technology Assessment in Health Care* 1986; **2**: 83–98.

526. Paul-Shaheen P, Clark J, Williams D. Small area analysis: a review and analysis of the North American literature. *Journal of Health Politics, Policy and Law* 1987; **12**: 741–792.

527. Peckham M. Research and development for the National Health Service. *Lancet* 1991; **33**: 367–371.

528. Peddecord K M, Janon E A, Robins J M. Substitution of magnetic resonance imaging for computed tomography. *International Journal of Technology Assessment in Health Care* 1988; **4**: 573–591.

529. Pena J. Distributing and transferring medical technology, a view from Latin America and the Caribbean. *International Journal of Technology Assessment in Health Care* 1987; **187**: 281–292.

530. Perissat J, Collet D, Belliard R. Gallstones: laparoscopic treatment—cholecystectomy, cholecystostomy, and lithotripsy. *Surgical Endoscopy* 1990; **4**: 1–5.

531. Perrow C. *Complex organizations: A critical essay*. Glenview, Illinois: Scott, Foresmen, 1972.
532. Perry S. The brief life of the National Center for Health Care Technology. *New England Journal of Medicine* 1982; **307**: 1095−1100.
533. Perry S, Wilkinson S. The Technology Assessment and Practice Guidelines Forum: a modified group judgement method. *International Journal of Technology Assessment in Health Care* 1992; **89**: 289−300.
534. Peters J, Ellison, EC, Innes J, *et al*. Safety and efficacy of laparoscopic cholecystectomy: a prospective analysis of 100 initial patients. *Annals of Surgery* 1991; **213**: 3−12.
535. Pharmaceutical Manufacturers Association (PMA). *Annual Survey*. Washington, DC, 1991.
536. Pharmaceutical Manufacturers Association (PMA). *Personal communication*, 1992.
537. Phelps C, Parente S. Priority setting in medical technology and medical practice assessment. *Medical Care* 1990; **28**: 703−723.
538. Piene H, Heggestad T, Skolbekken J A, Nilsen G. *Medical consequences of MRI diagnosis*. Presented at the 1990 meeting of the International Society for Technology Assessment in Health Care, Houston, May 21−23, 1990.
539. Pirsig R M. *Zen and the art of motorcycle maintenance*. New York: Bantam Books, 1975.
540. Pocock S. *Clinical trials, a practical approach*. New York: John Wiley & Sons, 1983.
541. Pocock S, *et al*. Statistical problems in the reporting of clinical trials: a survey of three medical journals. *New England Journal of Medicine* 1987: **317**: 426−432.
542. Preston T. *Coronary artery surgery: a critical review*. New York: Raven Press, 1977.
543. Pryor G, Williams D, Myles J, Anand J. Team management of the elderly patient with hip fracture. *The Lancet* 1988; **1**: 401−403.
544. Prystowsky J, Nahrwold D. Extracorporeal shock wave lithotripsy for biliary stones. *Surgical Clinics of North America* 1990; **70**: 1231−1248.
545. Racoveanu N. Towards a basic radiological service. *World Health Forum* 1981; **2**: 521−524.
546. Rada R. Automated medical diagnosis—a summary. In Schwartz M D ed. *Applications of computers in medicine*. A Publication of the IEEE Engineering in Medicine and Biology Society, 1982: 188−197.
547. Ratib O. *Current views on the functionalities of PACS*. Presented at the International Workshop on Technology Assessment of PACS, Enkhuizen, The Netherlands, May 26−27, 1991.
548. Read J, Quinn R, Berwick D, *et al*. Preferences for health outcomes: comparisons of assessment methods. *Medical Decision Making* 1984; **4**: 315−329.
549. Read J, Quinn R, Hoefer M. Measuring overall health: an evaluation of three important approaches. *Journal of Chronic Disease* 1987; **40**: 7S−22S.
550. Reddick E, Olsen D. Laparoscopic laser cholecystectomy: a comparison with mini-laparotomy cholecystectomy. *Surgical Endoscopy* 1989; **3**: 101−103.
551. Reddick E, Olsen D. Outpatient laparoscopic laser cholecystectomy. *American Journal of Surgery* 1990; **160**: 485−487.
552. Redisch M. *Hospital inflationary mechanisms*. Presented at the Meeting of the Western Economic Association. Las Vegas, Nevada, 10−12 June, 1974.

553. Reerink E ed. *Report on quality assurance programs in different countries.* Presented to the Institute of Medicine, Washington, DC, 1992.

554. Reid M. *The diffusion of four prenatal screening tests across Europe.* London: King's Fund Centre, 1991.

555. Reiser S J. *Medicine and the reign of technology.* London: Cambridge University Press, 1978.

556. Relman A. Dealing with conflicts of interest. *New England Journal of Medicine* 1985; **313**: 749–752.

557. Relman A. More on the Ingelfinger rule. *New England Journal of Medicine* 1988; **318**: 1125–1126.

558. Relman A. Reporting the aspirin study: the Journal and the media. *New England Journal of Medicine* 1988; **318**: 918–920.

559. Revicki D. Health-related quality of life in the evaluation of medical therapy for chronic illness. *Journal of Family Practice* 1989; **29**: 377–380.

560. Revicki D. Relationship between health utility and psychometric health status measures. *Medical Care* 1992; **30**(suppl).

561. Revicki, D, Allen H. Bungay K, *et al. Self-reported clinical symptoms and general well-being in patients with hypertension.* Washington, DC: Battelle Medical Technology Assessment and Policy Research Center, 1991.

562. Revicki D, Brown R, Adler M, Corea J. *Recombinant human erythropoietin and health-related quality of life of AIDS patients with anemia.* Battelle Medical Technology Assessment and Policy Research Center, Washington, DC, 1992.

563. Revicki D, Brown R, Corea J, Adler M. *Health-related quality of life associated with recombinant human erythropoietin therapy for predialysis renal disease patients.* Battelle Medical Technology Assessment and Policy Research Center, Washington, DC, 1991.

564. Revicki D, Rothman M, Luce B. Health-related quality of life assessment and the pharmaceutical industry. *Pharmacoeconomics* 1992; **1**.

565. Revicki D, Weinstein M, Alderman M, Allen H, Bungay K. *Health utility and health status outcomes of antihypertensive treatment.* Washington, DC: Battelle Medical Technology Assessment and Policy Research Center, 1992.

566. Rice D P. *Estimating the cost of illness.* Washington, DC: US Government Printing Office, Health Economics Series, 1966.

567. Rivero C C, Beaumont G F, Arredondo A, del Carmen Sánchez E, Sánchez J J, Hernández B. *Proyecto de investigación sobre la oferta de aparatos médicos en México: Directoria preliminar de empresas productoras, distribuidoras, importadores y de servicio de aparatos y equipo médico, en D.F. y Zona Metropolitana.* Mexico City: Instituto Nacional de Salud Pública, 1989.

568. Roberts E B. Technological innovation and medical devices. In: Ekelman K B ed. *New medical devices, invention, development, and use.* Washington, DC: National Academy Press, 1988: pp. 35–47.

569. Robinson R, Appleby J. *A review of capital and capital charges: cutting through the confusion.* National Association of Health Authorities and Trusts, 1991.

570. Rockette H, Redmond C, Fisher B, *et al.* Impact of randomized clinical trials on therapy of primary breast cancer: the NSABP overview. *Controlled Clinical Trials* 1982; **3**: 209–226.

571. Rodriguez Dominguez J, Toney S, Duran J, McNally A, Lopez M. Disponibilidad y utilizacion de innovaciones tecnologicas en atencion medica en Mexico. *Boletin de la Oficina Sanitaria Panamerican* 1984; **97**: 283–295.

572. Rogers A. European Community: health policy after Maastricht. *Lancet* 1992; **339**: 171–172.

573. Rogers E M, Shoemaker F F. *Communication of innovations, a cross-cultural approach*. New York: The Free Press, 1971.

574. Roland M, Morris R. A study of the natural history of back pain: development of a reliable and sensitive measure of disability in low-back pain. *Spine* 1983; **8**: 141–144.

575. Romeo A. *The hemodialysis equipment and disposables industry*. Office of Technology Assessment. Washington, DC: US Government Printing Office, 1984.

576. Romm L F J, Hulka B S. Peer review in diabetes and hypertension: the relationship between care process and patient outcome. *Southern Medical Journal* 1980; **73**: 564–568.

577. Rosser R, Kind P. A scale of valuations of state of illness: is there a social consensus? *International Journal of Epidemiology* 1978; **7**: 347–358.

578. Rossum W van. Besluitvorming en Medische Technologisch Aspectenonderzoek, Een analyse van de Gebruikswaarde van TA-Studies naar Hart- en Levertransplantaties en In Vitro Fertilisatie (*Decision-making and Medical Technology Assessment, An Analysis of the Utility of TA Studies of Heart and Liver Transplant and In Vitro Fertilization*). Appeldoorn: Ziekenfondsraad, 1990.

579. Rossum W van. Medical technology assessment, an analysis of the perceived value of the Dutch technology assessments of heart and liver transplantation and in vitro fertilization (in Dutch). *Medisch Contact* 1990; **45**: 509–511.

580. Rost K, Smith G, Burnam M, Burns B. Measuring the outcomes of care for mental health problems: the case of depressive disorders. *Medical Care* 1992; **30**(suppl).

581. Rostow V, Bulger R eds. *Medical professional liability and the delivery of obstetrical care*, volume 2, *an interdisciplinary review*. Washington, DC: National Academy Press, 1989.

582. Rothman M, Hedrick S, Bulcroft K, Hickman D, Rubenstein L. The validity of proxy-generated scores as measures of patient health status. *Medical Care* 1991; **29**: 115–124.

583. Rozynski E. *Global overview*. Presented at a Workshop at the Pan American Health Organization, Washington, DC, May 15, 1991.

584. Rublee D, Schneider M. International health spending: comparisons with the OECD. *Health Affairs* 1991; **10**: 187–201.

585. Russell L B. *Is prevention better than cure?* Washington, DC: The Brookings Institution, 1986.

586. Russell L B. *Technology in hospitals, medical advances and their diffusion*. Washington, DC: The Brookings Institution, 1979.

587. Russell L B, Sisk J E. Medical technology in the United States: the last decade. *International Journal of Technology Assessment in Health Care* 1988; **4**: 269–286.

588. Rutstein D D, Berenberg W, Chalmers T C, *et al.* Measuring the quality of care: a clinical method. *New England Journal of Medicine* 1976; **294**: 582–588.

589. Rutten F, Banta D. Health care technologies in The Netherlands: assessment and policy. *International Journal of Technology Assessment in Health Care* 1988; **4**: 229–238.

590. Rutten F, van der Werff A. Health policy in The Netherlands. In: McLachlan G, Maynard A eds. *The public/private mix for health*. London: The Nuffield Provincial Hospitals Trust, 1982:167–206.

591. Sackett D L. Bias in analytic research. *Journal of Chronic Disease* 1979; **32**: 51–63.

592. Sackett D, Chambers L, McPhearson A, Goldsmith A, Mcauley R. The development and application of indices of health: general methods and a summary of results. *American Journal of Public Health* 1977; **67**: 423–427.

593. Sacks B. Is the rising rate of Cesarean Sections a result of more defensive medicine? In: Rostow V, Bulger R eds. *Medical professional liability and the delivery of obstetrical care*, volume 2, *an interdisciplinary review*. Washington, DC: National Academy Press, 1989: pp. 27–40.

594. Sacks H, Berrier J, Reitman D *et al.* Meta-analysis of randomized clinical trials. *New England Journal of Medicine* 1987; **316**: 450–455.

595. Safran C. Using routinely collected data for clinical research. *Statistics in Medicine* 1991; **10**: 559–564.

596. Salkever D, Bice T. *Hospital certificate-of-need controls: impact on investment, costs and use*. Washington, DC: American Enterprise Institute of Public Policy Research, 1979.

597. Schersten T, Byringer H, Karlberg I, Jonsson E. Cost-effectiveness analysis of organ transplantation. *International Journal of Technology Assessment in Health Care* 1986; **2**: 545–552.

598. Schieber G, Poullier J-P, Greenwald L. Health care systems in twenty-four countries. *Health Affairs* 1991; **10**: 22–38.

599. Schifrin L, Tayan J. The drug lag: an interpretative review of the literature. *International Journal of Health Services* 1977; **7**: 359–386.

600. Schipper H, Clinch J, McMurray A, Levitt M. Measuring the quality of life of cancer patients: the functional living index—cancer: develoment and validation. *Journal of Clinical Oncology* 1984; **2**: 472–483.

601. Schipper H, Clinch J, Powell V. Definitions and conceptual issues. In: Spilker B ed. *Quality of life assessments in clinical trials*. Raven Press, New York, 1990.

602. Schmiedl U, Rowberg A. Literature review: Picture Archiving and Communications Systems. *Journal of Digital Imaging* 1990; **3**: 238–245.

603. Schor S, Karten I. Statistical evaluation of medical journal manuscripts. *Journal of the American Medical Association* 1966; **195**: 1123–1128.

604. Schroeder S. ReViews: a medical educator. *Health Affairs* 1984; **3**: 55–62.

605. Schroeder S. Strategies for reducing medical costs by changing physicians' behavior. *International Journal of Technology Assessment in Health Care* 1987; **3**: 39–50.

606. Schroeder S A, Marton K I, Strom B L. Frequency and morbidity of invasive procedures. *Archives of Internal Medicine* 1978; **138**: 1809–1811.

607. Schwartz D, Flamant R, Lellouch J. *Clinical trials*. New York: Academic Press, 1980.

608. Scitovsky A A. Changes in the costs of treatment of selected illnesses, 1971–1981. *Medical Care* 1985; **23**: 1345–1357.

609. Scitovsky A A. Changes in the use of ancillary services for 'common' illness. In: Altman S H, Blendon R, eds. *Medical technology: the culprit behind health care costs?* Washington, DC: US Government Printing Office, 1979: pp. 39–56.

610. Scitovsky A A. Estimating the direct costs of illness. *Milbank Memorial Fund Quarterly/Health and Society* 1982; **60**: 4623–4691.

611. Scitovsky A A. The high cost of dying: what do the data show? *Milbank Memorial Fund Quarterly/Health and Society* 1984; **62**: 591–607.

612. Scitovsky A, McCall N. *Changes in the cost of treatment of selected illness, 1951–1964–1971*. Washington, DC: National Center for Health Services Research, 1976. (DHEW Publication No. (HRA) 77-361).

613. Scott W R. Professionals in hospitals: technology and the organization of work. In: Georgopoulos B S ed. *Organization research on health institutions* 1972; pp. 139–202.

614. Secretaria de Salud, Consejo Nacional de Ciencia y Tecnologia. Encuesta nacional de investigacion en salud. Ano de captacion 1983–1984. *Serie de estudios 3*. Mexico: Edit. Litografia Electronica, Secretariat of Public Education, 1986.

615. Secretaria de Salud, Sistema Nacional de Informacion en Salud. *Folleto de difusion de publicaciones estadisticas*. Mexico: Secretariat of Health, 1991.

616. Sesso R, Eisenberg J M, Stabile C, Draibe S, Ajzen H, Ramos O. Cost-effectiveness analysis of the treatment of end-stage renal disease in Brazil. *International Journal of Technology Assessment in Health Care* 1990; **6**: 107–114.

617. Shaw B F. *The role of the interaction between the manufacturer and the user in the technological innovation process*. Sussex, United Kingdom: University of Sussex, PhD Dissertation, 1986.

618. Shaw C, Brooks T. Health services accreditation in the United Kingdom. *Quality Assurance in Health Care* 1991; **3**: 133–140.

619. Shepard D S. *Costs and benefits of health programs in developing countries: an annotated bibliography*. Boston: Harvard School of Public Health, 1981.

620. Shepard D S, Cash R A. *Manual for assessing the cost-effectiveness of oral rehydration therapy in the treatment of diarrhoeal disease*. Boston: Harvard School of Public Health, 1983.

621. Shepard D, Durch J S. *International comparison of resource allocation in health sciences: an analysis of expenditures on biomedical research in 19 industrialized countries*. Supported by the Fogarty International Center, National Institutes of Health. Boston: Harvard School of Public Health, 1985 (manuscript).

622. Showstack J A, Hughes Stone M, Schroeder S A. The role of changing clinical practices on the rising costs of hospital care. *New England Journal of Medicine* 1985; **313**: 1201–1207.

623. Showstack J A, Schroeder S A, Matsumoto M F. Changes in the use of medical technologies, 1972–1977. A study of 20 inpatient diagnoses. *New England Journal of Medicine* 1982; **306**: 706–712.

624. Shyrock R. *The development of modern medicine*. New York: Hafner Publishing Co., 1969.

625. Sigerist H E. *Man and medicine*. College Park, Maryland: McGrath Publishing Company, 1970 (Copyright 1932).

626. Silva L. *Technology assessment of different levels of neonatal care*. Thesis. University of Birminghan, Birmingham, UK, March 1992.

627. Silverman M. *The drugging of the Americas*. Berkeley: University of California Press, 1976.

628. Silverman M, Lee P. *Pills, profits, and politics*. Berkeley, California: University of California Press, 1974.

629. Silverman M, Lee P, Lydecker M. Drug promotion: the Third World revisited. *International Journal of Health Services* 1986; **16**: 659–667.

630. Silverman M, Lee P, Lydecker M. *Prescription for death: the drugging of the Third World*. Berkeley: University of California Press, 1982.

631. Silverman W A. *Human experimentation: a guided step into the unknown*. Oxford: Oxford University Press, 1985.

632. Sisk J. Introduction to measuring health care effectiveness. *International Journal of Technology Assessment in Health Care* 1990; **6**: 181–182.

633. Smith D, Kaluzny A. *The white labyrinth*. Berkeley, California: McCuktchan Publishing Corporation, 1975.
634. Smith G, Monson R, Ray D. Psychiatric consultation in somatization disorder: a randomized controlled study. *New England Journal of Medicine* 1986; **314**: 1407–1413.
635. Smith R. Doctors and the drug industry. *British Medical Journal* 1986; **293**: 905–906.
636. Soberon G. *Palabras de inauguracion*. Memorias de la Conferencia Latin-americana sobre Politicas Farmaceuticas y Medicamentos Essenciales. Mexico: National Institute of Public Health/World Health Organization, 1988.
637. Society of American Gastrointestinal Endoscopic Surgeons. *Granting of privileges for laparoscopic (peritoneoscopic) general surgery*. Los Angeles, Cal., 1990.
638. Society of American Gastrointestinal Endoscopic Surgeons. *The role of laparoscopic cholecystectomy: guidelines for clinical application*. Los Angeles, Cal., 1990.
639. Soto H K. *Proyecto de sustitucion de importaciones en cuanto a aparatos medico quirurgicos*. Mexico: Secretariat of Health, 1984 (mimeo).
640. Southern Surgeons Club. A prospective analysis of 1518 laparoscopic cholecystectomies. *New England Journal of Medicine* 1991; **324**: 1073–1078.
641. Sox H ed. *Common diagnostic tests: use and interpretation*. Philadelphia, Pa.: American College of Physicians, 1990.
642. Spath P ed. *Innovations in health quality management*. Chicago: American Hospital Publishing, 1989.
643. Spilker B ed. *Quality of life assessments in clinical trials*, Raven Press, New York, 1990.
644. Spilker B, Molinek F, Johnston K, Simpson R, Tilson H. Quality of life bibliography and indexes. *Medical Care* 1990; **29**(suppl): 1–77.
645. Spitzer W O. Report of the task force on the periodic health examination. *Canadian Medical Association Journal* 1979; **121**: 1193–254.
646. Spitzer W, Dobson A, Hall J, *et al.* Measuring the quality of life of cancer patients: a concise QL-index for use by physicians. *Journal of Chronic Disease* 1981; **34**: 585–557.
647. Starr P. *The social transformation of American medicine*. New York: Basic Books, 1982.
648. Stason W, Weinstein M. Allocation of resources to manage hypertension. *New England Journal of Medicine* 1977; **296**: 732–739.
649. State Secretary of Health. *Top-clinical care and investigational medicine* (in Dutch). Letter to Parliament, February 6, 1992.
650. Steel K, Gertman P M, Crescenzi C, Anderson J. Iatrogenic illness on a general medical service at a university hospital. *New England Journal of Medicine* 1981; **304**: 638–642.
651. Steinberg E P, Sisk J E, Locke K E. The diffusion of magnetic resonance imagers in the United States and worldwide. *International Journal of Technology Assessment in Health Care* 1985; **1**: 499–514.
652. Stevens R. *American medicine and the public interest*. New Haven, Connecticut: Yale University Press, 1971.
653. Stevens R. *Medical practice in modern England*. New Haven: Yale University Press, 1966.
654. Stewart A, Greenfield S, Hays R, *et al.* Functional status and well-being of patients with chronic conditions. Results from the Medical Outcomes Study. *Journal of the American Medical Association* 1989; **262**: 907–913.

655. Stewart A, Ware J. *Measuring Functioning and Well-Being: The Medical Outcomes Study Approach*. Durham, NC: Duke University Press, 1992.

656. Stocking B. Budgetary control of health resources policy: the situation in the United Kingdom. In: Banta D ed. *Resources for health: technology assessment for policy making*. New York: Praeger, 1982: pp. 203–205.

657. Stocking B. Factors affecting the diffusion of three kinds of innovative medical technology in European Community countries and Sweden. In: Bos M A. *The diffusion of heart and liver transplantation across Europe*. London: King's Fund Centre, 1991: pp. 129–168.

658. Stocking B. First consensus development conference in United Kingdom: on coronary artery bypass grafting. *British Medical Journal* 1985; **291**: 713–716.

659. Stocking B. *The image and the reality: a case study of the impacts of medical technology*. London: Nuffield Provincial Hospitals Trust, 1978.

660. Stocking B. *Initiative & inertia, case studies in the NHS*. London: The Nuffield Provincial Hospitals Trust, 1985.

661. Stocking B. Management of medical technology in the United Kingdom. In: Banta H D and Kemp K B eds. *The management of health care technology in nine countries*. New York: Springer Publishing Company, 1982: pp. 10–28.

662. Stocking B. Medical technology in the United Kingdom. *International Journal of Technology Assessment in Health Care* 1988; **4**: 171–183.

663. Straub W, Gur D. The hidden costs of delayed access to diagnostic imaging information: impact on PACS implementation. *American Journal of Radiology* 1990; **155**: 613–616.

664. Strom B ed. *Pharmacoepidemiology*. Churchill Livingstone, 1989.

665. Stross J K, Harlan W R. The dissemination of new medical information. *Journal of the American Medical Association* 1979; **241**: 2622–2624.

666. Swazey J, Fox R. The clinical moratorium. In Fox F. *Essays in medical sociology: journeys into the field*. New York: John Wiley & Sons, 1979.

667. Swedish Council for Technology Assessment in Health Care (SBU). *Bone-anchored implants in the head and neck region*. Proceedings of a conference. Stockholm, 1989.

668. Swedish Council for Technology Assessment in Health Care (SBU). *Critical analysis in medicine*. Proceedings of a conference. Stockholm, 1991 (ISBN 91-87890-12-7).

669. Swedish Council for Technology Assessment in Health Care (SBU). *Preoperative routines*. Stockholm, 1989. (ISBN 91-87890-04- 6).

670. Swedish Council for Technology Assessment in Health Care (SBU). *Prioritization and rationing in health care—trends in the U.S.A.* Proceedings of a conference. Stockholm, 1991. (ISBN 92-87890-11-9).

671. Swedish Council for Technology Assessment in Health Care (SBU). *The problem of back pain*. Proceedings from a conference. Stockholm, 1989. (ISBN 91-87890-04-6).

672. Talamini M, Gadacz T. Gallstone dissolution. *Surgical Clinics of North America* 1990; **70**: 1217–1230.

673. Tannon C, Rogers E. Diffusion research methodology: focus on health care organizations. In: Gordon G, Fisher L eds. *The diffusion of medical technology*. Cambridge, Massachusetts: Ballinger Publishing Company, 1975: pp. 51–77.

674. Teasdale G M, *et al.* Comparison of MRI and CT in suspected lesions in the posterior fossa. *British Medical Journal* 1989; **299**: 349–355.

675. Testa M, Hollenberg N K, Anderson R B, Williams G H. Assessment of quality of life by patient and spouse during antihypertensive therapy with atenolol and nifedipine gastrointestinal therapeutic system. *American Journal of Hypertension* 1991; **4**: 363–373.

676. Teutsch S M. A framework for assessing the effectiveness of disease and injury prevention. *Mortality and Morbidity Weekly Reports* (MMWR) March 27, 1992; **44**, No. 44-3.

677. Thacker S B. The efficacy of intrapartum electronic fetal monitoring. *American Journal of Obstetrics and Gynecology* 1987; **156**: 24–30.

678. Thacker S. The impact of technology assessment and medical malpractice on the diffusion of medical technologies: the case of electronic fetal monitoring. In: Rostow V, Bulger R eds. *Medical professional liability and the delivery of obstetrical care*, volume 2, *an interdisciplinary review*. Washington, DC: National Academy Press, 1989: pp. 9–26.

679. Thacker S, Kaplan J, Taylor W, Hinman A, Katz M, Roper W. *Assessing the effectiveness of preventive activities in health*. (unpublished 1992).

680. Thier S. Future developments in the transfer of technology assessment information. *International Journal of Technology Assessment in Health Care* 1988; **4**: 109–110.

681. Thomas K. *Religion and the decline of magic*. New York: Charles Scribner & Sons, 1971.

682. Thomas L. *The lives of a cell*. New York: The Viking Press, 1974.

683. Thomas L J. Federal support of medical device innovation. In: Ekelman K B ed. *New medical devices, invention, development, and use*. Washington, DC: National Academy Press, 1988: pp. 51–61.

684. Thornbury J R, Masters S J, Campbell J A. Imaging recommendations for head trauma: a new comprehensive strategy. *American Journal of Radiology* 1987; **149**: 781–783.

685. Tierney W, McDonald C. Practice databases and their use in clinical research. *Statistics in Medicine* 1992; **10**: 541–557.

686. Timmer E J, Kovar M G. *Expenses for hospital and institutional care during the last year of life for adults who died in 1964 and 1965*. Vital and Health Statistics, series 22, no. 11, March. Hyattsville, Maryland: US Department of Health, Education, and Welfare, 1971.

687. Torrance G. Measurement of health state utilities for economic appraisal. *Journal of Health Economics* 1986; **5**: 1–30.

688. Torrance G, Feeny D. Utilities and quality-adjusted life years. *International Journal of Technology Assessment in Health Care* 1989; **5**: 559–575.

689. Tsevat J, Goldman L, Lamas G, *et al*. Functional status versus utilities in survivors of myocardial infarction. *Medical Care* 1991; **29**: 1153–1159.

690. Tugwell P, Bombardier C, Bell M, *et al*. Current quality-of-life research challenges in arthritis relevant to the issue of clinical significance. *Controlled Clinical Trials* 1991; **12**: 217S–225S.

691. Tuhrim S, Reggia J. Feasibility of physician-developed expert systems. *Medical Decision Making* 1986; **6**: 23–26.

692. Tygstrup N, Lachin Jm, Juhl E. *The randomized clinical trial and therapeutic decisions*. New York: Marcel Dekker, 1982.

693. United Nations Industrial Development Organization (UNIDO). *Global study of the pharmaceutical industry*. Vienna, 1980. Report no. (ID/WG.331/6).

694. US Department of Health, Education and Welfare (USDHEW), Office of the Assistant Secretary: NCHCT Fact Sheet, n.d.

695. US Department of Health and Human Services, Health Care Financing Administration. *Federal Register*, Vol. 54, No. 18, Jan 30, 1989.

696. University of California at Los Angeles School of Public Health. *The effect of third party reimbursement on expenditures for medical care*. Prepared for the National Center for Health Care Technology. Rockville, Maryland: National Center for Health Care Technology, 1981.

697. US Preventive Services Task Force. *Guide to clinical preventive services: an assessment of the effectiveness of 169 interventions*. Baltimore: Williams & Wilkins, 1989.

698. Vanden Brink J, Cywinski J. *Investment alternative: the status quo or PACS?* Proceedings Medical Imaging Conference SPIE IV. 1990; **1234**: 881–886.

699. Vang J. The consensus development conference and the European experience. *International Journal of Technology Assessment in Health Care* 1986; **2**: 65–76.

700. Velez Gil, A, Tulio M, Guerrero R, Pardo de Velez G, Peterson O, Bloom B L. Surgeons and operating rooms: underutilized resources. *American Journal of Public Health* 1983; **73**: 1361–1365.

701. Villegas, C. *Conference on assessment of modern technologies in the Americas*, Pan American Health Organization, Brasilia, Brazil. November, 1983.

702. von Hippel E. The dominant role of users in the scientific instrument innovation process. *Research Policy* 1976; **5**: 212–239.

703. de Vries M J. *The redemption of the intangible in medicine*. London: Institute of Psychosynthesis, 1981.

704. Vrolijk H. *Hoe soft is de laser in de fysiotherapie?* Apeldoorn, The Netherlands: Studiecentrum voor Technologie en Beleid TNO, 1989.

705. Wade V, Mansfield P, McDonald P. Drug companies' evidence to justify advertising. *Lancet* 1989; **2**: 1261–1264.

706. Wagner J L, Krieger M J, Lee R H, Romeo A A, Stassen M. *Final report, a study of the impact of reimbursement strategies on the diffusion of medical technologies*. Washington, DC: The Urban Institute, 1982.

707. Walan A. Clinical evaluation of cimetidine with special reference to socioeconomic effects. In: Culyer A, Horisberger B eds. *Economic and medical evaluation of health care technologies*. Berlin: Springer-Verlag, 1983: pp. 171–180.

708. Waldman S. *The effect of changing technology on hospital costs*. Research and Statistics Note, US Department of Health, Education, and Welfare, Washington, DC, February 28, 1972.

709. Walsh J, Warren K. Selective primary health care, an interim strategy for disease control in developing countries. *New England Journal of Medicine* 1979; **301**: 967–974.

710. Warburton R. *Economic evaluation of digital imaging: what is important?* Presented at the International Workshop on Technology Assessment of PACS, Enkhuizen, The Netherlands, May 26–27, 1991.

711. Ware J E. Methodologic considerations in the selection of health status assessment procedures. In: Wenger N, Mattson M, Furberg C, Elinson L eds. *Assessment of quality of life in clinical trials of cardiovascular therapies*. New York: Le Jacq, 1984.

712. Ware J. Personal communication, 1992.

713. Ware J. *The use of health status and quality of life measures in outcomes and effectiveness research*, Prepared for the National Agenda Setting Conference on Outcomes and Effectiveness Research, Agency for Health Care Policy and Research, Alexandria, Va., April, 1991.

714. Ware J, Brook R, Lohr K. Choosing measures of health status for individuals in general populations. *American Journal of Public Health* 1981; **71**: 620–625.
715. Warner K. 'Desperation-reaction' model of medical diffusion. *Health Services Research* 1975; **10**: 369–379.
716. Warner K. The need for some innovative concepts of innovations: an examination of research on the diffusion of innovations. *Policy Sciences* 1974; **5**: 433–451.
717. Warner K. Treatment decision making in catastrophic illness. *Medical Care* 1977; **15**: 19–33.
718. Warner K, Luce B R. *Cost-benefit and cost-effectiveness analysis in health care, principles, practice, and potential.* Ann Arbor, Michigan: Health Administration Press, 1982.
719. Wastell C. Laparoscopic cholecystectomy, better for patients and the health service. *British Medical Journal* 1991; **302**: 30–31.
720. Weinstein M C, Fineberg H V. *Clinical decision analysis.* Philadelphia: WB Saunders Co., 1980.
721. Weinstein M, Stason W. Foundations of cost-effectiveness analysis for health and medical practices. *New England Journal of Medicine* 1977; **296**: 716–721.
722. Weisbrod B. The health care quadrilemma: an essay on technological change, insurance, quality of care, and cost containment. *Journal of Economic Literature* 1991; **29**: 523–552.
723. Welch H G, Fisher E. Cost-containment efforts in the public sector: Oregon's priority list. In: Gelijns A ed. *Technology and health care in an era of limits.* Washington, DC: National Academy Press, 1992: pp. 63–75.
724. Wells K, Stewart A, Hays R, *et al.* The functioning and well-being of depressed patients: results from the Medical Outcome Study. *Journal of the American Medical Association* 1989; **262**: 914–919.
725. Wenger N, Furberg C. Cardiovascular disorders. In: Spilker B ed. *Quality of life assessments in clinical trials.* New York: Raven Press, 1990.
726. Wenger N, Mattson M, Furberg C, Elinson L eds. *Assessment of quality of life in clinical trials of cardiovascular therapies.* New York: Le Jacq, 1984.
727. Wennberg J E. Dealing with medical practice variations: a proposal for action. *Health Affairs* 1984; **3**: 6–32.
728. Wennberg J. What is outcomes research? In: *Modern methods of clinical investigation*, Vol. 1, *Medical innovation at the crossroads.* Washington, DC: National Academy Press, 1990: pp. 33–46.
729. Wennberg J E, Gittelsohn A. Small area variations in health care delivery. *Science* 1973; **182**: 1102–1108.
730. Wennberg J E W, Blowers L, Parker R, Gittelsohn A M. Changes in tonsillectomy rates associated with feedback and review. *Pediatrics* 1977; **59**: 821–826.
731. Werko L. Personal communication, 1992.
732. White L J, Ball J R. The Clinical Efficacy Assessment Project of the American College of Physicians. *International Journal of Technology Assessment in Health Care* 1985; **1**: 169–174.
733. White S J K. Statistical errors in papers in the British Journal of Psychiatry. *British Journal of Psychiatry* 1979; **135**: 336–342.
734. Wickham J. The new surgery. *British Medical Journal* 1987; **295**: 1581–1582.
735. Willems J S, Banta H D. Improving the use of medical technology. *Health Affairs* 1982; **1**: 86–102.
736. Willems J, Sanders C, Riddiough M. Cost effectiveness of vaccination against pneumococcal pneumonia. *New England Journal of Medicine* 1980; **303**: 553–559.

737. Williams A. Economics of coronary artery bypass grafting. *British Medical Journal* 1985; **291**: 326–329.
738. Williamson J W. *Assessing and improving health care outcomes: the health accounting approach to quality assurance.* Cambridge, Massachusetts: Ballinger Publishing Co., 1978.
739. de Wit A. Hysteroscopy: an evolving care of MIT in gynecology. *Health Policy* (in press).
740. Witte J J, Axnik N W. *The benefits from 10 years of measles immunizations in the United States,* Public Health Report, 1985; **90**: 205–207.
741. Wittenberg J, Fineberg H V, Black E B, Kirkpatrick R H, Schaffer D L, Ikeda M K, Ferruci J T. Clinical efficacy of computed body tomography. *American Journal of Roentgenology* 1978; **131**: 5–14.
742. Wittenberg J, Fineberg H V, Ferruci J T, Simeone J F, Mueller P R, Sonnenberg E van, Kirkpatrick R H. Clinical efficacy of computed body tomography, II. *American Journal of Roentgenology* 1980; **134**: 1111–1120.
743. Woolf S, Battista R, Anderson O, *et al.* Assessing the clinical effectiveness of preventive maneuvers: analytic principles and systematic methods in reviewing evidence and developing clinical practice recommendations. The Canadian Task Force on the Periodic Health Examination. *Journal of Clinical Epidemiology* 1990; **43**: 891–905.
744. The World Bank. *Financing health services in developing countries.* Washington, DC, 1987.
745. The World Bank. *Poland, health system reform, meeting the challenge.* Washington, DC, February 19, 1991.
746. The World Bank. *Staff appraisal report, China, Integrated Regional Health Development Report.* Washington, April 3, 1989.
747. The World Bank. *Staff appraisal report, Romania, health rehabilitation project.* Washington, DC, July 5, 1991.
748. The World Bank. *World development report 1991. The challenge of development— world development indicators.* Oxford: Oxford University Press, 1991.
749. World Health Organization. *The selection of essential drugs.* Geneva: WHO, 1977.
750. World Health Organization. *The world drug situation.* Geneva: WHO, 1988.
751. World Health Organization. *World Health Organization Constitution.* Basic Documents. Geneva: World Health Organization, 1948.
752. World Health Organization. *Action Programme on Essential Drugs and Vaccines.* Progress report by the Executive Board Ad Hoc Committee on drugs policies. Geneva: WHO/DAP/84.4, 1984.
753. World Health Organization. Regional Office for Europe. *Having a baby in Europe, report on a study.* Copenhagen: The World Health Organization, 1985.
754. World Health Organization. Regional Office for Europe. *Quality assurance of health services.* Thirty-eighth Session, Technical Discussions, Copenhagen, 12–17 September 1988. (Document no. EUR/RC38/Tech.Disc./1)
755. World Health Organization. Regional Office for Europe. *Targets for health for all.* Targets in support of the European Regional Strategy for Health for All. Copenhagen: The World Health Organization, 1985.
756. Wortman P M, Saxe L. *Assessment of medical technology: methodological considerations.* Appendix C in Office of Technology Assessment. Strategies for medical technology assessment. Washington, DC: US Government Printing Office, 1982: pp. 127–149.

757. Wortman P M, Vinokur A. *Evaluation of NIH consensus development process. Phase I: final report.* Ann Arbor, Michigan: Center for Research on Utilization of Scientific Knowledge, University of Michigan, 1982.

758. Wortman P M, Yeaton W H. Using research synthesis in medical technology assessment. *International Journal of Technology Assessment in Health Care* 1987; **3**: 509–522.

759. Wu A, Rubin H, Matthews W, *et al.* A health status questionnaire using 30 items from the medical outcomes study. *Medical Care* 1991; **29**: 786–798.

760. Wu A, Mathews W, Brysk L, *et al.* Quality of life in a placebo-controlled trial of zidovudine in patients with AIDS and AIDS-related complex. *Journal of Acquired Immune Deficiency Syndrome* 1990; **3**: 683–690.

761. Wu A, Rubin H, Mathews W, *et al. Functional status and well-being in a placebo-controlled trial of zidovudine in early ARC.* Presented at the Sixth International Conference on AIDS, San Francisco, Cal., June 1990.

762. Wulff H R, Pedersen S A, Rosenberg R. *Philosophy of medicine, an introduction.* Oxford: Blackwell Scientific Publications, 1986.

763. Yeaton W H, Wortman P M. Medical technology assessment: the evaluation of coronary artery bypass graft surgery using data synthesis techniques. *International Journal of Technology Assessment in Health Care* 1985; **1**: 125–146.

764. Young D A. Communications linking clinical research and clinical practice. In Roberts E G, Levy R I, Moskowitz J, Sondik E J eds. *Biomedical innovations.* Cambridge, Massachusetts: MIT Press, 1981:177–199.

765. Zucker K, Bailey K, Gadacz T. Laparoscopic guided cholecystectomy. *American Journal of Surgery* 1991; **161**: 36–42.

Acronyms and abbreviations

ACP	American College of Physicians
AHA	American Hospital Association
AHCPR	Agency for Health Care Policy and Research
AHMAC	Australian Health Ministers Advisory Panel
AIDS	Acquired Immune Deficiency Syndrome
AIM	Advanced Informatics in Medicine
AMA	American Medical Association
ANDEM	Agence pour le Developpement de l'Evaluation Medicale
APED	Action Programme on Essential Drugs
BCBS	Blue Cross/Blue Shield (Association)
BCOHTA	British Columbia Office of Health Technology Assessment
BRS	Basic Radiology System
CABG	Coronary Artery Bypass Graft
CBA	Cost-Benefit Analysis
CCC	Copenhagen Collaborating Centre
CCOHTA	Canadian Co-ordinating Office for Healthcare Technology Assessment
CDC	Centers for Disease Control
CEA	Cost-Effectiveness Analysis
CEAP	Clinical Efficacy Assessment Project
CETS	Conseil d'Evaluation des Technologies de la Sante
CON	Certificate-of-Need
CRDC	Central Research and Development Committee
CSAG	Clinical Standards Advisory Group
CT	Computed Tomography
CUA	Cost-Utility Analysis
CVA	Cerebro-Vascular Accident
DATTA	Diagnostic and Therapeutic Technology Assessment
DES	Diethylstilbestrol

DH	Department of Health
DHHS	Department of Health and Human Services
DHSS	Department of Health and Social Security
DNA	Deoxyribonucleic Acid
DRG	Diagnosis-Related Groups
EAC	European–American Centre (for Policy Analysis)
EC	European Community
EEG	Electroencephalogram
EFM	Electronic Fetal Monitoring
EMA	European Medicines Agency
EMRC	European Medical Research Council
EORTC	European Organization for Research on Treatment for Cancer
ESWL	Extra-corporeal Shock Wave Lithotripsy
FAST	Forecasting and Assessment of Science and Technology
FCC	Federation of County Councils
FDA	Food and Drug Administration
FHSA	Family Health Services Authorities
GATT	General Agreement on Tariffs and Trade
GP	General Practitioner
HCFA	Health Care Financing Administration
HIAA	Health Insurance Association of America
HIV	Human Immunodeficiency Virus
HMO	Health Maintenance Organization
HRQOL	Health-Related Quality Of Life
HSA	Health Systems Agencies
IDE	Investigational Device Exemption
IMF	International Monetary Fund
IMTA	Institute of Medical Technology Assessment
IND	Investigational New Drug
IOM	Institute of Medicine
JAMA	*Journal of the American Medical Association*
MOPH	Ministry of Public Health
MRC	Medical Research Council
MRI	Magnetic Resonance Imaging

NCHCT	National Center for Health Care Technology
NCHSR	National Center for Health Services Research
NDA	New Drug Application
NHS	National Health Service
NHTAP	National Health Technology Advisory Panel
NIH	National Institutes of Health
NMR	Nuclear Magnetic Resonance
OECD	Organization for Economic Co-operation and Development
OHTA	Office of Health Technology Assessment
OMAR	Office of Medical Applications of Research
OTA	Office of Technology Assessment
PACS	Picture Archiving and Communication Systems
PAHO	Pan American Health Organization
PAR	Population-Attributable Risk
PECT	Prospective Economic Clinical Trial
PET	Positron Emission Tomography
PF	Prevented Fractions
PMS	Post-Marketing Surveillance
PORTs	Patient Outcomes Research Teams
PPO	Preferred Provider Organization
PPRC	Physician Payment Review Commission
PPS	Prospective Payment System
ProPAC	Prospective Payment Assessment Commission
PSRO	Professional Standards Review Organizations
PTCA	Percutaneous Transluminal Coronary Angioplasty
QALY	Quality-Adjusted Life Years
QWB	Quality of Well-Being (scale)
R&D	Research and Development
RAND (Corporation)	Research and Development Corporation
RBRVS	Resource-Based Relative Value Scale
RCT	Randomized Controlled Trial
RLF	Retro Lental Fibroplasia
SENIC	Study on the Efficacy of Nosocomial Infection Control
SPAC	State Pharmaceutical Administration
SPIE	Society of Photo-optical Instrumentation Engineers
SPRI	Swedish Planning and Rationalization Institute

TAC	Technology Advisory Committee
TAPSS	Technology Assessment Priority-Setting System
TNO (Organisatie voor)	Toegepast Natuureten-Schappelijk Onderzoek
UCLA	University of California at Los Angeles
UK	United Kingdom
UNICEF	United Nations Children's Fund
USA	United States of America
VA	Veterans Administration

Name and organization index

Subject index

abortion 1, 3
absorbent materials 208
academic inputs 18, 32, 40, 42, **198–202,** 206, 259
accessibility 12, 137, 141, 191–3, 209
accidents 96, 240
  cerebrovascular 145
Activities of Daily Living Scale 122
acupuncture 10, 255
administration 10, 42, 51–2, 192, 210
adoption of technology 4, **35–45,** 46, **207–11,** *see also* diffusion; use of technology
adverse events **145–6,** 177–9, 218, 223
advertising 53–6, 225, 288
Africa 54
ageing retardation 59
AIDS
  Audit Commission 211
  NIH 227
  quality of life 114, 116, 119, 121, 126
  social attitudes 133
alcohol withdrawal treatment 78–9
alternative therapy 10, 250–6, 289
ambulances 251
ambulatory care 143, 147, 171
anabolic hormones 54
anaemia 119, 121
anaesthesia 17, 170
angina pectoris 168, 180
angiography 190
angioplasty 170–2, 233
animal tests 87
Annals of Internal Medicine 234
antibiotics 18, 28, 84, 254
antihistamines 177
antisepsis 15, 17
appendix 47, 84, 96, 170
Argentina 276, 287
arthritis 78, 116, 119–20, 126, 130, 179
arthroscopy 164
artificial organs 31, 59, 73, 243
Asia 54
aspirin 15, 56

assessment
  drugs 21, 176–87, 199–201
  informal 87
  quantitative 20
  social 137–9
  surgical practice 167–75
  see also health care technology assessment; technology assessment
Assessment of Biomedical Technology in the Health Care Field: International Perspectives in Methodology 279
audit 143, 208–11
auranofin 120, 179
Australia 44, 79, 128, 163, 186, **273–4**
auto-analysers 95, 251, 274

babies 84–5, 96, 119, 125, 214, 288, *see also* children
back problems 44, 116, 119, 143, 164–5, 202, 274
bacteriology 14, 15
Battelle studies 56–7
bed sores 81
bed utilization 211
behaviour modification 59, 151
benefits 59, 62, 69, 87, 282–3, *see also* cost-benefit; efficacy
biomaterials 16, 31
biomechanics 31
biomedical engineering 30, 277
biomedical literature, *see* literature
biomedical research, *see* research
biosensors 31
biotechnology 16, 28, 29, 260, 272
bladder, *see* gall bladder; urinary tract
blood banks 17, 95
blood pressure cuff 14, *see also* hypertension
blood products 217–18
blood transfusion 81
body scanner 25, 159–60, 253, *see also* computed tomography
brain 136, 137, 164–5, 274
Brazil 276, 287, 288, 289
bureaucracy 51–2